Alcohol, Drugs, Genes and the Clinical Laboratory

Alcohol, Drugs, Genes and the Clinical Laboratory

Alcohol, Drugs, Genes and the Clinical Laboratory

An Overview for Healthcare and Safety Professionals

Amitava Dasgupta

McGovern Medical School
The University of Texas
Health Science Center at Houston
Houston, TX, USA

AMSTERDAM • BOSTON • HEIDELBERG • LONDON
NEW YORK • OXFORD • PARIS • SAN DIEGO
SAN FRANCISCO • SINGAPORE • SYDNEY • TOKYO
Academic Press is an imprint of Elsevier

Academic Press is an imprint of Elsevier
125 London Wall, London EC2Y 5AS, United Kingdom
525 B Street, Suite 1800, San Diego, CA 92101-4495, United States
50 Hampshire Street, 5th Floor, Cambridge, MA 02139, United States
The Boulevard, Langford Lane, Kidlington, Oxford OX5 1GB, United Kingdom

Notices
Knowledge and best practice in this field are constantly changing. As new research and experience broaden our
understanding, changes in research methods, professional practices, or medical treatment may become necessary.

Practitioners and researchers must always rely on their own experience and knowledge in evaluating and using any
information, methods, compounds, or experiments described herein. In using such information or methods they should
be mindful of their own safety and the safety of others, including parties for whom they have a professional
responsibility.

To the fullest extent of the law, neither the Publisher nor the authors, contributors, or editors, assume any liability for
any injury and/or damage to persons or property as a matter of products liability, negligence or otherwise, or from any
use or operation of any methods, products, instructions, or ideas contained in the material herein.

British Library Cataloguing-in-Publication Data
A catalogue record for this book is available from the British Library

Library of Congress Cataloging-in-Publication Data
A catalog record for this book is available from the Library of Congress

ISBN: 978-0-12-805455-0

For Information on all Academic Press publications
visit our website at https://www.elsevier.com

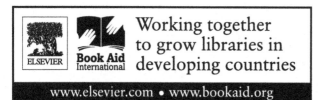

Working together
to grow libraries in
developing countries

www.elsevier.com • www.bookaid.org

Publisher: Mica Haley
Acquisition Editor: Erin Hill-Parks
Editorial Project Manager: Tracy Tufaga
Production Project Manager: Stalin Viswanathan
Designer: Greg Harris

Typeset by MPS Limited, Chennai, India

Contents

Preface

Alcohol is a double-edged sword. There are many health benefits of drinking in moderation (up to 2 drinks a day for a male and up to 1 drink a day for female), including protection against cardiovascular diseases, stroke, type 2 diabetes, and many others. In addition, moderate drinking may also increase longevity. Drinking red wine may provide protection against Alzheimer's disease and age-related dementia. However, drinking in excess is associated with many health hazards. Even binge drinking once a month (4 or more drinks in a 2 h period for females and 5 or more drinks in a 2 h period for males) may be harmful. Moreover, driving with a blood alcohol level of 0.08% or more is against the law and if stopped by the police, the driver may be charged with driving while intoxicated. As a result, drug and alcohol abuse is a serious public health issue and many factors play an important role in the development of drug and alcohol abuse.

Clinical laboratories play an important role in diagnosis of alcohol and drug abuse because false positive test results may cause severe emotional stress to a patient. There are many excellent reference books on alcohol and drug abuse as well as reference books on laboratory based methods for drugs of abuse testing. The purpose of this book is to provide a through overview of this topic, which will be useful for healthcare professionals including family physicians (who are responsible for identifying patients who may have drug or alcohol abuse issues), pathologists (who are involved with drug and alcohol testing), emergency room physicians (treating drug and alcohol overdose), psychiatrists (involved in drug and alcohol rehab centers), public health professionals, and nurse practitioners. In addition, safety professionals who are involved in workplace drug testings such as human resources managers, lawyers, and professionals working in alcohol/drug rehabilitation facilities will also benefit from reading this book. This book will cover all important aspects of drug and alcohol abuse including genetic aspects along with laboratory methods for analysis of alcohol and abused drugs with emphasis on false positive test results.

In Chapter 1, Alcohol a Double-Edged Sword: Health Benefits with Moderate Consumption but Health Hazard with Excess Alcohol Intake, the health benefits of drinking in moderation and the health hazards of alcohol abuse are discussed, with guidelines. In Chapter 2, Drugs of Abuse: An Overview, overview of abuse of illicit and prescription drugs (barbiturates, benzodiazepines, and opioids) is provided. Chapter 3, Designer Drugs Including Bath Salts and Spices, is devoted to the discussion of designer drugs, including the more recently introduced bath salts and spices (synthetic cannabinoids). Combining alcohol with drug abuse is a deadly combination because alcohol decreases the threshold of drug toxicity and severe overdose and even fatality may occur with much lower drug concentration if alcohol is also present. This is discussed in Chapter 4, Combined Alcohol and Drug Abuse: A Potentially Deadly Mix. In Chapter 5, Link Between Environmental Factors, Personality Factors, and Addiction, environmental and personality traits that may increase susceptibility of alcohol and/or drug abuse is discussed. Chapter 6, Genetic Polymorphisms of Alcohol Metabolizing Enzymes Associated With Protection From or Increased Risk of Alcohol Abuse, addresses how certain polymorphisms of genes that encode alcohol dehydrogenase and aldehyde dehydrogenase may protect an individual against alcohol abuse. However, certain genetic polymorphisms may increase susceptibility to alcohol abuse. Chapter 7, Pharmacogenomics of Abused Drugs, discusses pharmacogenetic issues with abused drugs.

Unlike monogenic disorder, there is no single gene identified that is associated with alcohol and drug addiction. In general it is considered that alcohol and drug addictions are polygenic disorders where genes may account for approximately 50% vulnerability while another 50% is due to environmental factors. Association between polymorphisms of various receptors and transporter genes with alcohol and/or drug addiction is addressed in Chapter 8, Association between Polymorphisms in Genes Encoding Various Receptors, Transporters, and Enzymes and Alcohol/Drug Addiction. Methods of alcohol measurement are discussed in Chapter 9, Methods of Alcohol Measurement, with emphasis on interferences with breathalyzers. In Chapter 10, Laboratory Methods for Measuring Drugs of Abuse in Urine, Substance Abuse and Mental Health Services Administration guidelines for drug abuse testing in urine along with methods for screening and confirmation (using gas chromatography/mass spectrometry or liquid chromatography combined with tandem mass spectrometry) are addressed. In Chapter 11, Analysis of Drugs of Abuse in Serum, Hair, Oral Fluid, Sweat, and Meconium, drug testings in alternative matrixes such as hair, oral fluid, sweat, and meconium are discussed.

I would like to thank my wife Alice for putting up with me during the long evening and weekend hours I devoted to preparing this manuscript. Robert L. Hunter, MD, PhD, chairman of Pathology and Laboratory Medicine supported me during the preparation of the manuscript and I also thank him for his support. If readers find this book useful, my hard work will be duly rewarded.

Respectfully submitted by
Amitava Dasgupta
Houston, TX
USA

Alcohol a double-edged sword: health benefits with moderate consumption but a health hazard with excess alcohol intake

1

Introduction

Alcohol has health benefits if consumed in moderation but alcohol acts as a toxin in heavy drinkers. Alcohol content of various alcoholic beverages varies widely, e.g., beer contains approximately 4−7% alcohol while the average alcohol content of vodka is 40−50%. However, due to wide differences between serving size, 1 drink (often called 1 standard drink) contains approximately 0.6 ounces of alcohol which is equivalent to 14 g of pure alcohol. In the United States, a standard drink is defined as a bottle of beer (12 fluid ounces) containing 5% alcohol, 8.5 fluid ounces of malt liquor containing 7% alcohol, a 5 fluid ounce glass of wine containing 12% alcohol, 3.5 fluid ounces of fortified wine like sherry or port containing about 17% alcohol, 2.5 fluid ounces of cordial or liqueur containing 24% alcohol, or 1 shot (1.5 fluid ounces) of a distilled spirits such as gin, rum, vodka, or whiskey.

Currently, in the United States, the alcohol content of a drink is measured by the percentage of alcohol by the volume. The code of Federal Regulations requires that the label of alcoholic beverages must state the alcohol content by volume. Alcoholic drinks primarily consist of water, alcohol, and variable amounts of sugars and carbohydrates (residual sugar and starch left after fermentation) but negligible amounts of other nutrients such as proteins, vitamins, or minerals. However, distilled liquors such as cognac, vodka, whiskey, and rum contain no sugars. Red wine and dry white wines contain 2−10 g of sugar per liter while sweet wines and port wines may contain up to 120 g of sugar per liter of wine. Beer and dry sherry contain 30 g of sugar per liter [1].

Guidelines for alcohol consumption

United States Department of Agriculture (USDA) and Department of Health and Human Services jointly publish "Dietary Guidelines for Americans" every 5 years, suggesting to Americans what constitutes a balanced diet. These guidelines also include suggestions for drinking in moderation. However, alcohol is not a component in the USDA food pattern. If alcohol is consumed, the calories from alcohol must be

Alcohol, Drugs, Genes and the Clinical Laboratory. DOI: http://dx.doi.org/10.1016/B978-0-12-805455-0.00001-4

accounted for when other foods are consumed so that daily calorie intake does not exceed the recommended limit (1600–2400 calories per day for women and 2000–3000 calories per day for men). The latest Dietary Guidelines for Americans, 2015–2020, eighth edition, suggests that if alcohol is consumed it should be consumed in moderation following these guidelines:

- Up to 1 drink per day for women and up to 2 drinks per day for men—and only by adults of legal drinking age (21 years or older).

One drink is defined by the guidelines as containing 14 g (0.6 fluid ounces) of pure alcohol. One alcoholic drink is equivalent to 12 fluid ounces of regular beer (5% alcohol), 5 fluid ounces of wine (12% alcohol), or 1.5 fluid ounces of 80 proof distilled spirits (40% alcohol). If light beer is consumed (4.2% alcohol) it should be considered as 0.8 drink. Mixed drinks (including fruit drinks mixed with spirits) with more than 1.5 fluid ounces of alcohol should be considered as more than 1 drink. The formula for calculating drink equivalent is:

Drink equivalent = Volume of alcoholic beverage $\times$ Alcohol content$/0.6$

For example, drinking 16 fluid ounces of beer containing 5% alcohol is equivalent to 1.33 drinks.

Federal Food and Drug Administration has determined that mixing alcohol and caffeine is not a safe practice and recommended four manufacturers of alcoholic beverages containing caffeine to discontinue using caffeine in alcoholic drinks. People who mix alcohol and caffeine may drink more alcohol and become more intoxicated than they realize, increasing the risk of alcohol-related adverse events. Energy drinks are gaining popularity among young adults as well as among underage drinkers. Studies have indicated that energy drinks may increase craving for alcohol and binge drinking. When an energy drink, which often contains caffeine, is combined with alcohol, the desire to drink alcohol is more pronounced compared to drinking alcohol without consumption of an energy drink. Moreover, pleasurable experience of drinking alcohol is also enhanced by consuming energy drinks at the same time [2].

National Institute of Alcohol Abuse and Alcoholism (NIAAA) considers high risk drinking as consuming 4 or more drinks in any day or 8 or more drinks per week for women and 5 or more drinks in any day or 15 or more drinks per week for men. Binge drinking is defined by NIAAA as the consumption of 5 drinks in 2 h for men and 4 drinks in the same time period for women and such drinking patterns always produce a blood alcohol level of 0.08% or higher. However, another government agency Substance Abuse and Mental Health Services Administration (SAMHSA) defines binge drinking as consuming 5 or more alcoholic beverages on the same occasion in the past 30 days. SAMHSA also defines heavy drinking as consuming 5 or more drinks on the same occasion on each of 5 or more days in the past 30 days. However, National Institute for NIAAA investigators have shown that if women consume 3 drinks on a single day, not exceeding 7 drinks per week, and men consume 4 drinks on a single occasion but not exceeding 14 drinks per week,

Table 1.1 Definition of moderate, high risk, heavy, and binge drinking

Type of drinking	Definition/guideline
Moderate drinking (Dietary Guidelines for Americans 2015—2020, eighth edition)	Up to 1 drink per day for women and up to 2 drinks per day for men.
High risk drinking (NIAAA)	Consumption of 4 or more drinks on any day or 8 or more drinks per week for women and 5 or more drinks on any day or 15 or more drinks per week for men.
Heavy drinking (SAMHSA) guideline	Consuming 5 or more drinks in the same occasion on each of 5 or more days in the past 30 days in both females and males.
Binge drinking (NIAAA)	Consuming 5 drinks in a 2 h period for men and four drinks in a 2 h for women. Such drinking practice produces a blood alcohol level of 0.08% or more.
Binge drinking (SAMHSA)	Consuming 5 or more drinks in the same occasion at least 1 day in the past 30 days for both men and women.
Underage drinking	Legal age of drinking in all States in United States is 21 years. Anyone drinking below that age is considered to be underage drinking.

NIAAA, National Institute on Alcohol Abuse and Alcoholism; SAMHSA, Substance abuse and Mental Health Services Administration.

the possibility of developing alcohol use disorder (AUD) is approximately 2%, a relatively low risk for developing AUD. Definitions of moderate drinking, binge drinking, heavy drinking, and underage drinking are listed in Table 1.1.

Alcohol use and abuse

According to the 2014 National Survey on Drug Use and Health (published in September 2015) conducted by SAMHSA (an agency of the US government), 139.7 million Americans had consumed alcohol during the past 30 days when contacted for the survey, including 16.3 million Americans who were heavy alcohol users (drinking 5 or more drinks in one occasion on 5 or more days in the past 30 days). It was also estimated that 60.9 million Americans were binge drinkers. The World Health Organization (WHO) estimated that 5.1% global burden of disease and injuries are related to alcohol abuse [3]. Drinking more than the recommended amount can cause serious problems because the health benefits of drinking in moderation disappear fast with consuming more than 3—4 drinks a day. Heavy consumption of alcohol not only leads to increased domestic violence, decreased productivity, increased risk of motor vehicle as well as job related accidents, but also to increased mortality from liver cirrhosis, stoke, and cancer. Alcohol poisoning may also cause fatality.

Alcohol is involved in many fatal car accidents and according to US Highway National Traffic and approximately 30% of traffic fatalities are linked to excessive alcohol consumption. Excessive alcohol consumption is responsible for 10−18% of injured patients who are admitted to emergency departments in United States. Moreover, economic cost of excessive alcohol consumption is estimated to be $223.5 billion annually in the United States [4].

Physiological effects of various blood alcohol levels

Blood alcohol depends on many factors including number of drinks, gender (females show higher blood alcohol than males for consuming same amounts of alcohol when body weights are comparable), and body weight. Moreover, peak blood alcohol level is lower if alcohol is consumed with food and if alcohol is sipped instead of consumed rapidly. The presence of food not only reduces blood alcohol level but also stimulates its elimination through the liver. Alcohol is first metabolized to acetaldehyde by the enzyme alcohol dehydrogenase and then by aldehyde dehydrogenase into acetate. Acetate finally breaks down into carbon dioxide and water. For higher alcohol consumption, liver CYP2E1 plays a role in alcohol metabolism.

Substantial research has established that the effect of alcohol on the human depends on the blood alcohol concentration. At a very low blood alcohol level people usually feel relaxation and mild euphoria and some loss of inhibition or shyness. However, at blood alcohol levels that exceed the legal limit for driving in United States, significant impairment of motor skills may occur. At a blood alcohol level of 0.3% and higher, complete loss of consciousness may occur and a blood alcohol level of 0.5% and higher may even cause death (Table 1.2). Drinking excessive alcohol in one occasion may cause alcohol poisoning which if not treated promptly may be fatal. Celik et al. reported that postmortem blood alcohol levels ranged from 136 to 608 mg/dL in 39 individuals who died due to alcohol overdose. Most of those deceased were male [5]. The mechanism of death from alcohol poisoning is usually attributed to paralysis of respiratory and circulatory centers in the brain causing asphyxiation.

Impairment of motor skills may occur at blood alcohol levels lower than 0.08%. Phillips and Brewer commented that accident severity increases when the driver is merely "buzzed" compared to sober drivers because buzzed drivers are significantly more likely to speed, and the greater the blood alcohol, the greater the speed as well as the severity of the accident. Moreover, a buzzed driver may not put the seatbelt on properly. Usually alcohol-related traffic accidents are more likely to take place on weekends, in the months of June−August, and from 8 pm to 4 am [6].

Table 1.2 **Physiological effects of various blood alcohol levels**

Blood alcohol level	Physiological effect
0.01–0.04% (10–40 mg/dL)	Mild euphoria, relaxation, and increased social interactions.
0.05–0.07% (50–70 mg/dL)	Euphoria with loss of inhibition making a person more friendly and talkative. Some impairments of motor skills may take place in some individuals, and as a result, in some countries, e.g., Germany, the legal limit of driving is 0.05%.
0.08% (80 mg/dL)	Legal limit of driving in United States. Some impairment of driving skills may be present in some individuals.
0.08–0.12% (80–120 mg/dL)	Moderate impairment to significant impairment of driving skills depending on drinking habits. Emotional swings and depression may be observed in some individuals.
0.12–0.15% (120–150 mg/dL)	Motor function, speech, and judgement are all severely affected at this height of blood alcohol. Staggering, and slurred speech, may be observed. Severe impairment of driving skills.
0.15–0.2% (150–200 mg/dL)	This is the blood alcohol level where a person appears drunk and may have severe visual impairment.
0.2–0.3% (200–300 mg/dL)	Vomiting, incontinence, symptoms of alcohol intoxication.
0.3–0.4% (300–400 mg/dL)	Signs of severe alcohol intoxication and a person may not be able to move without the help of another person. Stupor, blackout, and total loss of consciousness may also happen.
0.4–0.5% (400–500 mg/dL)	Potentially fatal and a person may be comatose.
Above 0.5% (500 mg/dL)	Highly dangerous/fatal blood alcohol level.

Falleti et al. demonstrated that cognitive impairment associated with 0.05% blood alcohol is similar to staying awake for 24 h [7]. Moreover, many industrialized countries such as Austria, France, Germany, and Italy have set legal limit of driving at 0.05%. Although the legal limit of driving in Canada is 0.08%, in some Canadian provinces, 0.05% blood alcohol is considered as the "warning range" limit at which officers may suspend a driver's license for 1–7 days. The National Transportation Safety Board in 2014 recommended lowering the legal limit of driving in the United States to 0.05%, but it is not adopted as the law. Scientific research has shown that even at 0.05% blood alcohol virtually all drivers are impaired regarding at least some driving practices [8]. For avoiding driving while intoxicated in United States, consumption of alcohol with food is highly recommended. For men, up to 2 standard drinks consumed with food in a 2 h period (1 drink per hour) and for women up to 1 drink with food consumed in a 2 h period should produce blood alcohol levels below 0.08%.

Benefits of drinking in moderation

Consuming alcohol in moderation has many health benefits, including increased longevity. These health benefits are summarized in Table 1.3. Some of these benefits
are attributable to alcohol while many other benefits are due to the combined effect
of both alcohol and many beneficial phytochemicals present in beer and wine that
are excellent antioxidants. More than 400 different phytochemicals are present in
beer; some of these compounds originate from raw materials while others are generated during fermentation process. Melatonin is generated during the brewing process.

Table 1.3 **Physical health benefits of consuming alcohol in moderation**

Health benefit	Type of alcoholic beverage and quantity	Comments
Reduced risk of cardiovascular diseases	Beer and wine provide better protection than liquors. One author has suggested drinking one glass of red wine before or with evening meal. Women may get protection from drinking as little as 1 drink per week.	Alcohol in moderate concentration increases HDL cholesterol. Resveratrol present in red wine prevents oxidation of LDL. Protection is more significant in men of 50 years of age and older but women of any age may get benefits from consuming alcohol in moderation.
Reduces mortality in survivors of myocardial infarction	Any type of alcoholic beverage (beer, wine, or liquor) can reduce mortality after surviving a myocardial infarction.	Alcohol is responsible for protection.
Reduced risk of ischemic stroke	In one study, the authors observed maximum protection from daily consumption of 1.2 standard drinks. Any alcoholic beverage (beer, wine, or liquor) can provide the protection if consumed in moderation.	Drinking more than 2 standard drinks a day may increase the risk of hemorrhagic stroke.
Reduced risk of type 2 diabetes	Any alcoholic beverage (beer, wine, or liquor) can provide the protection if consumed in moderation (half a drink to up to 2 drinks a day).	Alcohol reduces blood glucose after a meal by stimulating insulin secretion but also may improve insulin sensitivity. However, for individuals taking sulfonylurea medication alcohol may cause hypoglycemia.

(Continued)

Table 1.3 (Continued)

Health benefit	Type of alcoholic beverage and quantity	Comments
Reduced risk of certain type of cancer	Red wine (1 drink a day) may reduce risk of lung cancer even in smokers. One drink a day (beer, wine) reduces risk of head and neck cancer as well as renal cell carcinoma.	Oxidative stress increases cancer risk but both beer and wine contain antioxidants as well as anticarcinogen (e.g., xanthohumol in beer, resveratrol in red wine).
Reduced risk of developing rheumatoid arthritis	Moderate consumption of any type of alcoholic beverage reduces the risk of rheumatoid arthritis.	Alcohol has antiinflammatory effects.
Reduced risk of forming kidney stones	Beer may be more effective than wine.	Probably both alcohol and polyphenolic compounds present in beer and wine protects from developing kidney stones.
Reduced risk of forming gallstone	Consuming 5–7 drinks (any type of alcoholic beverage) per week reduces risk of gallstone disease.	People who are light drinkers (consuming 1–2 drinks per week) may not get any protection from gallstone disease.
Protection from the common cold	Only wine may provide protection against the common cold.	Probably some specific polyphenolic compounds present in wine provide the protection.
Increased longevity	One or two drinks a day may increase longevity but drinking more than 2 drinks a day may reduce longevity.	Overall effect of alcohol and antioxidants present in beer and wine may be responsible for longer life in moderate drinkers. Drinking wine may have additional benefit for longevity.
Better perception of good health	Only wine is associated with better perception of good health.	Mechanism is not clear.

Beers with higher alcoholic content usually have higher amounts of melatonin [9]. More than 1600 phytochemicals are present in wine prepared from grapes [10].

Hazards of alcohol abuse

In general there is a U-shape curve correlating alcohol consumption with a diseased state. With lower alcohol consumption, risk of disease is significantly reduced, while with heavy consumption, risk of the same disease is significantly increased. Adverse effects of heavy consumption of alcohol are listed in Table 1.4.

Table 1.4 **Health hazards of alcohol abuse**

Disease/condition	Comments
Alcohol liver disease and alcoholic cirrhosis	Alcohol has toxic effect on hepatocytes. Moreover, in alcoholics, a part of the alcohol is metabolized by liver enzyme CYP2E1 which produces free radicals. Although alcohol in low concentration is an antioxidant due to presence of many antioxidants in beer and wine, at high concentration especially with consumption of distilled liquors such as vodka or whiskey, alcohol is a prooxidant and significantly increases oxidative stress.
Increased risk of cardiovascular disease	Alcohol at high concentration is toxic to the heart, causing alcohol induced cardiomyopathy and heart failure.
Psychiatric illness including anxiety/ mood disorder as well as major depression	Alcohol at higher blood alcohol level is a central nervous system depressant and may cause mood disorder.
Neurological damage	Alcohol is toxic to the developing brain and teenagers are susceptible to adverse effects of alcohol from any amount of drinking.
Fetal alcohol syndrome	Any amount of alcohol is toxic to the fetus and in order to avoid fetal alcohol syndrome or fetal alcohol spectrum disorders, a pregnant woman must practice total abstinence.
Increased risk of cancer	Alcohol may act as a carcinogen. Heavy alcohol consumption also increases oxidative stress.
Increased violence and domestic abuse	By modulating serotonin and testosterone concentration, alcohol may exert its effect in inducing aggressive and violent behavior when consumed in excess.
Reduced life span	Alcohol is related to fatal car accidents, increased hospitalization due to injury, as well as increased burden of risk of developing various diseases including myocardial infarction. As a result, life span is reduced.

In general, liver is the major site of adverse effects of alcohol abuse. Alcoholic liver diseases represent a spectrum of liver pathologies ranging from fatty changes in the liver to fibrosis and alcoholic cirrhosis. Heavy drinking for as little as a few days may produce fatty changes in the liver (steatosis), which are reversed after abstinence. However, if a person continues to drink heavily, fatty changes may lead to fibrosis and even cirrhosis. Women are at greater risk of developing alcoholic liver diseases. Obesity as well as smoking may increase the risk of alcoholic liver diseases [11].

The amount of alcohol consumed is one of the determining factors in developing alcoholic liver cirrhosis. In one report the authors commented that cirrhosis of the liver does not develop below a lifetime ingestion of 100 kg of alcohol (1 standard drink is approximately 14 g of alcohol; therefore a lifetime consumption of 7143 drinks). This amount corresponds to an average of 5 drinks a day for about 4 years. The authors also commented that consuming alcohol with food lowers the risk of developing cirrhosis of the liver compared to if alcohol is consumed on an empty stomach [12]. Consumption of coffee may protect males against alcohol induced liver damage but no such data is currently available for females [13]. Hepatitis C is a liver disease caused by hepatitis C virus. Even moderate consumption of alcohol may cause adverse effects in individuals infected with hepatitis C [14].

Early diagnosis of alcoholic liver diseases is important in order to avoid cirrhosis and hepatocellular carcinoma. Liver biopsy is the gold standard for diagnosis but a series of biochemical tests and measuring stiffness of the liver are also widely used for diagnosis of alcoholic liver diseases. Although supportive care including complete abstinence is necessary to treat alcoholic liver diseases, cirrhosis may be fatal and liver transplantation remains the ultimate therapy [15].

The mechanism of alcohol induced liver disease is complex. Although alcohol has direct toxic effects on hepatocytes, alcohol induced oxidative stress also plays an important role in the pathophysiology of alcoholic liver diseases. While in moderate drinkers alcohol is mostly metabolized by alcohol dehydrogenase in the liver, in alcoholics CYP2E1, a member of the cytochrome P-450 drug metabolizing family of enzymes in the liver becomes activated. In this process reactive oxygen species are generated. Hydroxyethyl radicals are probably involved in the alkylation of proteins found in hepatocytes. Formation of nitric oxide and elevated concentrations of stable metabolites; nitrites; and nitrates have been documented in alcoholics [16].

Alcohol consumption and cardiovascular disease

Cardiovascular diseases including myocardial infarction are the number one killer in the United States and other industrialized countries. The beneficial effects of moderate alcohol consumption in reducing the risk of various cardiovascular diseases, including reducing the risk of myocardial infarction, have been well characterized. However, alcohol abuse is associated with increased risk of cardiovascular diseases.

Moderate alcohol consumption reduces risk of cardiovascular diseases

The relationship between alcohol consumption and coronary heart disease was examined in the original Framingham Heart Study which showed a U-shape curve with reduced risk of cardiovascular diseases with moderate drinking but a higher risk of cardiovascular diseases with heavy drinking. Smoking is a risk factor for developing coronary heart disease but moderate alcohol consumption may also provide some protection against coronary heart disease among smokers [17]. Interestingly, women may get beneficial effects of alcohol from consuming lower amounts as well as consuming alcohol less frequently than men. In one study with 28,448 women and 25,052 men between 50 and 65 years of age who were free from cardiovascular diseases at the time of enrollment, the authors observed that during a 5.7 year follow-up, women who consumed alcohol at least 1 day per week had lower risk of coronary heart disease than those who drank alcohol less than 1 day per week. However, little difference was found between women who consumed at least 1 drink per week compared to women who consumed 2−4 drinks per week, 5−6 drinks per week, or even 7 drinks per week. For men lowest risk was found in individuals who consumed 1 drink per day [18]. Moderate alcohol consumption can also provide protective effects against heart failure [19]. Gemes et al., based on a study of 58,827 individuals and an 11.6-year follow-up, observed that light to moderate consumption of alcohol was associated with lower risk of myocardial infarction [20].

O'Keefe et al. reviewed effects of alcohol on the health of the human heart and commented that habitual light to moderate drink lowers the rate from death due to coronary artery disease, diabetes mellitus, congestive heart failure, and stroke. However, excessive alcohol consumption is the third leading cause of premature death in United States. In general men older than age 50 get more favorable effects of consuming alcohol in moderation than younger men but women of any age get favorable effects of consuming alcohol in moderation. Unfortunately, the cardioprotective effect of alcohol has not been documented in epidemiological studies of populations from India and China. The authors advise people to drink one glass of red wine (5−6 ounces glass) daily immediately before or during dinner. However, authors also advise individuals who are teetotalers not to initiate light to moderate alcohol consumption for health benefits because of paucity of randomized outcome data and the potential for developing a problem drinking practice [21].

There are several hypotheses on how moderate drinking can reduce the risk of developing heart disease. Many studies have demonstrated increased high-density lipoprotein cholesterol (HDL cholesterol) levels in drinkers compared to nondrinkers. Alcohol also diminishes thrombus formation on damaged walls of the coronary artery due to inhibition of platelet aggregation mediated through inhibiting phospholipase A2. Studies have also indicated that the level of increase in HDL cholesterol in blood may explain 50% of protective effects of alcohol against cardiovascular disease and the other 50% may be partly related to inhibition of platelet aggregation and antioxidant effects of various polyphenolic compounds present in alcohol beverages. The polyphenolic antioxidant compounds found in abundance in red wine can further reduce platelet activity via other mechanisms [22]. Significant research to understand the epidemiological phenomenon known as "the French paradox," (low incidence of cardiovascular diseases in the French population despite coexistence of high risk factor is postulated to be associated with regular consumption of wine), indicates the superiority of wine in reducing risk of cardiovascular diseases compared to other alcoholic beverages [23].

Some studies indicate that red wine may be superior to white wine, beer, or spirits for cardioprotection because resveratrol, found in higher amounts in red wine, is very effective in preventing low-density lipoprotein (LDL) oxidation. Oxidized LDL has a higher tendency to deposit on coronary arteries causing plaque formation (atherosclerosis). Moreover, other polyphenolic components of red wine can further inhibit platelets, reduce inflammation, and activate proteins that prevent cell death. The effects are weaker in the case of white wine or beer due to lower concentrations of polyphenols compared to red wine [24].

Chiva-Blanch et al. compared the effects of wine, spirits, and beer on protection against cardiovascular diseases and concluded that wine and beer (but especially red wine) seem to confer greater cardiovascular protection than spirits because of their polyphenolic content [25]. Rimm and Stampfer commented that beer and wine may have similar cardioprotective effects although in one study, the authors observed a 32% risk reduction in wine drinkers and a 22% risk reduction in beer drinkers, but other studies observed no difference between beer and wine drinkers. In another study, the authors observed 25% risk reduction in wine drinkers and a 23% risk reduction in beer drinkers [26].

In an interesting study Barefoot et al. concluded that the apparent health benefits of wine compared to other alcoholic beverages as reported by other investigators may be a result of cofounding by dietary habits and other lifestyle factors. The authors observed that subjects who preferred wine had healthier diets than those who preferred beer or sprits or had no preference. Wine drinkers also reported eating more servings of fruits and vegetables and fewer servings of red or fried meat. In addition, wine drinkers were less likely to smoke [27].

Only beer is a rich source of folate and drinking beer is associated with a good blood level of folate and vitamin B12, which lower homocysteine concentration in blood. Higher blood level of homocysteine is associated with increased risk of cardiovascular diseases. Mayer concluded that moderate beer consumption may help to maintain the homocysteine level within the normal range in blood due to its high folate content [28]. This is a unique feature of beer because wine and spirits may slightly increase the blood homocysteine level.

Light to moderate consumption of alcohol also increases the chance of survival after first heart attack. Based on a study of 1253 women who survived first acute heart attack, Rosenbloom et al. observed that compared to women who did not drink at all, women who consumed less than 1 drink per week, 1−3 drinks per week, or more than 3 drinks per week, all showed lower mortality in a 10 year follow-up. All types of alcoholic beverages (beer, wine, or liquor) were associated with the protection. The authors estimated that light to moderate consumption of alcohol by women after first heart attack was associated with approximately 35% lower chance of dying compared to women who did not consume any alcohol [29].

Heavy alcohol consumption and increased risk of cardiovascular diseases

Unfortunately, protective effect of alcohol on the heart disappears with excessive drinking and people who abuse alcohol have a much higher chance of heart diseases compared to nondrinkers or moderate drinkers. Chronic alcohol abuse over several years may result in alcoholic cardiomyopathy and heart failure, systematic hypertension, heart rhythm disturbances, and hemorrhagic stroke [30]. Alcoholics who consume 90 g or more of alcohol a day (7–8 drinks) for 5 years are at high risk of developing alcoholic cardiomyopathy and if they continue drinking alcohol, cardiomyopathy may proceed to heart failure, a potentially fatal medical condition. Without complete abstinence, 50% of these patients will die within the next 4 years of developing heart failure [31]. Women are at higher risk of alcoholic cardiomyopathy than men. Chronic consumption of excess alcohol is also associated with higher risk of death after heart attack [32].

Alcohol consumption and stroke

Another beneficial effect of consuming alcohol in moderation is reduction in the risk of stroke among both men and women regardless of age or ethnicity. The Copenhagen City Heart Study, with 13,329 eligible men and women aged between 45 and 84 years, with 16 years of follow-up, indicated a U-shaped relation between intake of alcohol and risk of stroke. People who consumed low to moderate alcohol experienced protective effects of alcohol against stroke but heavy consumers of alcohol were at higher risk of suffering from a stroke compared to moderate drinkers or nondrinkers [33].

Heavy drinking also increases risk of stroke, particularly the risk of hemorrhagic stroke. In one study, the authors observed that risk of hemorrhagic stroke increases in an individual drinking 300 g or more of alcohol weekly (21 or more drinks) [34].

Alcohol consumption and type 2 diabetes

Moderate consumption of alcohol reduces the risk of developing type 2 diabetes by reducing oxidative stress and increasing insulin sensitivity. Based on 15 studies conducted in the United States, Finland, Netherlands, Germany, United Kingdom, and Japan with 369,862 men and women and an average follow-up of 12 years, light drinkers and moderate drinkers had lower risk of developing type 2 diabetes compared to nondrinkers. It made little difference whether an individual consumes beer, wine of spirit and it is better to consume alcohol frequently (such as daily or several times in week) rather than occasionally. The authors concluded that observational studies suggest an approximately 30% reduced risk of developing type 2 diabetes in moderate drinkers whereas no risk reduction was observed in people who consumed alcohol in excess (more than 48 g/day) [35]. Baliunas et al., based on reviewing 20 studies, observed a U-shape relationship between alcohol consumption and risk of developing type 2 diabetes, where moderate alcohol consumption decreased the risk of developing diabetes, but heavy alcohol consumption increased the risk [36].

Alcohol consumption and human brain

Moderate alcohol consumption can dramatically reduce the risk of age related dementia and Alzheimer's disease. The triggering agent for Alzheimer's disease is β-amyloid peptide (Aβ-aggregates) which alters the synaptic activity and disrupts neurotransmission mediated by cholinergic and N-methyl-D-aspartate receptors. Alcohol in low dosage can prevent formation of Aβ-aggregates thus delaying or preventing onset of Alzheimer's disease. Moreover, low to moderate consumption of alcohol is also associated with reduced risk of other neurodegenerative diseases as evidenced from data of several large clinical trials [37].

However, onset of drinking at an early age (13 or earlier) has devastating effects on the brain and such adverse effects may last a lifetime in such individuals. Underage drinkers are also susceptible to immediate ill effects of alcohol use such as blackouts, hangover, and alcohol poisoning and these individuals are also at higher risk of neurodegeneration, impairment of functional brain activity, and neurocognitive deficits [38]. Women are more susceptible to alcohol-related neurological damage than men, because a female adolescent brain is more vulnerable to alcohol exposure than a male adolescent brain. Consistent with adult literature, alcohol use during adolescence is associated with prefrontal volume abnormality including differences in white matter but girls are more affected than boys by adverse effects of alcohol [39].

The two major alcohol-related brain damages are alcoholic Korsakoff's syndrome and alcoholic dementia. When Wernicke's encephalopathy accompanies Korsakoff's syndrome in an alcoholic, it is called Wernicke–Korsakoff syndrome. Wernicke's encephalopathy and Korsakoff syndrome are two related diseases, both caused by thiamine deficiency, but clinical symptoms may be different. The Royal College of Physicians in London recommends that patients admitted to the hospital who show evidence of chronic misuse of alcohol and poor diet should be treated with B vitamins [40].

Alcohol consumption and cancer

Moderate consumption of alcohol may reduce the risk of certain types of cancer because wine and beer (e.g., xanthohumol) contain anticarcinogenic compounds and also antioxidants. In the California Men's Health Study using 84,170 men aged between 45 and 69, consumption of 1 or more drink of red wine per day was associated with approximately 60% reduced risk of lung cancer even in smokers [41]. Consumption of up to 1 drink per day reduced the risk of head and neck cancer in both men and women but consuming more than three alcoholic beverages increased the risk of cancer. In an Italian study the authors observed that moderate consumption of alcohol reduced the risk of developing renal cell carcinoma in both males and females [42]. Beer is slightly more effective in lowering risk of kidney stones than other alcoholic beverages. In one study based on 194,095 participants, the authors concluded that consumption of sugar-sweetened sodas and punch was associated with a higher risk of kidney stone formation whereas moderate consumption of beer was associated with 41% lower risk of developing kidney stones. Consuming wine was associated with 31−33% lower risk while orange juice reduced the risk by 12%. Drinking caffeinated coffee may lower the risk by 26% while decaffeinated coffee may lower the risk by 16% and tea may lower the risk by 11% [43].

Epidemiological research has demonstrated a dose dependent relationship between consumption of alcohol and certain types of cancers and the strongest link was found between alcohol abuse and cancer of the mouth, pharynx, larynx, and esophagus. Pancreatitis and gallstone are common findings among alcohol abusers. In alcohol abusers, endotoxin may be released from gut bacteria by action of excess alcohol and such a process may trigger progression of acute pancreatitis into chronic pancreatitis. Chronic pancreatitis may lead to pancreatic cancer [44].

There is a consensus that heavy alcohol consumption significantly increases the risk of breast cancer. In general having 1 additional drink per day increases the risk from 2% to 12%. However, relation between moderate alcohol consumption and risk of breast cancer is controversial because there are conflicting reports in the medical literature. Pelucchi et al. concluded that consumption of fewer than 3 alcoholic drinks per week is not associated with increased risk of breast cancer, but consuming 3−6 drinks per week may be associated with a small increase in risk [45]. Lowry et al. based on a study of 7835 women who had breast cancer concluded that consumption of alcohol before and after breast cancer diagnosis did not increase the risk overall or cause specific mortality [46]. Interestingly, alcohol is not associated with an increased risk of all types of breast cancer. Strumylaite et al. observed that moderate alcohol consumption (up to 5 drinks per week to more than 5 drinks per week) is associated with the risk of estrogen receptor positive breast cancer particularly in postmenopausal women [47].

Beverage type is not associated with increased risk of breast cancer because alcohol acts as a weak breast carcinogen. Moreover, alcohol may increase responsiveness of estrogen receptors present in breast. Acetaldehyde, a metabolite of alcohol, is also a carcinogen. However, there are many other factors that may increase the risk of breast cancer, including family history (BRCA1 and BRCA2 gene mutation are the most common inherited factors), being older (only 10−15% breast cancer diagnosis among women 45 years or younger), using hormone replacement therapy, used or using birth control pills, not having a child, or having a dense breast.

Other benefits of moderate alcohol consumption

Moderate alcohol consumption reduces the risk of developing rheumatoid arthritis. Results from two Scandinavian studies indicated that among moderate drinkers, the risk of rheumatoid arthritis was significantly reduced [48]. Nissen et al. reported, based on a study using 2908 patients suffering from rheumatoid arthritis, that occasional or daily consumption of alcohol reduced the progression of the disease based on radiological studies (x-ray). The best results were observed in male patients [49].

Relation between moderate alcohol consumption and reduced risk of common cold has been studied. In a large study using 4272 faculty and staff of 5 Spanish Universities as subjects, the investigators observed that total alcohol intake from drinking beer and spirits had no protective effect against common cold whereas moderate wine consumption was associated with reduced risk of common cold [50].

Because moderate consumption of alcohol can prevent many diseases, it is expected that moderate drinkers may live longer than lifetime abstainers of alcohol. Klatsky et al. studied 10 year mortality rates in relation to alcohol in 8060 subjects and observed that persons who consumed 2 drinks or less daily fared best and had significant reductions in mortality rate than nondrinkers. The heaviest drinkers (6 or more drinks a day) had much higher mortality rate than moderate drinkers while people who drink 3−5 drinks per day had a similar mortality rate as nondrinkers. Therefore consuming 2 or less drinks per day is the best practice [51].

Poikolainen commented that the lowest risk of death seems to be at the average intake of 1 drink per day. However, there is no major difference between beer, wine, or liquor [52]. In another cohort study, the authors concluded that low frequent use of any alcoholic beverage was associated with lower all-cause mortality as well as mortality from cardiovascular diseases [53]. However, based on a study of 13,064 men and 11,459 women, Gronbaek et al. observed that compared to nondrinkers, light drinkers who avoided wine had a 10% lower chance of mortality but wine drinkers had 34% lower chance of mortality [54]. In another study, the authors concluded that light drinkers of any kind of wine had lower mortality risk than beer or liquor drinkers [55]. Gronbaek et al. based on results of Copenhagen Health City Survey, Denmark (12,039 subjects) concluded that light to moderate wine intake is related to good self-perceived health whereas this is not the case for beer and spirits [56].

Other health hazards of heavy drinking

Alcohol abuse is associated with increased risk of bacterial and viral infection due to impairment of the immune system by alcohol. Exposure to alcohol can result in reduced cytokine production. Mast cells produce a variety of compounds including cytokines, histamine, eicosanoid, and tumor narcosis factor-alpha which play important roles in defense against bacteria, and parasite. Alcohol reduces viability of mast cells and may cause cell death and alcohol induced reduction of the viability of mast cells could contribute to impaired immune system associated with alcohol abuse [57].

Alcohol abuse can have adverse effects on human endocrine system. Alcohol abuse may lead to a disease known as pseudo Cushing's syndrome which is indistinguishable from Cushing's syndrome characterized by excess production of cortisol causing high blood pressure, muscle weakness, diabetes, obesity, and a variety of other physical disturbances. Diminished sexual function in alcoholic men has been described. Administration of alcohol in healthy young male volunteers caused diminished level of testosterone. Guthauser et al. reported a case of a man who had azoospermia due to alcohol abuse but was able to father a child following assisted reproduction technique 2 years after complete withdrawal from alcohol [58]. Even drinking 3 or more drinks a day may cause significant problems in women including delayed ovulation or failure to ovulate, and menstrual problems but such problems were not noticed in women who consumed 2 or fewer drinks a day. This may be related to alcohol induced estrogen levels in women. Alcoholic women often experiences reproductive problems. Chronic consumption of alcohol may reduce bone mass through a complex process of inhibition of hormonal balance needed for bone growth including testosterone in men which is diminished in alcoholics. Alcohol abuse may also interfere with pancreatic secretion of insulin causing diabetes [59].

Alcohol in a higher dosage is a central nervous system depressant and as a result higher blood alcohol may cause depression, anxiety, and other related symptoms. Psychiatric illness may also be associated with alcohol abuse. Alcohol abuse is associated with all causes of decreased longevity compared to abstainers. Even occasional heavy drinking may be detrimental to health. Dawson reported an increased risk of mortality among individuals who usually drink more than five drinks per occasion but consumed alcohol less than once a month [60].

Alcohol also accelerates disease progression in patients with HIV infection due to impairment of the immune system. In one study using 231 patients with HIV infection who were undergoing antiretroviral therapy, the authors observed that even consumption of 2 or more drinks daily can cause a serious decline in CD4+ cell count (lower CD4+ counts indicates progression of AIDS) [61]. Irregular heavy drinking even once a month (5 or more drinks per occasion) increases risk of heart disease rather than protecting the heart as observed in moderate drinkers. The cardioprotective effect of moderate drinking also disappears when on average light to moderate drinking is mixed with occasional heavy drinking episodes [62].

Alcohol abuse and violent behavior/homicide

Many investigators reported a close link between violent behavior, homicide, and alcohol intoxication. Studies conducted on convicted murders suggested that about half of them were under heavy influence of alcohol at the time of murder [63]. Alcohol may induce aggression and violent behavior by disrupting normal brain function when consumed in high dosage. By impairing normal information processing capability of the brain, a person can misjudge a perceived threat and may react more aggressively than warranted. Serotonin, a neurotransmitter, is considered as a behavioral inhibitor. Alcohol abuse may lead to decreased serotonin activity causing aggressive behavior. By modulating serotonin and testosterone concentration, alcohol may exert its effect in inducing aggressive and violent behavior when consumed in excess. Alcohol abuse by husbands may be related to marital violence [64]. According to US Bureau of Justice, approximately 37% state prison inmates and 21% federal prison inmates serving time for violent crimes were under the influence of alcohol when they committed crimes.

Fetal alcohol syndrome

Fetal alcohol syndrome due to prenatal alcohol exposure was first reported by Jones and Smith in 1973 [65]. Since then many publications have documented teratogenic effects of alcohol in both human and animal studies. This syndrome is the most common noninherited cause of mental retardation in the United States. "Fetal alcohol spectrum disorders" was a term described in 2004 to convey that exposure of the fetus to alcohol produces a continuum of effects and that many babies who do not fulfill all criteria for diagnosis of fetal alcohol syndrome may nevertheless be profoundly impacted negatively throughout their lives due to exposure to alcohol. Approximately 1−4.8 of every 1000 children born in the United States has fetal alcohol syndrome while as many as 9.1 out of 1000 babies born has fetal alcohol spectrum disorder [66].

Conclusion

Although moderate alcohol consumption has many health benefits, heavy consumption of alcohol is detrimental to health. In moderation alcohol use can increase longevity, reduce risk of heart disease, stroke, and certain type of cancers. In addition, moderate alcohol consumption also has neuroprotective effect and reduces the risk of dementia including Alzheimer's type. However, alcohol consumption in excess produces intoxication, withdrawal, brain trauma, central nervous system infection, and hepatic failure. Moreover, a pregnant woman should not drink at all in order to avoid adverse outcomes of pregnancy.

References

[1] Liber CS. Relationship between nutrition, alcohol use and liver disease. Alcohol Res Health 2003;2003(27):220−31.
[2] Marczinski CA. Can energy drinks increase the desire for more alcohol? Adv Nutr 2015;6:96−101.

[3] Erol A, Karpyak VM. Sex and gender related differences in alcohol use and its consequences: contemporary knowledge and future research considerations. Drug Alcohol Depend 2015;156:1–13.

[4] Lotfipour S, Cisneros V, Ogbu UC, McCoy CE, et al. A retrospective analysis of ethnic and gender differences in alcohol consumption among emergency department patients: a cross-sectional study. BMC Emerg Med 2015;29:24.

[5] Celik S, Karapirli M, Kandemir E, Ucar F, Kantarci MN, Gurler M, et al. Fatal ethyl and methyl alcohol related poisoning in Ankara: a retrospective analysis of 10,720 cases between 2001 and 2011. J Forensic Leg Med 2013;20:151–4.

[6] Phillips DP, Brewer KM. The relationship between serious injury and blood alcohol concentration (BAC) in fetal motor vehicle accidents: BAC = 0.01% is associated with significantly more dangerous accidents than BAC = 0.00%. Addiction 2011;106:1614–22.

[7] Falleti MG, Maruff P, Collie A, Darby DG, et al. Qualitative similarities in cognitive impairment associated with 24 g of sustained wakefulness and blood alcohol concentration of 0.05%. J Sleep Res 2003;12:265–74.

[8] Fell JC, Voss RB. The effectiveness of a 0.05% blood alcohol concentration (BAC) limit for driving in the United States. Addiction 2014;109:869–74.

[9] Garcia-Moreno H, Calvo JR, Maldonado MD. High levels of melatonin generated during the brewing process. J Pineal Res 2013;55:26–30.

[10] Murch SJ, Hall BA, Le CH, Saxena PK. Changes in the levels of indoleamine phytochemicals during veraison and ripening of wine grapes. J Pineal Res 2010;49:95–100.

[11] Orman ES, Odena G, Bataller R. Alcoholic liver disease: pathogenesis, management and novel targets for therapy. J Gastroenterol Hepatol 2013;28(Suppl 1):77–84.

[12] Belentani S, Tribelli C. Spectrum of liver disease in general population. Lessons from Dionysus study. J Hepatol 2001;2001(35):531–7.

[13] Walsh K, Alexander G. Alcoholic liver disease. Postgrad Med J 2000;281:280–6.

[14] Hezode C, Lonjon I, Roudot-Thorval F, Pawlotsky JM, Zafrani ES, Dhumeaux D. Impact of moderate alcohol consumption on histological activity and fibrosis in patients with chronic hepatitis C, and specific influence of steatosis, a prospective study. Aliment Pharmacol Ther 2003;17:1031–7.

[15] Dugum M, McCullough A. Diagnosis and management of alcoholic liver disease. J Clin Transl Hepatol 2015;28:109–16.

[16] Zima T, Fialova L, Mestek O, Janebova M, Crkovska J, Malbohan I, et al. Oxidative stress, metabolism of ethanol and alcohol related disease. J Biomed Sci 2001;8:59–70.

[17] Friedman LA, Kimball AW. Coronary heart disease mortality and alcohol consumption in Framingham. Am J Epidemiol 1986;124:481–9.

[18] Tolstrup J, Jensen MK, Tjonneland A, Overvad K, Mukamal KJ, Gronbaek M. Prospective study of alcohol drinking patterns and coronory heart disease in women and men. BMJ 2006;332:1244–8.

[19] Bryson CL, Mukamal KJ, Mittleman MA, Fried LP, Hirsch CH, Kitzman DW, et al. The association of alcohol consumption and incident heart failure: the cardiovascular health study. J Am Coll Cardiol 2006;48:305–11.

[20] Gemes K, Janszky I, Laugsand LE, Laszlo KD, et al. Alcohol consumption is associated with a lower incident of acute myocardial infarction: results from a large prospective population based study in Norway. J Intern Med 2016;279:365–75.

[21] O'Keefe JH, Bhatti SK, Bajwa A, DiNicolantonio J, et al. Alcohol and cardiovascular health: the dose makes the poison or the remedy. Mayo Clin Proc 2014;89:382−93.

[22] Ruf JC. Alcohol, wine and platelet function. Biol Res 2004;37:209−15.

[23] Wu JM, Hiieh TC. Resveratrol: a cardioprotective substance. Ann N Y Acad Sci 2011;1215:16−21.

[24] Wu JM, Wang ZR, Hsieh TC, Bruder JL, et al. Mechanism of cardioprotection by resveratrol, a phenolic antioxidant present in red wine (review). Int J Mol Med 2001;8:3−17.

[25] Chiva-Blanch G, Arranz S, Lamuela-Raventos RM, Estruch R. Effects of wine, alcohol and polyphenols on cardiovascular disease risk factors: evidences from human studies. Alcohol Alcohol 2013;48:270−7.

[26] Rimm EB, Stampfer MJ. Wine, beer and spirits: are they really horses of a different color? Circulation 2002;15:2806−7.

[27] Barefoot JC, Gronbaek M, Feaganes JR, McPherson RS, et al. Alcoholic beverage preference, diet, and health habits in UNC Alumni Heart Study. Am J Clin Nutr 2002;76:466−72.

[28] Mayer Jr O, Simon J, Rosolova H. A population study of the influence of beer consumption on folate and homocysteine concentrations. Eur J Clin Nutr 2001;55:605−9.

[29] Rosenbloom JI, Mukamal KJ, Frost LE, Mittleman MA. Alcohol consumption patterns, beverage type, and long term mortality among women survivors of acute myocardial infarction. Am J Cardiol 2012;109:147−52.

[30] Klatsky AL. Alcohol and cardiovascular health. Physiol Behav 2010;100:76−81.

[31] Laonigro I, Correale M, Di Biase M, Altomare E. Alcohol abuse and heart failure. Eur J Heart Fail 2009;11:453−62.

[32] Yedlapati SH, Mendu A, Stewart SH. Alcohol related diagnoses and increased mortality in acute myocardial infarction patients: an analysis of nationwide inpatient sample. J Hosp Med 2016;11:563−7.

[33] Truelsen T, Gronbaek M, Schnohr P, Boyen G. Intake of beer, wine and spirits and risk of stroke: the Copenhagen city heart study. Stroke 1998;29:2467−72.

[34] Ikehara S, Iso H, Yamagishi K, Yamamoto S. Alcohol consumption, social support and risk of stroke and coronary heart disease among Japanese men: the JPHC study. Alcohol Clin Exp Res 2009;33:1025−32.

[35] Koppes LL, Dekker JM, Hendriks HF, Bouter LM, Heine RJ. Moderate alcohol consumption lowers the risk of type 2 diabetes: a meta-analysis of prospective observational studies. Diabetes Care 2005;28(3):719−25.

[36] Baliunas DO, Taylor BJ, Irving H, Roereke M, Patra J, Mohapatra S, et al. Alcohol as a risk factor for type 2 diabetes: a systematic review and meta-analysis. Diabetes Care 2009;32:2123−32.

[37] Parodi J, Ormeno D, Ochoa-de laPaz LD. Amyloid pore channel hypothesis: effect of ethanol on aggregation state using frog oocytes for an Alzheimer's disease study. BMB Rep 2015;48:13−18.

[38] Zeigler DW, Wang CC, Yoast RA, Dickinson BD, McCaffree MA, Robinowitz CB, et al. The neurocognitive effects of alcohol on adolescents and college students. Prev Med 2005;40:23−32.

[39] Medina KL, McQueeny T, Nagel BJ, Hanson KL, Schweinsburg AD, Tapert SE. Prefrontal cortex volumes in adolescents with alcohol use disorders: unique gender effects. Alcohol Clin Exp Res 2008;32:386−94.

[40] Harper C. The neurotoxicity of alcohol. Hum Exp Toxicol 2007;26(3):251−7.

[41] Chao C, Slezak JM, Caan BJ, Quinn VP. Alcoholic beverage intake and risk of lung cancer: the California Men's Health Study. Cancer Epidemiol Biomarkers Prev 2008;17:2692−9.

[42] Pelucchi C, Galeone C, Montella M, Polesel J, Crispo A, Talamini R, et al. Alcohol consumption and renal cell cancer risk in two Italian case controlled study. Ann Oncol 2008;19:1003−8.

[43] Ferraro PM, Taylor EN, Cambaro G, Curhan GC. Soda and other beverages and the risk of kidney stones. Clin J Am Soc Nephrol 2013;8:1389−95.

[44] Apte M, Pirola R, Wilson J. New insights into alcoholic pancreatitis and pancreatic cancer. J Gastroenterol Hepatol 2009;24(3, Suppl 3):S351−6.

[45] Pelucchi C, Tramacere I, Boffetta P, Negri E, et al. Alcohol consumption and cancer risk. Nutr Cancer 2011;63:983−90.

[46] Lowry SJ, Kappahahn K, Chlebowski RT, Li CI. Alcohol use and breast cancer survival among participants in the women's health initiative. Cancer Epidemiol Biomarkers Prev 2016;25:1268−73.

[47] Strumylaite L, Sharp SJ, Kregzdyte R, Poskiene L, et al. The association of low to moderate alcohol consumption with breast cancer subtypes defined by hormone receptor status. PLoS One 2015;10:e0144680.

[48] Kallberg H, Jacobsen S, Bengtsson C, Pedersen M, et al. Alcohol consumption is associated with decreased risk of rheumatoid arthritis: results from two Scandinavian studies. Ann Rheum Dis 2009;68:222−7.

[49] Nissen MJ, Gabay C, Scherer A, Finchk A. The effect of alcohol on radiographic progression in rheumatoid arthritis. Arthritis Rheum 2010;62:1265−72.

[50] Takkouch B, Regueira-Mendez C, Garcia-Closas R, Figueiras A, Gestal-Oterro JJ, Hernan MA. Intake of wine, beer, and spirits and the risk of clinical common cold. Am J Epidemiol 2002;155:853−8.

[51] Klatsky AL, Friedman GD, Siegekaub AB. Alcohol and mortality: a ten year Kaiser-Permanente experience. Ann Int Med 1981;95:139−45.

[52] Poikolainen K. Alcohol and mortality: a review. J Clin Epidemiol 1995;48:455−65.

[53] Graff-Iversen S, Jansen MD, Hoff DA, Hoiseth G, et al. Divergent associations of drinking frequency and binge consumption of alcohol with mortality within same cohort. J Epidemiol Community Health 2013;67:350−7.

[54] Gronbaek M, Becker U, Johansen D, Gottschau A, et al. Type of alcohol consumed and mortality from all causes, coronary heart disease and cancer. Ann Intern Med 2000;133:411−19.

[55] Klatsky AL, Friedman CD, Armstrong MA, Kipp H. Wine, liquor, beer and mortality. Am J Epidemiol 2003;158:585−95.

[56] Gronbaek M, Mortensen EL, Mygind K, Andersen AT, et al. Beer, wine, spirits and subjective health. J Epidemiol Community Health 1999;53:721−4.

[57] Numi K, Methuen T, Maki T, Lindstedt KA, Kovanen PT, Sandler C, et al. Ethanol induces apoptosis in human mast cells. Life Sci 2009;85:678−84.

[58] Guthauser B, Boitrelle F, Plat A, Thiercelin N, et al. Chronic excessive alcohol consumption and male fertility: a case report on reversible azoospermia and a literature review. Alcohol Alcohol 2014;49:42−4.

[59] Emanuele N, Emanuele MA. Alcohol alters critical hormonal balance. Alcohol Health Res World 1997;21:53−64.

[60] Dawson DA. Alcohol and mortality from external causes. J Stud Alcohol Drug 2001;62 (6):790−7.

[61] Baum MK, Rafie C, Lai C, Sales S, Page JB, Campa A. Alcohol use accelerates HIV disease progression. AIDS Res Hum Retroviruses 2010;26:511—18.
[62] Roerecke M, Rehm J. Irregular heavy drinking occasions and risk of ischemic heart disease: a systematic review and meta-analysis. Am J Epidemiol 2010;171 (6):633—44.
[63] Palijan TZ, Kovacevic D, Radeljak S, Kovac M, Mustapic J. Forensic aspects of alcohol abuse and homicide. Coll Antropol 2009;33:893—7.
[64] Quigley BM, Leonard KE. Alcohol and the continuation of early marital aggression. Alcohol Clin Exp Res 2000;24:1003—10.
[65] Jones KL, Smith DW. Recognition of the fetal alcohol syndrome in early infancy. Lancet 1973;302:999—1001.
[66] Sampson PD, Streissguth AP, Bookstein FL. Incidence of fetal alcohol syndrome and prevalence of alcohol related neurodevelopmental disorder. Teratology 1997;56:317—26.

Drugs of abuse: an overview

2

Introduction

Drug and alcohol abuse is not only an important public health issue in the United States but also worldwide. According to the latest 2014 National Survey of Drug Use and Health conducted by the Substance Abuse and Mental Health Services Administration (SAMHSA) of the US government published in September 2015, and estimated 27.0 million people in the United States (10.2% of the American population) of 12 years or older used an illicit drug in the past 30 days of the survey. The percentage was higher than those in every year of survey from 2002 to 2013. The major drug abused in 2014 survey was marijuana (estimated 22.2 million current users) followed by nonmedical use of prescription pain medication (4.3 million users). In addition there are 1.9 million individuals abusing tranquilizers, 1.5 million people abusing cocaine, and 0.4 million people abusing heroin. Substance abuse alone is estimated to cost Americans $600 billion each year. It is also estimated that 17.0 million people in United States suffer from alcohol use disorder [1].

Drug overdose is the leading cause of injury and death in the United States. In 1999, the death rate was 6.0 per 100,000 people but increased to 13.8 per 100,000 people in 2013. The increase in drug overdose death rate in United States is mostly attributable to abuse of prescription drugs, especially opioids, sedatives, tranquilizers, and stimulants [2]. Commonly abused drugs in United States include amphetamine, methamphetamine, cocaine, barbiturates, benzodiazepines, opioids, marijuana, and phencyclidine. In addition, various designer drugs including bath salts (synthetic cathinone) and spices (synthetic cannabinoids) are also abused. Certain drugs such as 3,4-methylenedioxymethamphetamine (MDMA, a designer drug), gamma-hydroxybutyric acid (GHB), ketamine, and Rohypnol (flunitrazepam) are used in rave parties. GHB and Rohypnol are encountered in date rape situations. Less commonly abused drugs include the abuse of magic mushrooms, and peyote cactus. This chapter provides an overview of commonly abused drugs as well as brief discussion on the abuse of magic mushrooms, and peyote cactus. Designer drugs including bath salts (synthetic cathinone) and spices (synthetic cannabinoids) are discussed in Chapter 3, Designer Drugs Including Bath Salts and Spices. Commonly abused drugs in United States are listed in Table 2.1. Street names of commonly abused drugs are summarized in Table 2.2.

Alcohol, Drugs, Genes and the Clinical Laboratory. DOI: http://dx.doi.org/10.1016/B978-0-12-805455-0.00002-6

Table 2.1 Abused drugs in the United States

Class of drug	Commonly abused	Less commonly abused
Stimulants	Amphetamine, methamphetamine, MDMA, MDA, synthetic cathinone, cocaine	Designer drugs other than MDMA and MDA which are related to amphetamine structure
Opioids	Heroine, morphine, codeine, oxycodone, hydrocodone, hydromorphone, methadone, meperidine, propoxyphene	Fentanyl and structurally related designer drugs
Cannabinoid	Marijuana (tetrahydrocannabinol), Hashish along with synthetic cannabinoids	Abuse of hemp product is rare
Anesthetics	Phencyclidine, ketamine	None
Benzodiazepines	Alprazolam, lorazepam, temazepam, diazepam, flunitrazepam, etc.	None
Barbiturates	Pentobarbital, secobarbital	Phenobarbital
Hallucinogens	Lysergic acid diethylamide (LSD)	Magic mushroom, peyote cactus
Club drugs	MDMA, ketamine, gamma-hydroxybutyric acid (GHB), Rohypnol (flunitrazepam)	
Prescription drugs	Oxycodone, hydromorphone, methadone, propoxyphene, benzodiazepines, zolpidem, zaleplon, methylphenidate, dextro-amphetamine	Hydrocodone, mephobarbital, phenmetrazine

Table 2.2 Street names of commonly abused drugs

Drug	Street names
Amphetamine	Black Beauties, Crosses, Hearts, Speed, Truck Drivers, Uppers
Methamphetamine	Ice, Meth, Speed, Crystal, Fire, Glass, Go Fast, Ice
MDMA	Ecstasy, Molly, Adam, Clarity, Lover's Speed, Peace
MDA	Eve, Sally, Sass
Cocaine	Blow, Bump, C, Candy, Charlie, Coke, Crack, Rock, Snow
Heroin	Brown Sugar, Horse, White Horse, Junk, Smack
Oxycodone	O.C., Oxycet, Oxy, Hillbilly Heroin
Barbiturates	Barbs, Pennies, Red Birds, Reds, Yellow Jackets, Yellows
Benzodiazepines	Candy, Downers, Sleeping Pills, Tranks
Marijuana	Bud, dope, Ganja, Grass, Green, Joint, Mary Jane, Pot, Reefer, Smoke, Trees, Weed, Hashish, Gangster, Hash, Hemp
Phencyclidine (PCP)	Angel Dust, Boat, Hog, Love Boat, Peace Pill
Ketamine	Cat Valium, K, Special K, Vitamin K
Gamma-hydroxybutyric acid (GHB)	G, Georgia Home Boy, Bodily Harm, Liquid Ecstasy, Liquid X, Soap
Rohypnol	Date Rape Drug, Forget Pill, Forget-Me Pill, Mexican Valium, R2, Reynolds, Rib, Roach, Roofies, Rope
Synthetic cathinone	Bath Salts, Cloud Nine, Ivory Wave, Lunar Wave, Vanilla Sky
Synthetic cannabinoids	K2, Spice, Black Mamba, Bliss, Bombay Blue, Fake Weed, Fire, Genie, Moon Rocks, Skunk, Smacked

Drugs of abuse: historical perspective

Substances capable of changing mood and producing euphoria are found in many plants. Some of these psychoactive plants were known to ancient people. The history of the cultivation of poppy plants dates back to 3400 BC, in Mesopotamia. Poppy plants were cultivated by Egyptians and then the poppy plants were introduced in India and China. Arabian physicians used opium very extensively around 1000 AD [3]. Opium addiction was widespread in China and, following the 1799 ban on opium in there, the smuggling of the substance became a common industry that led to the Opium War between Britain and China in 1839.

During the 19th century, opium was grown in the United States as well as imported. Use of opium in many tonics, and the unhindered smoking of opium, together resulted in an epidemic of opiate addiction by the late 1800s. The generous use of morphine in treating wounded soldiers during the Civil War also produced many addicts. Heroin was first synthesized in 1874. Heroin was considered as a highly effective medicine for treating the cough, chest pains, and discomfort of tuberculosis, but later the addictive property of heroin was recognized.

The psychoactive plant *Cannabis sativa* (hemp plant) was known in ancient China and India 5000 years ago. The earliest reference was found in a pharmacy book written in 2737 BC during the time of Chinese Emperor Shen Nung. Around 1000 AD, hemp products were widely used in the Middle East and Africa [4]. Most likely in the 16th century, cannabis reached South America. In the 1800s cannabis was used in medicine due to its narcotic effect. In the second half of the 19th century, many scientific articles were published in Europe and the United States regarding the therapeutic values of cannabis, but in the beginning of the 20th century the use of cannabis in medicine was reduced significantly [5].

Cocaine is a naturally occurring alkaloid in the leaves of the coca plant (*Erythroxylon coca*). Coca leaves were chewed by native people of South America (Peru, Bolivia, and Ecuador). Chewing coca leaves was also a part of religious ceremonies of Incas. In the mid-19th century, cocaine became known to Western Civilizations and after 1885 pharmaceutical companies started selling cocaine. Cocaine was used in local anesthesia and in many tonics designed for regaining strength and vigor. In earlier days, extract of coca leaves was used in Coca Cola, but in the beginning of 20th century, coca extract was removed from Coca Cola drink and was replaced by a higher amount of caffeine [4].

Lysergic acid is a naturally occurring alkaloid found in the ergot fungus (*Claviceps purpurea*). Lysergic acid diethylamide (LSD) is a potent hallucinogen synthesized in 1938 by Dr. Albert Hoffman, a chemist of Sandoz Laboratories who later discovered its hallucinogenic effect. LSD is also abused throughout the world today.

Abused drugs: regulatory issues

In most countries drugs with high abuse potential are strictly regulated by the Government. In the United States, The Drug Abuse Control Act of 1956 provided guidelines for pharmaceutical industries for manufacturing and dispensing controlled

Table 2.3 **Classification of commonly abused drugs as schedule drugs**

Class	Abuse potential	Examples
Schedule I	Highest	Heroin, MDMA, marijuana, LSD, methaqualone, mescaline (active ingredient of magic mushroom), active ingredient of peyote cactus (psilocybin and psilocin), gamma-hydroxybutyric acid (GHB), synthetic cathinone (bath salts), synthetic cannabinoids (spices), and various designer drugs, methaqualone
Schedule II	High	Cocaine, methadone, morphine, meperidine, codeine, oxycodone, hydrocodone, amphetamine, methamphetamine, phencyclidine
Schedule III	Moderate to low	Products containing less than 90 mg of codeine per dose (tylenol with codeine), ketamine, testosterone, anabolic steroids
Schedule IV	Low	Diazepam, alprazolam, lorazepam, triazolam, tramadol, propoxyphene, phenobarbital
Schedule V	Lowest	Codeine containing cough mixtures (less than 200 mg of codeine per 100 mL)

substances. Then, in 1970, the Controlled Substances Act was passed for further regulating drugs with high abuse potential. The major focus of this law was the scheduling of drugs into five different classes based on abuse potential, harmfulness, and development of drug dependence as well as potential benefits when used medically. Several amendments were later added in order to provide power to the Attorney General of the United States and subsequently to Drug Enforcement Administration to classify a drug with high abuse potential in "Schedule I" prior to completion of formal review. The two other well-known amendments to the drug act were Anti-Drug Abuse Acts of 1986 and 1988 [6]. Controlled substances are categorized in five groups depending on the medical need and abuse potential. Schedule I drugs have no known medical use but very high abuse potential. Schedule II drugs may have known medical use but are also highly addictive. Schedule III drugs are used medically but may have some abuse potential. However, abuse potential of Schedule III drugs is lesser in magnitude compared to Schedule II drugs. Schedule IV drugs are used in medical practice but may have low potential of abuse. Schedule V drugs are widely used in medical practice and some drugs may have very low abuse potential. Example of a Schedule V drug is cough mixture containing low level of codeine. Classifications of various abused drugs as controlled substances are given Table 2.3.

Abuse of stimulants

Amphetamine, methamphetamine, along with the popular designer drugs MDMA, and 3,4-methylenedioxyamphetamine (MDA), are widely abused in the United

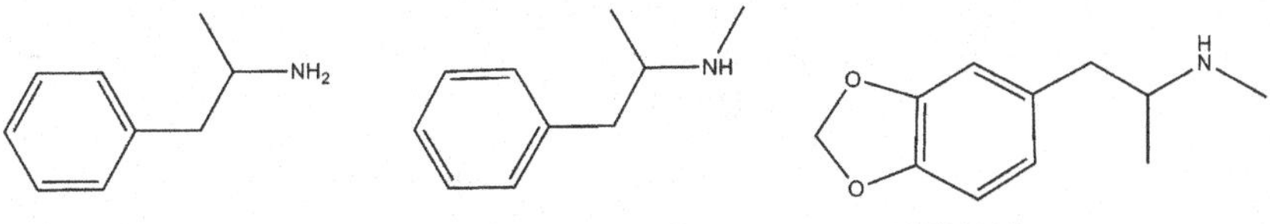

Amphetamine   **Methamphetamine**   **MDMA/ecstasy**

Figure 2.1 Chemical structure of amphetamine, methamphetamine, and MDMA/ecstasy. *Source*: Figure courtesy of Matthew D. Krasowski, MD, PhD, Clinical Professor of Pathology, University of Iowa Carver College of Medicine. All figures (Figs. 2.1–2.9) in this chapter were drawn by Dr. Krasowski using ChemDraw program.

States. Amphetamine was first synthesized in 1887 and was introduced clinically in 1932. Today, common medical use of amphetamines like drugs (amphetamine, methamphetamine, and methylphenidate) is in the treatment attention deficit hyperactive disorder (ADHD). However, due to central nervous system (CNS) stimulant effects, these drugs are also abused. On the clandestine market, methamphetamine is more readily available than amphetamine due to ease of synthesis of methamphetamine from ephedrine or pseudoephedrine. Moreover, both drugs are equally potent as CNS stimulants [7]. The chemical structure of amphetamine, methamphetamine, and MDMA are given in Fig. 2.1.

Amphetamine and related compounds have structural similarities with phenylethylamine. These drugs produce their clinical effects via modulation of peripheral and central catecholamine neurotransmitter system thus causing sympathomimetic effects. Clinical symptoms of toxicity include hyperthermia, hypertension, tachycardia, hyperarousal, agitation, hallucination, and paranoia. Seizure and coma may result from serious overdose and electrolyte abnormalities may also be observed. Diagnosis can be confirmed by using urine drug screening which includes testing for amphetamine/methamphetamine. Care is mostly supportive and benzodiazepines are first line agents to control agitation. However, beta-blockers must be avoided in treating amphetamine induced hypertension due to potential alpha-receptor stimulation that may worsen toxicity [8].

Hepatic and renal clearance contribute to elimination of amphetamine and methamphetamine with an approximate half-life of 6–12 h. A significant amount of both amphetamine and methamphetamine are excreted as parent drug in the urine. However, methamphetamine is metabolized to amphetamine by the action of cytochrome P 450 mixed function enzymes most noticeably by the action of CYP2D6. Amphetamine is also metabolized to 4-hydroxy amphetamine (para-hydroxyamphetamine), benzoic acid including its glycine conjugate. MDMA is metabolized to MDA and a variety of other metabolites including 4-hydroxy-3-methoxyamphetamine (major metabolite also excreted in urine as glucuronide or sulfate conjugate), 3,4-dihydroxy-methamphetamine, and 3-hydroxy-4-methoxymethamphetamine. The approximate half-life of MDMA is 7 h. Metabolites of amphetamine, methamphetamine, and MDMA are summarized in Table 2.4.

Table 2.4 **Metabolites of commonly abused drugs**

Drug	Metabolites
Amphetamine	Para-hydroxyamphetamine, benzoic, acid, and conjugates
	Significant amount of amphetamine is also recovered in the urine
Methamphetamine	Amphetamine, 4-hydroxyamphetamine, 4-hydroxymethamphetmine, benzoic acid; unchanged methamphetamine also recovered in the urine
MDMA	3,4-Methylenedioxyamphetamine (MDA), 4-hydroxy-3-methoxyamphetamine (major metabolite also excreted in urine as glucuronide or sulfate conjugate), 3,4-dihydroxy-methamphetamine, and 3-hydroxy-4-methoxymethamphetamine
Cocaine	Benzoylecgonine, ecgonine methyl ester, nor-cocaine (minor metabolite)
Heroin	6-Monoacetyl morphine (also known as 6-acteyl morphine; marker of heroin abuse), morphine
Morphine	Morphine-3-glucuronider (major metabolite; inactive) and morphine-6-glucuronide (active metabolite)
Codeine	Morphine, morphine-3-glucuronide
Hydrocodone	Hydromorphone
Oxycodone	Oxymorphone
Methadone	2-Ethylidine-1,5-diemethyl, 3,3-diphenylpyrrolidine (EDDP)
Propoxyphene	Nor-propoxyphene
Marijuana (Δ^9-tetrahydrocannabinol)	11-Nor-9-carboxy-Δ^9-tetrahydrocannabinol
Phencyclidine (PCP)	*Cis* and *trans*-1-(1-phenylcyclohexyl)-4-hydroxypiperidine, 4-phenyl-4-piperidinocyclohexanol, and their conjugates
Amobarbital	3-Hydroxy amobarbital
Pentobarbital	3-Hydroxy pentobarbital
Secobarbital	3-Hydroxy secobarbital
Lysergic acid diethylamide (LSD)	2-Oxo-3-hydroxy lysergic acid diethylamide (O-H-LSD)

Fatalities from abuse of amphetamine and related compounds have been reported. De Letter et al. examined fatalities between January 1976 and December 2004 due to amphetamine overdose in their district and concluded that in addition to amphetamine, abuse of MDMA, 3,4-methylenedioxyethylamphetamine, MDA, 4-methylthioamphetamine, and para-methoxyamphetamine also caused fatalities. The authors reported 24 fatalities due to overdose with amphetamines and related drugs. Most victims were male and under 25 years of age [9]. In another study, the authors detected 146 fatalities related to use of methamphetamine and determined that 52 fatalities were primarily related to the direct toxic effect of methamphetamine and other fatalities were drug related. The authors determined the blood level of methamphetamine using gas chromatography/mass spectrometry (GC/MS) and commented that methamphetamine blood levels varied from 0.05 to 9.30 mg/L in these individuals. Most methamphetamine related deaths were associated with blood methamphetamine levels greater than 0.5 mg/L but lower levels were also encountered in methamphetamine related fatalities [10]. Wollner et al. recently reported two fatal cases (a 19-year old man and a 39-year old man) due to abuse of MDMA and amphetamine, respectively. A 19-year old man died from MDMA overdose and femoral vein postmortem blood showed MDMA level of 4.27 mg/L. A 39-year old man collapsed at the workplace and later died in the hospital. His femoral vein blood showed amphetamine level of 1.08 mg/L. In his rucksack, a small bag was found containing 1.6 g of amphetamine [11]. Amphetamine, methamphetamine, and MDMA are routinely detected in clinical laboratory using immunoassays. Results may be confirmed by using GC/MS. For confirming methamphetamine in urine, its metabolite amphetamine must also be present.

Abuse of cocaine

Cocaine is a natural alkaloid found in the plant *E. coca* that grows naturally in South America and, to a lesser extent, in other parts of the world. Cocaine was extracted from coca leaves in the mid-1800s by Albert Neimann who then evaluated the anesthetic properties of cocaine. Today cocaine has a limited medical use during surgical procedures involving the manipulation of the mucous membranes, particularly those of upper respiratory track, as a topical anesthetic agent. The anesthetic effect is believed to be the result of a reversible blocking of nervous impulse conduction, itself a result of restricting sodium movement within cell membranes [12].

Cocaine is sold in illegal markets as hydrochloride salt that is usually cut with agents such as mannitol, lactose, and sugar, in order to make more profit. As a result preparations usually contain around 50% cocaine. Cocaine is also sold in the street as crack cocaine and cocaine powder. Crack is a freebase of cocaine that produces a characteristic sound when smoked. Cocaine can also be snorted, taken orally or intravenously. People abuse cocaine to get desired effects, which include euphoria, elevated mood, and enhanced sexual energy. However, cocaine also has many undesirable effects including paranoia, hallucination, and psychosis. Cocaine induced delirium is also common.

Unfortunately cocaine abuse is a serious public health issue not only in United States but worldwide. It has been estimated that 25−30 million Americans have used cocaine and an estimated 5−6 million people are using cocaine on a regular basis. Abuse of cocaine may cause sudden death due to cardiac toxicity of cocaine. Moreover, the cardiotoxic effect of cocaine in any individual is unpredictable. A large number of cardiovascular diseases including acute myocardial infraction, arrhythmias, myocarditis, cardiomyopathy, endocarditis, and hypertension have been associated with regular abuse of cocaine. Cerebrovascular aneurysm may also result from cocaine abuse. Cocaine blocks the reuptake of catecholamines, including norepinephrine and dopamine, at the presynaptic level in the central and peripheral nervous systems. Increased serum catecholamine in patients suffering from cocaine cardiotoxicity has been reported. Accumulation of catecholamines in the myocardium stimulates beta-adrenergic receptors thus causing increased heart rate. Cocaine also affects the heart due to its anesthetic effect causing negative ionotropic effect [13]. Besides cardiovascular complications, psychiatric, and neurological abnormalities are also serious complications of cocaine abuse. Such complications include stroke, subarachnoid, and intracerebral hemorrhages as well as cerebral ischemia. Cocaine induced vasospasm, impaired platelet function, and decreased cerebral blood flow may contribute to neurological complications associated with cocaine abuse [14]. Cocaine abuse during pregnancy has a devastating effect on the fetus and may cause preterm birth, impaired fetal growth, and poor neurological development of the child (learning and behavioral problems). As a result pregnant women must avoid cocaine abuse [15]. Much lower concentration of cocaine may be associated with fatality of the users if an individual abuses simultaneously both cocaine and alcohol. This is due to formation of cocaethylene, a metabolite of cocaine observed only in conjunction with alcohol abuse. Unlike benzoylecgonine, which is inactive, cocaethylene is an active metabolite of cocaine. Please see Chapter 4, Combined Alcohol and Drug Abuse: A Potentially Deadly Mix for more detail.

Cocaine is readily absorbed after snorting with a short half-life of 0.5−1.5 h. Cocaine is spontaneously metabolized by plasma butylcholinesterase into ecgonine methyl ester. However, the major metabolite of cocaine, benzoylecgonine, is formed due to spontaneous hydrolysis of cocaine in vivo. A small amount of cocaine is also excreted unchanged in urine. Nor-cocaine, another minor metabolite of cocaine, is formed due to the action of liver enzymes. Other minor metabolites include para-hydroxy-benzoylecgonine, metahydroxy-benzoylecgonine, and metahydroxy cocaine. The chemical structures of cocaine and benzoylecgonine are given in Fig. 2.2. The chemical structure of cocaethylene is given in Fig. 2.3. Major metabolites of cocaine are listed in Table 2.4.

Maximal urinary excretion of unchanged cocaine is observed within 2 h of intranasal absorption while excretion of benzoylecgonine is maximal between 4 and 8 h. In one study after intranasal administration of cocaine (1.5 mg/kg of bodyweight) in subjects, peak cocaine, and benzoylecgonine concentrations in urine were 24 and 75 μg/mL, respectively. Although cocaine was detected for 8 h, benzoylecgonine was detected for 48−72 h by chromatographic or enzyme immunologic assay [16]. The presence of benzoylecgonine in urine is accepted as a proof of cocaine abuse.

Wide ranges of cocaine and benzoylecgonine concentrations have been reported in individuals who have died due to cocaine overdose. In one report the authors commented that significantly more men (95−98%) abused cocaine than women (2−5%) but mean age did not differ between men (29 years) and women (30 years). In drug induced deaths, the median cocaine concentration was 0.13 mg/L but other illicit drugs and alcohol were also abused by some subjects prior to death [17].

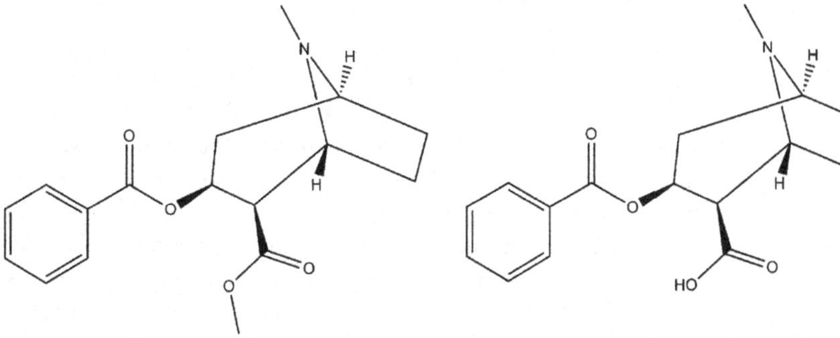

Cocaine   **Benzoylecgonine**

Figure 2.2 Chemical structure of cocaine and benzoylecgonine.
Source: Figure courtesy of Matthew D. Krasowski, Clinical Professor of Pathology,
University of Iowa Carver College of Medicine.

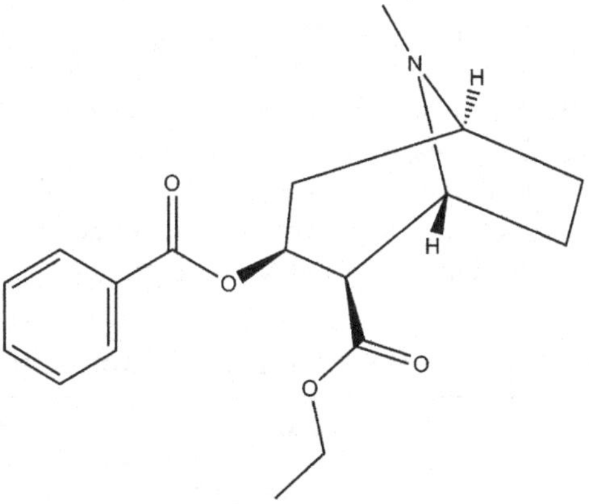

Cocaethylene

Figure 2.3 Chemical structure of cocaethylene.
Source: Figure courtesy of Matthew D. Krasowski, MD, PhD, Clinical Professor of
Pathology, University of Iowa Carver College of Medicine.

However, blood concentration of cocaine may be very high in subjects who died
from cocaine abuse. In one study, the authors reported the death of a 26-year old
Caucasian woman who was a known cocaine abuser. Her cocaine level in postmortem blood was 330 mg/L and benzoylecgonine concentration was 50 mg/L. High concentration of cocaine (215 mg/L) and benzoylecgonine (250 mg/L) were also
detected in her urine [18]. Cocaine is routinely measured in clinical laboratories
using immunoassay that targets benzoylecgonine. Confirmation may be conducted
using GC/MS.

Abuse of opioids

Opium has been used in ancient medicine but from a technical point of view only morphine, codeine, and the thebaine are natural opiates. Morphine and codeine are used for pain management while several semisynthetic opiates such as thebaine are used as the starting material for synthesis of oxycodone, oxymorphone, buprenorphine, naloxone, and related semisynthetic opiates. Opioids are synthesized compounds that are pharmacologically related to action of natural opiates. Common synthetic opioids are meperidine, methadone, and fentanyl. However, sometimes the term "opioids" is used to refer all compounds that render their pharmacological effects by acting as agonists of opiate receptors. Opioids are widely used in pain management in both cancer and noncancer patients. Commonly prescribed opioids are listed in Table 2.5. Naloxone and naltrexone are common opioid antagonists used medically to treat patients with opiate overdose. Sometimes naloxone or naltrexone is combined with an opioid to lower abuse potential of prescription opioid.

Heroin was synthesized from morphine but today heroin is a Schedule I drug with no known medical use. However, heroin is a popular drug of abuse and often this drug is abused in addition to other prescription opioids. Heroin is metabolized into 6-monoacetylmorphine (also known as 6-acetylmorphine) and finally to morphine by hydrolysis of ester linkage. Serum pseudocholinesterase and liver enzymes carboxylesterase 1 and 2 are responsible for metabolism of heroin. Detection and confirmation of 6-monoacetylmorphine is a proof of heroin abuse (marker of heroin abuse). The chemical structures of codeine, morphine, heroin, and oxycodone are given in Fig. 2.4. Heroin metabolites are listed in Table 2.4.

Table 2.5 Commonly prescribed common opioids in United States

Drug	Nature	Schedule drug
Codeine	Natural opiate	Schedule II
Morphine	Natural opiate	Schedule II
Dihydrocodeine	Semisynthetic	Schedule II
Hydrocodone	Semisynthetic	Schedule II
Hydromorphone	Semisynthetic	Schedule II
Oxycodone	Semisynthetic	Schedule II
Oxymorphone	Semisynthetic	Schedule II
Buprenorphine	Semisynthetic	Schedule III
Fentanyl/alfentanil/sufentanil	Synthetic	Schedule II
Meperidine	Synthetic	Schedule II
Methadone	Synthetic	Schedule II
Levorphanol	Synthetic	Schedule II
Pentazocine	Synthetic	Schedule IV
Propoxyphene	Synthetic	Schedule IV
Tapentadol	Synthetic	Schedule II
Tramadol	Synthetic	Schedule IV

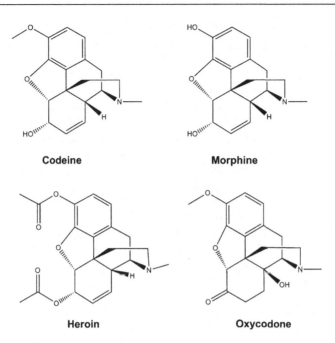

Figure 2.4 Chemical structure of codeine, morphine, heroin, and oxycodone.
Source: Figure courtesy of Matthew D. Krasowski, MD, PhD, Clinical Professor of Pathology, University of Iowa Carver College of Medicine.

In 2014, a total of 10.3 million Americans abused opioids that were not prescribed to them. In addition, death from overdose of prescription opioids is also troublesome as the rate increased from 1.5 deaths per 100,000 people in 2000 to 5.9 deaths per 100,000 people in 2014 according to latest data available. The pattern of nonprescription opioids abuse varies from once or twice per year to daily abuse as well as heavy abuse. Unfortunately, available data indicate that nonprescription abuse of prescription opioids is a strong risk factor for heroin abuse [19]. Most opioids abusers take opioids orally but also through other routes of administration including inhalation (snorting or smoking, second most common route after oral), and injection.

The pharmacological effects of opioids are due to their complex interactions with three types of opioid receptors (mu, delta, and kappa) found presynaptically or postsynaptically (depending on cell type) in the brain stem, thalamus, cortex, and the spinal cord dorsal horn. The endogenous opioids (beta-endorphin, met and leu-enkephalins, and dynorphins) also interact with opioid receptors [20]. Animal studies have indicated that euphoria induced by opioids as well as opioid addictions are related to their action on the mesolimbic dopamine system which appears to be different than interactions between opioid and opiate receptors that produce analgesic effect. Morphine and morphine-like opioids (hydromorphone, methadone, levorphanol, oxycodone, meperidine, and codeine) interact primarily with mu-receptor for their pharmacological actions. Buprenorphine is a partial agonist of opiate receptors while pentazocine, nalbuphine, and butorphanol are mixed opiate receptor agonists. Naloxone, which is used in reversing the clinical effects of opioid overdose, is an opioid antagonist that binds with all three opiate receptors.

Morphine's oral bioavailability is variable (35–75%) and duration of analgesic effect is 4–6 h. Morphine-6-glucuronide is an active metabolite, which is excreted in urine but may accumulate in blood in patients with renal insufficiency. However, the major metabolite of morphine (morphine 3-glucuronide) is inactive and is also secreted in urine. The major isoform of uridine diphosphate glucurono-syltransferase enzyme responsible for conjugation of morphine with glucuronic acid (both 3- and 6-morphine glucuronide) is UGT2B7. Codeine is metabolized into morphine by the liver due to action of CYP2D6 isoenzyme. Codeine may be considered as a pro-drug because most of the analgesic action of codeine is due to its active metabolite morphine. People who are deficient in CYP2D6 enzyme active may not get adequate pain relief from codeine therapy. Hydromorphone is excreted in urine mostly in the conjugated form but a small amount of parent drugs may also be recovered in the urine. Metabolites of opiates are given in Table 2.4.

Levorphanol is a long acting opioid which is an alternative to morphine therapy. However, hydromorphone is a short acting opioid. Oxymorphone is structurally similar to morphine but not used widely at this time. The oral bioavailability of methadone is 85%. Methadone can be used as an analgesic or in drug rehabilitation to reduce symptoms of withdrawal. Oxycodone is a widely used prescription pain medication, which is available as immediate release or extended release form. Oxycodone is metabolized into oxymorphone that is then further conjugated by the liver enzyme. A minor mostly inactive metabolite of oxycodone is nor-oxycodone. Fentanyl is 80–100 times as potent as morphine but with a short duration of action. This drug is administered by intravenous, or epidural route but transdermal patch is also available. Adverse effects of opioids include respiratory depression, nausea and vomiting, sedation, constipation, etc. Opioid tolerance may also develop where higher dosage is needed for pain relief. Physical dependence may also develop where abrupt withdrawal from opioid results in various withdrawal symptoms. Nonprescription abuse of opioids is common. Overdose from opioids may also cause fatality [21]. Even prescription use of opioids during pregnancy may be associated with poor fetal growth, preterm birth, birth defects, and neonatal abstinence syndrome [22].

Strong opioids such as buprenorphine, fentanyl, methadone, morphine, and oxycodone are used for treating severe pain whereas relatively weak opioids such as codeine, propoxyphene, and tramadol are used to treat mild or moderate pain. However, opioids are frequently associated with fatal poisoning due to oversedation, and respiratory depression. Unfortunately there are overlaps between therapeutic and toxic blood concentrations of opioids. Although poisoning due to use of weak opioids such as codeine and tramadol are associated with large and often suicidal overdoses resulting in high drug concentrations in blood, poisoning from a strong opioids such as methadone may be associated with blood methadone concentration in therapeutic levels. Sedative drugs and/or alcohol are frequently associated with fatal opioid poisoning [23].

Methadone is used in drug rehabilitation programs but methadone is also used as an analgesic. For treatment of heroin abuse, methadone may be administered once daily but for analgesic effects a more than once daily dosage may be needed. The analgesic effect of methadone lasts for 4–6 h although approximate half-life is 15–55 h. Methadone is mostly metabolized in the liver by N-demethylation by the action of enzyme CYP3A4. However, both the parent drug and the major metabolite (2-ethylidine-1,5-diemethyl, 3,3-diphenylpyrrolidine; inactive metabolite) can be recovered in the urine.

Methadone related death is common. In one study, the authors examined 76 cases of methadone related deaths in Vermont between 2001 and 2006. The manners of the deaths were 84% accident, 4% suicide, and 12% undetermined. The mean methadone blood level was 457 ng/mL (range: 50–3793 ng/mL) [24]. Heroin is a Class I schedule drug with no known medical use. However, heroin is abused, and fatality from heroin abuse has been reported. Gambaro et al. examined 14 cases of fatal heroin overdose, including 7 cases of poly drug use, and reported that concentrations of morphine in blood varied from 33 to 688 ng/mL. The brain morphine concentrations varied from 86 to 396 ng/g [25]. However, fentanyl associated fatalities were associated with a mean blood concentration of 0.02 μg/mL [26].

Loperamide (Imodium) is an over–the-counter antidiarrheal medicine which has poor bioavailability thus making it a safe drug for therapeutic use. However, intentional overdose of loperamide in order to achieve euphoria may cause serious toxicity and even death. Dierksen et al. reported a case of a young man who died from loperamide overdose. The authors detected 63 ng/mL of loperamide in postmortem blood, a concentration significantly higher than the therapeutic peak concentration. In addition, fluoxetine and alprazolam were also detected in his blood. Cause of death was determined as toxic effects of loperamide with fluoxetine and alprazolam [27]. Eggleston et al. also reported two fatalities associated with loperamide overdose. The postmortem cardiac blood showed loperamide concentration of 77 ng/mL (therapeutic: 0.24–3.1 ng/mL) along with 7-aminoclonazepam (180 ng/mL; therapeutic: 23–137 ng/mL), free buprenorphine (1.8 ng/mL; therapeutic: 1–8 ng/mL), and free nor-buprenorphine (2.9 ng/mL; therapeutic: 0.33–3.5 ng/mL) in the first patient (24 year old man). The cause of death was due to mixed drug overdose. In the second deceased patient (a 39-year old man) the postmortem femoral blood showed the presence of high concentration of loperamide (140 ng/mL), but no other drug was detected. The likely cause of death was loperamide overdose [28].

Opiate immunoassay can detect the presence of codeine and morphine but cannot detect the presence of many opioids including oxycodone, oxymorphone, hydromorphone, hydrocodone propoxyphene methadone, meperidine, and fentanyl due to poor cross-reactivity. However, specific immunoassays are available for detecting oxycodone, hydrocodone/hydromorphone, methadone, and fentanyl. Heroin is widely abused but heroin is metabolized to morphine and heroin abusers show the presence of morphine in urine. Eating poppy seeds contained in food may produce positive results even at 2000 ng/mL using opiate immunoassays. However, both codeine and morphine should be present in urine.

Cannabinoid abuse

The *C. sativa* plant has been smoked for its psychoactive properties since prehistoric times. Today cannabis (marijuana) is the most commonly abused drug in the United States. Over the past decade, some states in the United States, e.g., Colorado and Washington, have legalized use of cannabis for medicinal or recreational purposes, which has resulted in the increased use of marijuana by youths in these states. The most common route of administration is smoking but edible forms of marijuana are also available (including marijuana tea). Cannabinoids are present in the stalks, leaves, flowers, and seeds of the plant but are also found in resin secreted by the female plant. More than 100 cannabinoid like compounds have been isolated from the plant but delta-9-tetrahydrocannabinol (Δ^9-THC) is the major psychoactive component. The Δ^9-THC is a partial agonist at both cannabinoid receptors (cannabinoid receptor 1 and cannabinoid receptor 2) located in the brain, thus rendering its pharmacological action. However, cannabidiol is the major nonpsychoactive cannabinoid present in the cannabis plant and it has a low affinity for cannabinoid receptors. The amount of Δ^9-THC may vary significantly depending on the strain of the plant, cultivating factors, and methods of preparation (extract contain more material than dry plant material). However, a single joint smoke may contain approximately 150 cannabinoids. Hashish which is prepared from the resin of the female plant contains higher amounts of cannabinoids, approximately 300 mg in a single dosage. Although Hashish and marijuana joints (prepared from flowers leaves and stems of *C. sativa*) contain same cannabinoids, in general more active components are present in Hashish.

The major medical use of cannabis is for treating cancer patients and patients with AIDS but it may also be used in noncancer patients. However, a limited number of clinical trials have been reported assessing efficacy and safety of medical use of cannabis. Synthetic marijuana (Marinol) is available for medical use for treating nausea and vomiting produced by chemotherapy. In addition, various derivatives of Δ^9-THC have also been introduced clinically [29]. Although cannabis is often perceived as a harmless drug with potential therapeutic benefits by the general public, cannabis has detrimental effects on brain development, psychiatric health (may cause anxiety, depression, psychosis, and schizophrenia), lung function (bronchitis and lung cancer), and heart (arrhythmia and myocardial infarction). Acute medical complications of marijuana use are primarily cardiovascular and respiratory depression in nature [30].

After smoking a joint, approximately 50% of Δ^9-THC is present in the mainstream smoke, which is absorbed rapidly through the lungs and enters the bloodstream. The effects such as euphoria, change in perception, etc., are observed within minutes of smoking. However, if cannabis is taken orally bioavailability is poor

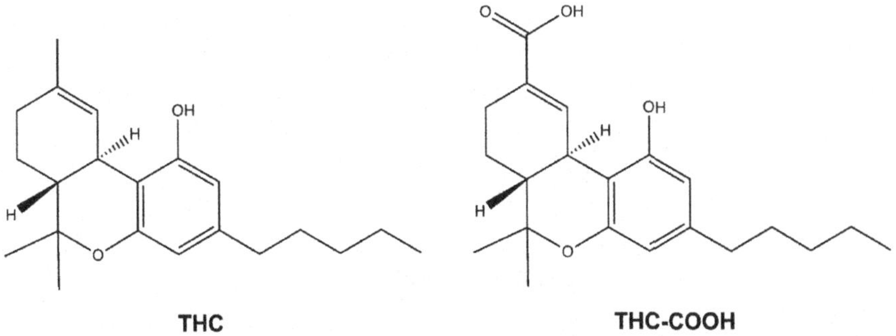

Figure 2.5 Chemical structure of THC and THC-COOH.
Source: Figure courtesy of Matthew D. Krasowski, MD, PhD, Clinical Professor of Pathology, University of Iowa Carver College of Medicine.

(approximately 25−30%). After smoking, the maximum effect can be observed in 15−30 min but the effect may last 2−3 h. The elimination half-life is about 7 days, due to the lipophilic nature of the molecule, and complete elimination may take up to 30 days. The major inactive metabolite of Δ^9-THC is 11-nor-9-carboxy-Δ^9-tetrahydrocannabinol (THC-COOH) but another metabolite 11-hydroxy-Δ^9-tetrahydrocannabinol is active. These metabolites are formed in the liver by the cation of CYP3A4, CYP2C9, and CYP2C11 isoenzymes. Chemical structure of tetrahydrocannabinol (THC) and THC-COOH are given in Fig. 2.5. Major metabolite of marijuana is listed in Table 2.4.

Smoking marijuana also causes impairment as cognitive and psychomotor functions are impaired. Cannabinoid also impairs driving performance. Chronic heavy use of cannabinoid may cause impairment even when an individual is not smoking. Cannabinoids have effects on the cardiovascular system and respiratory system. Chronic smoking of marijuana may be associated with bronchitis and emphysema. Even bronchogenic carcinoma may be associated with long-term smoking of marijuana [31]. Heavy cannabis users are at elevated risk of stroke. In one study, the authors, based on a review of 153 cases of stroke/transient ischemic attack, concluded that cannabis users had 3.3 times higher incidents of stroke compared to nonusers [32]. Hadener et al. reported that median THC-COOH (metabolite of Δ^9-THC) concentration in blood was 25.7 ng/mL (range: <5.0−166 ng/mL) and median THC-COOH glucuronide concentration in blood was 87.1 ng/mL (range: <5.0−869 ng/mL) in 926 blood specimens collected from cannabis users [33]. Cannabinoid is routinely tested in urine toxicology screen as THC-COOH. However, confirmation requires GC/MS analysis.

Abuse of anesthetics

Major anesthetics abused are phencyclidine and ketamine, although their abuse is relatively less compared to abuse of cannabis, amphetamines, opioids, and cocaine. Phencyclidine (PCP), like ketamine, was initially used for preinduction anesthesia and animal tranquilizer. PCP is available in the underground market as crystalline

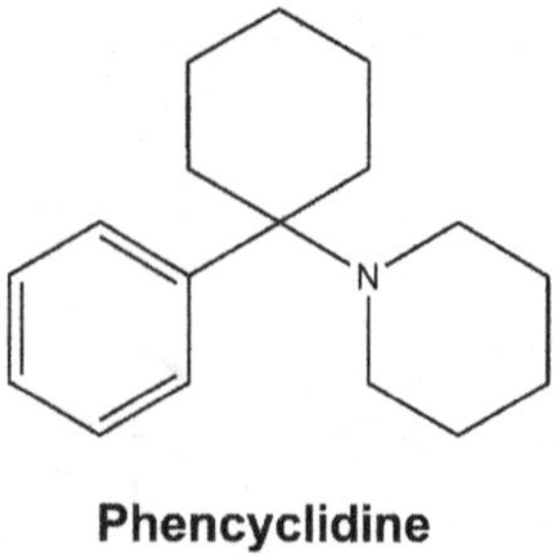

Phencyclidine

Figure 2.6 Chemical structure of phencyclidine (PCP).
Source: Figure courtesy of Matthew D. Krasowski, MD, PhD, Clinical Professor of
Pathology, University of Iowa Carver College of Medicine.

powder (angel dust), crystal, or liquid, and it can be snorted, smoked, ingested, or injected intravenously or subcutaneously. Onset of action is fast [2−5] if inhaled but effects may start 15−60 min after oral ingestion. PCP has several sites of action on the CNS but it has high affinity for the N-methyl-D-aspartate (NMDA) receptors complexes present in the hippocampus, neocortex, basal ganglia, and limbic system. A dose of 1−5 mg of PCP is capable of inhibiting dopamine, norepinephrine, and serotonin reuptake, thus increasing dopamine and norepinephrine production by stimulating tyrosine hydroxylase. As a result, PCP exerts its dopaminergic and sympathomimetic effects. PCP intoxication may cause violent behavior, nystagmus, tachycardia, and hypertension as well as reduced perception of pain. PCP intoxication may also cause acute schizophrenia, psychosis, audiovisual hallucinations, and paranoid delusions. PCP induced coma may be manifested as an unresponsive patient with open eyes. Cardiotoxicity of PCP has been reported [34]. Chemical structure of PCP is given in Fig. 2.6.

McCarron et al. reviewed 1000 cases of PCP intoxication and reported that nystagmus and hypertension only occurred in 57% of patients. The incidence of violent behavior was observed in 35% of patients, bizarre behavior in 29% patients, and agitation in 34% patients. Interestingly, 46% of patients were alert and oriented. A small percentage of patients were presented with severe disturbances in vital signs including three cases of cardiac arrest (0.3%) and 28 cases of apnea (2.8%). Hypoglycemia, elevated serum creatinine kinase, uric acid, and liver enzymes were common. Confirmation of the presence of PCP in urine could establish the diagnosis of PCP intoxication. Urine PCP results were available for 594 patients. Unconscious patients showed PCP concentrations between 200 and 142,000 ng/mL. However, urine PCP levels did not correlate with severity of clinical findings [35]. PCP is also metabolized in the liver by mostly by CYP3A4 into several hydroxy metabolites (Table 2.4). PCP is routinely tested in urine toxicology screen. Although the presence of PCP can be detected by using PCP immunoassay and automated analyzer, dextromethorphan an antitussive agent found in some over-the-counter cough and cold medications interferes with PCP immunoassay and may cause false positive test result [36].

Ketamine, a dissociative anesthetic, is a phencyclidine derivative first synthesized in 1962. Ketamine is available as a racemic mixture with S-isomer being three to four times more potent than R-isomer as an anesthetic. The clearance and volume of distribution is dependent of hepatic blood flow. In human CYP3A4 is primarily responsible for metabolism of ketamine into nor-ketamine. Ketamine is a noncompetitive antagonist of NMDA receptors. Ketamine may target other receptors such as alpha-amino-3-jydroxy-5-methyl-4-isoxazo-lepropionic acid receptors. Ketamine is mostly administered intravenously because oral bioavailability is poor due to first pass metabolism. Ketamine produces hemodynamically stable anesthesia via central sympathetic stimulation but does not affect respiratory function. Although ketamine is used for induction of anesthesia, ketamine is also used in pediatric pain control in emergency departments due to its antihyperalgesic and antiinflammatory effects. Ketamine may be useful in acute and chronic pain management. Ketamine also has potential antidepressive and antisuicidal effects. However, safety issues with long-term ketamine therapy has not yet been established [37,38]. Ketamine is widely used in veterinary medicine.

Ketamine is also abused. It can produce a dissociative state and hallucinations making it a recreational drug for abusers. Although death primarily due to ketamine abuse is rare, ketamine abuse can alter normal functions of the brain affecting memory, attention, cognition, reaction time, color perception, and sense of time. Ketamine abuse also produces gastrointestinal and urinary track dysfunction [39].

Ketamine can be detected up to 2 days after use in children in clinical environments. In one study the authors reported that concentration of ketamine varied from 29 to 1410 ng/mL while nor-ketamine levels varied from 0.1 to 1442 ng/mL using GC/MS. However, nor-ketamine in urine was detected for up to 14 days. Using more sophisticated liquid chromatography and MS, ketamine was detected for up to 11 days [40]. Unfortunately ketamine is misused as a date rape drug to induce amnesia in unsuspected victims. Although bioavailability is poor, approximately 16% of ketamine is absorbed after oral ingestion. As a result ketamine may be passed to a drink of a victim. One problem of the use of ketamine in date rape situations is that when the victim is brought to the emergency room, the urine drug test may be negative because ketamine is not routinely tested in most clinical laboratories. However specimens can be sent to a reference laboratory for detection of the presence of ketamine in urine or serum.

Abuse of benzodiazepines

Benzodiazepines were introduced in the 1960s as a sedative hypnotic which contributes to their anxiolytic effects. Although over 50 benzodiazepines were developed, many are not approved for use in the United States although they may be used clinically in other countries. Commonly used benzodiazepines in United States are listed in Table 2.6. Benzodiazepines are used as sedatives, anxiolytics, and also as muscle relaxants. Some benzodiazepines such as clonazepam and diazepam are

Table 2.6 Commonly used benzodiazepines in United States and their characteristics

Drug	Duration of action	Half-life (h)	Metabolites
Alprazolam	Short to intermediate	10–14	Inactive metabolite: 4-hydroxyalprazolam, alpha-hydroxy alprazolam
Chlordiazepoxide	Short to intermediate	5–15	Active metabolites: desmethylchlordiazepoxide, demoxepam, diazepam, oxazepam
Clobazam	Long acting	71–82	Active metabolite: N-desmethyl-clobazam, other metabolite: 4-hydroxyclobazam
Clonazepam	Long acting	18–50	Active metabolite: 7-aminoclonazepam
Clorazepate	Long acting	20–100	Active metabolite: desmethyldiazepam
Diazepam	Long acting	20–70	Nor-diazepam is the major active metabolite; minor active metabolites are oxazepam and temazepam
Estazolam	Short to intermediate	10–24	4-Hydroxy estazolam (major metabolite) and 1-oxo-estarzolam (minor metabolite) has some pharmacological properties
Flurazepam	Long acting	40–100	Active metabolite: N-desalkyl-flurazepam
Lorazepam	Short to intermediate	9–19	Inactive metabolite: lorazepam glucuronide
Midazolam	Short acting	3–8	Inactive metabolite: alpha-hydroxy midazolam glucuronide
Oxazepam	Short to intermediate	5–15	Inactive metabolite: oxazepam glucuronide
Temazepam	Short to intermediate	10–16	Inactive metabolite: temazepam glucuronide
Triazolam	Short acting	1.5–5.5	Active metabolite; alpha-hydroxy triazolam

used to treat seizures. Alprazolam is effective in treating panic disorder. Midazolam is used is used in induction of general anesthesia preoperatively. Chlordiazepoxide, clorazepate, diazepam, and oxazepam are used in treating alcohol withdrawal symptoms.

All benzodiazepines are CNS depressants and are indirect agonists of gamma-aminobutyric acid (GABA) receptors most noticeably GABA$_A$ receptors. As a result of GABA receptors the mediated opening of chloride channels is increased but benzodiazepines cannot open chloride channels without the aid of GABA receptors. In addition, certain benzodiazepines, e.g., clonazepam, may also interact with serotonin receptors. Benzodiazepines are lipophilic in nature and are strongly bound to serum proteins. Benzodiazepines are metabolized by the liver enzymes and some of the metabolites may be pharmacologically active.

Although benzodiazepines are used widely in clinical practice, these drugs are also habit forming if used on a long-term basis. Benzodiazepines with a shorter half-life, e.g., alprazolam, may be more prone to causing tolerance and dependence than benzodiazepines with a long half-life such as diazepam. Abrupt discontinuation of benzodiazepine may produce withdrawal symptoms. Therefore, discontinuation of therapy must be supervised by a physician. Risk of driving while on benzodiazepines is about the same as risk of driving with a blood alcohol level between 0.05% and 0.079% (legal limit of driving in all states is 0.08%). In summary, benzodiazepines increase the risk of addiction, withdrawal, cognitive decline, motor-vehicle accidents, and hip fracture. Moreover, risk of benzodiazepine overdose is very significant if combined with opioids and alcohol. As a result, in general benzodiazepines should not be prescribed continuously for more than 1 month [41].

The half-life of benzodiazepines varies widely depending on the particular drug. For example, the average half-life of alprazolam is 7−10 h but half-life of triazolam is 2 h. Benzodiazepines are extensively metabolized by the liver enzymes and are often excreted as glucuronide conjugates. Oxazepam, which is a drug by itself and also a common metabolite of both diazepam and temazepam, is pharmacologically active. Oxazepam is also conjugated and excreted in the urine as oxazepam glucuronide. Clorazepate is metabolized to nor-diazepam, an active metabolite. Chlordiazepoxide is metabolized into nor-chlordiazepoxide and demoxepam. Both metabolites are pharmacologically active. Demoxepam is further metabolized into nor-diazepam, which is then subsequently metabolized into oxazepam. Alprazolam is metabolized into alpha-hydroxy alprazolam and 4-hydroxyalprazolam (both active metabolites). Clonazepam is metabolized into 7-amino clonazepam. The chemical structures of diazepam, clonazepam, and flunitrazepam (a benzodiazepine not approved by Federal Food and Drug Administration but used in date rape) are given in Fig. 2.7. Metabolites of common benzodiazepines are listed in Table 2.6.

Benzodiazepines are also abused. Overdose from benzodiazepine alone rarely causes fatality but in one report the authors described a case of a 19-year old man who was overdosed with alprazolam (an empty strip was found in the room) and died few weeks after overdose due to leukoencephalopathy (selective cerebral white matter injury). On admission his urine benzodiazepine level was over 1000 ng/mL and THC level was over 100 ng/mL. Toxic leukoencephalopathy can occur following an overdose of benzodiazepine and respiratory failure. This syndrome has no successful treatment [42]. Isbister et al. reported that alprazolam is relatively more

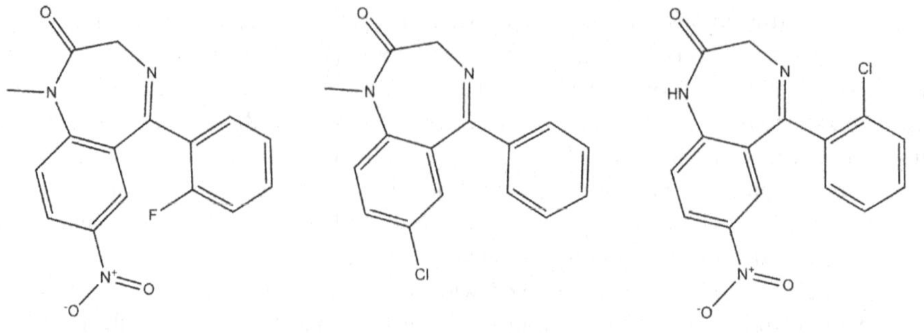

Flunitrazepam   **Diazepam**   **Clonazepam**

Figure 2.7 Chemical structure of diazepam, clonazepam, and flunitrazepam.
Source: Figure courtesy of Matthew D. Krasowski, MD, PhD, Clinical Professor of
Pathology, University of Iowa Carver College of Medicine.

toxic than other benzodiazepines in overdose. The authors studied 2063 single
benzodiazepine overdoses in admission where 131 cases were alprazolam overdoses, 823 diazepam overdoses, and 1109 other benzodiazepines overdoses.
The median length of stay in the hospital was longer with alprazolam overdoses
compared to other benzodiazepine overdose. The authors concluded that alprazolam
was more toxic than other benzodiazepines in overdoses [43].

Recently, S100B protein, a part of large calcium binding protein S100, has
gained interest as a neuro biochemical marker of brain injury. In one study, the
authors observed that there were significant differences in S100B levels between a
control group and patients with benzodiazepine overdose who were unresponsive to
verbal stimuli. All patients with benzodiazepine overdose showed elevated serum
S100B levels but S100B levels were further elevated in patients with depressed
levels of consciousness and respiratory insufficiency [44].

More recently, older benzodiazepines have been replaced with newer drugs with
more sedative and hypnotic properties for treating insomnia. These agents include
eszopiclone (Lunesta), zaleplon (Sonata), zolpidem (Ambien), and zopiclone
(Imovane). Although these drugs are structurally unrelated to benzodiazepines, their
pharmacological actions are due to interaction with GABA receptors. Although
these drugs are Schedule IV drugs, these drugs are also abused.

Abuse of barbiturates

Barbiturates are CNS depressants that are used clinically as sedative hypnotic drugs.
Barbituric acid, a pharmacologically inactive compound, was synthesized in 1864
while in the early 1900s barbital, the first barbituric acid derivative with pharmacological activity, was discovered. More than 2500 derivatives of barbituric acid have
been synthesized but approximately 50 drugs have been used clinically. Based on

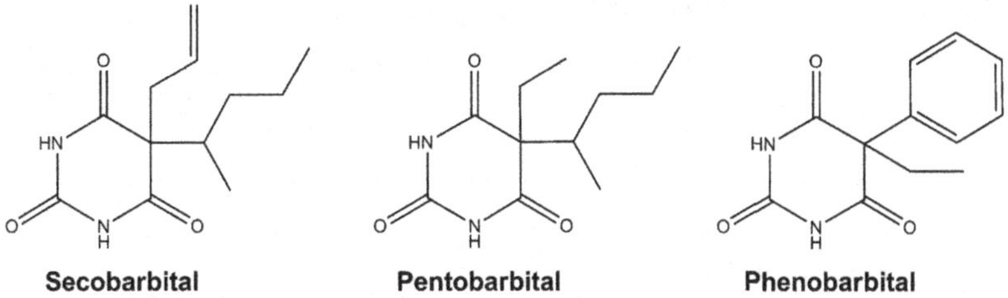

Figure 2.8 Chemical structure of secobarbital, pentobarbital, and phenobarbital.
Source: Figure courtesy of Matthew D. Krasowski, MD, PhD, Clinical Professor of Pathology, University of Iowa Carver College of Medicine.

the duration of action, barbiturates are classified as ultra-short acting, short acting, intermediate acting, and long acting barbiturates. Long acting barbiturates such as phenobarbital (Luminal) and mephobarbital (Mebaral) are classified as Schedule IV drugs and are medically used as anticonvulsants. These long acting barbiturates are rarely abused. The chemical structures of secobarbital, pentobarbital, and phenobarbital are given in Fig. 2.8.

The ultra-short acting barbiturates can produce anesthesia within minutes after intravenous administration. Currently thiopental (Pentothal), thiamylal (Surital), and methohexital (Brevital) are used medically. Other short and intermediate acting barbiturates include butalbital (Fiorinal), butabarbital (Butisol), talbutal (Lotusate), and aprobarbital (Alurate). These barbiturates are Schedule III drugs. After oral administration, usually the onset of action starts within 15–40 min. The effect of these barbiturates may last up to 6 h. These drugs are used for treating insomnia and may also be used to achieve preoperative sedation. The short and intermediate acting barbiturates which are Schedule II drugs include amobarbital (Amytal), pentobarbital (Nembutal), and secobarbital (Seconal). Drug abusers usually prefer amobarbital, pentobarbital, and secobarbital. A combination of amobarbital and secobarbital (Tuinal) is also abused. Many barbiturates are extensively metabolized by the liver enzymes. Secobarbital is metabolized into 3-hydroxy secobarbital and also into secodiol and 5-(1-methylbutyl) barbituric acid. Pentobarbital is mainly metabolized into 3-hydroxy pentobarbital which is inactive. A minor metabolite is N-hydroxy pentobarbital. Major metabolite of amobarbital is 3-hydroxy amobarbital which has some pharmacological activity. Major metabolites of amobarbital, pentobarbital, and secobarbital are given in Table 2.4.

The GABA system plays an important role in the pathophysiology of anxiety disorder. GABA is the major inhibitory neurotransmitter in the brain which activates various GABA receptors ($GABA_A$, $GABA_C$, and $GABA_B$). Upon activation, chloride ion influx is increased and the membrane becomes hyperpolarized causing neuronal inhibition. The mechanism of action of barbiturates is GABA-mediated inhibition of synaptic transmission. Barbiturates demonstrate anxiolytic effects at dosages which are close to producing hypnotic effects and such dosages also affect motor skills and mood. Chronic administration of barbiturates causes dependence [45].

Currently abuse of barbiturates is declining but barbiturate abuse is clinically challenging due to the narrow margin between therapeutic and toxic blood levels and high abuse potential. Routine urine toxicology can detect the presence of barbiturates in urine.

Abuse of hallucinogens

LSD was first synthesized by Albert Hofmann in 1938 and then its psychedelic effect was discovered in 1943. Lysergic acid is found naturally in the parasitic fungus *C. purpurea*. Although LSD was a popular recreational drug in 1960s, today its abuse is less common. A moderate dose of $75-150 \mu g$ of LSD can produce psychedelic effects (optimum dosage used for recreational purpose is $100-200 \mu g$). Traumatic experience (bad trips) may also occur from LSD abuse. LSD also alters the state of consciousness as well as impairing psychomotor functions. The biochemical action of LSD is due to its partial agonistic property of serotonin receptors 5-hydroxytryptamine (5-HT) especially $5\text{-}HT_{2A}$ receptors. Although LSD abuse can result in severe toxicity, there is no documented death due to abuse of LSD alone. LSD is completely absorbed after ingestion and psychological effects are observed $30-45$ min after ingestion. In humans, LSD is also rapidly metabolized into structurally similar metabolites [46]. The major metabolite is 2-oxo-3-hydroxy lysergic acid, which is present in human urine $16-43$ times greater than LSD [47].

Abuse of club drugs

Abuse of MDMA and ketamine has already been discussed. This section addresses abuse of GHB and Rohypnol (flunitrazepam), which are also encountered in date rape situations.

GHB is a minor metabolite and precursor of GABA, a neurotransmitter. GHB is also used for recreational purposes and is a Schedule I controlled substance in the United States. A 25-mg/kg of oral dose caused dizziness in adult subjects with an average plasma concentration of $80 \mu g/mL$. Blood GHB concentration over $260 \mu g/mL$ caused deep sleep, levels $156-260 \mu g/mL$ caused moderate sleep and levels $52-156 \mu g/mL$ caused light sleep [48]. GHB in lower doses may also produce euphoria. Abuse of GHB is widespread throughout the world and because GHB can make an individual unconscious, this illicit drug is widely used in drug induced sexual assaults and rapes. Because GHB has no distinct taste, it can be slipped into a drink and has been used in date rape situations. Abuse of GHB is also associated with high morbidity and mortality rate.

It is usually considered that the concentration of GHB in blood should not exceed 50 mg/L and in urine should not exceed 10 mg/L due to endogenous production of GHB. Yeatman and Reid studied the urinary concentrations of endogenous GHB in 55 volunteers and observed that the endogenous urinary concentrations of

GHB ranged from 0.9 to 3.5 mg/L with a mean urinary concentration of 1.56 mg/L. The authors concluded that their results confirm that the suggested 10 mg/L cut-off value for endogenous GHB concentration in forensic analysis is justified [49].

GHB if ingested is converted into succinic semialdehyde and then into succinic acid, which enters Kerbs cycle and is finally converted into water and carbon dioxide. For documenting GHB abuse blood and urine GHB level is measured. As expected, concentrations of GHB in blood and urine in subjects died from GHB overdose are significantly higher than the suggested cut-off values in blood and urine due to endogenous production of GHB. In one report the concentrations of GHB in the blood of eight patients who died from GHB overdose ranged from 77 to 370 mg/L [50]. In another report the femoral blood and urinary concentrations of GHB in a fatal overdose were 2937 and 33,727 mg/L, respectively [51]. Because GHB is cleared from both blood and urine relatively rapidly compared to other drugs, testing of hair specimens is useful to document exposure of a victim to GHB during sexual assault. Kintz et al. documented the presence of GHB in hair after single exposure and demonstrated that hair analysis is useful to document use of GHB during a sexual assault [52]. GHB is not detected in routine urine toxicology analysis but reference laboratories offer testing for GHB. The chemical structure of GHB and ketamine is given in Fig. 2.9.

Rohypnol (flunitrazepam) is a benzodiazepine which is not currently available in the United States. Flunitrazepam can cause rapid sedation and is used in date rape situations. A single 1 or 2 mg dose of flunitrazepam can produce significant sedative effect and this drug is more potent than diazepam. The effect of flunitrazepam can last up to 12 h. Regular use of this drug causes dependence [53]. Flunitrazepam is metabolized by the liver into 7-aminoflunitrazepam (major metabolite) and also to a lesser extent into desmethylflunitrazepam and 3-hydroxyflunitrazepam. The presence of flunitrazepam and its metabolites in urine may not be detected by using benzodiazepine immunoassays at 200 ng/mL cut-off but can be confirmed by GC/MS. Chemical structure of flunitrazepam is given in Fig. 2.7.

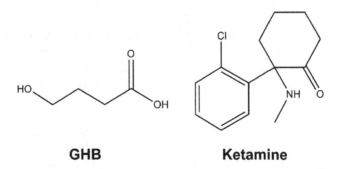

GHB   **Ketamine**

Figure 2.9 The chemical structure of GHB and ketamine.
Source: Figure courtesy of Matthew D. Krasowski, MD, PhD, Clinical Professor of Pathology, University of Iowa Carver College of Medicine.

Abuse of prescription drugs

Abuse of prescription drugs is a serious public health concern worldwide. Medications which belong to Schedules II−V are legally available from pharmacies based on valid prescriptions. People who abuse prescription drugs may obtain such drugs illegally from underground markets; illegal Internet based pharmacy, from friends or a family member or by doctor shopping, whereby they go from one doctor to another claiming intense pain and getting the same prescription from different physicians. Moreover, abusers also attempt to mislead the physician to legally obtain prescription medications that they do not need. The most common pain medications which are abused are oxycodone and hydrocodone with acetaminophen (Vicodin) [54]. Other opiate analgesics are also abused. In addition, various CNS depressants (such as benzodiazepines), CNS stimulants (such as phenmetrazine, dextro-amphetamine), and medications which are used in ADHD are also abused. In addition, muscle relaxants such as Carisoprodol (Soma) and drugs for treating erectile dysfunction Sildenafil (Viagra) are also abused. Carisoprodol is metabolized to meprobamate, a Schedule IV drug which has a sedative and hypnotic effect. Carisoprodol when ingested in high amounts can cause euphoria as well as impaired hand-eye coordination and balance. Sildenafil is abused by both men and women and its abuse among individuals using MDMA (ecstasy) is increasing because sildenafil can reverse the erectile dysfunction effect of ecstasy [55].

Abuse of nonprescription drugs

Dextromethorphan is present in many over the counter cough and cold medications (Robitussin DM, Vicks Formula 44). Although this drug is safe and effective in recommended dosage, at higher dosages dextromethorphan can produce euphoria. Teenagers abuse dextromethorphan containing products such as Coricidin HBP cough and cold medication (dextromethorphan hydrobromide 30 mg and chlorpheniramine malate 4 mg) in high dosage in order to achieve a high like state comparable to abuse of LSD. Other dextromethorphan containing over the counter medications are also abused. Cough syrup or capsules also may contain in addition to dextromethorphan, guaifenesin, ephedrine, or pseudoephedrine. Dextromethorphan in high dosage (5−10 times above that recommended) can cause psychosis, dependence, and physical withdrawal symptoms. At very high dose dextromethorphan can be life threatening.

Diphenhydramine (Benadryl), an antihistamine which is often used as a sleep aid, is also abused. Other over the counter sleeping aids such as Sominex and Nytol are also abused because these drugs can produce hallucination, delirium, and confusion when taken in excessive amounts. Cyclizine, an over the counter antihistamine in high dosage can produce some euphoric effects. There are also reports of abuse of decongestant medications ephedrine and pseudoephedrine. People abuse these medications for prolonging erection and sexual function [55].

Less commonly abused drugs

Methaqualone is a sedative hypnotic drug with pharmacological effects similar to barbiturates. Methaqualone was clinically introduced in the US market in 1954 but due to high abuse potential it was discontinued in 1984. Currently it is a Schedule I drug. Although abused in the past this drug is less commonly abused in United States. However, this drug is known as Mandrax in South Africa and is abused. Glutethimide was introduced in 1954 in United States an alternative to barbiturates. In 1991, it was classified as a Class II drug. Glutethimide combined with codeine produces euphoria [56]. This drug is less commonly abused now.

Abuse of magic mushroom and peyote cactus

Magic mushrooms (psychoactive fungi) that grow in the United States, Mexico, South America, and many other parts of the world contain psilocybin and psilocin, which are hallucinogens and are Class I controlled substances. Magic mushrooms can be eaten raw, cooked with food or dried, and then consumed. These mushrooms can be mistaken for other nonhallucinogenic mushrooms or even poisonous mushrooms such as Amanita class. After ingestion, psilocybin, often the major component of the mushroom, is rapidly converted by dephosphorylation into psilocin which has psychoactive effects similar to LSD. In general, duration of the trip after abusing magic mushrooms may be between 2 and 6 h and effects range from the intended feelings of relaxation, uncontrollable laughter, joy, euphoria, visual enhancement of colors, hallucinations, and altered perceptions, but some abusers may also experience negative effects such as depression or paranoia. Intoxication from use of magic mushroom is common. Some species of magic mushroom contain phenylethylamine which may cause cardiac toxicity. Fatality from abusing magic mushrooms alone is rare [57]. Currently there is no immunoassay for determination of psilocybin and psilocin in body fluids. Therefore, chromatographic methods must be employed for their analysis especially during a forensic investigation.

Peyote cactus (*Lophophora williamsii*) is a small spineless cactus that grows in the Southwestern part of the United States and Mexico. The top of the Peyote cactus, known as the "crown," contains the psychoactive compound mescaline. Mescaline is classified as a Class I controlled substance but approximately 300,000 members of Native Americans Church can ingest peyote cactus legally as a religious sacrament during all night prayer in the Native American Church [58]. The mescaline content of peyote cactus is usually 0.4% in fresh cactus and 3−6% in dried cactus. The highest psychedelic effect may be achieved within 2 h of ingestion but the effect may last up to 8 h [59]. The psychoactive effects of mescaline are similar to LSD including deeply mystical feelings. Abuse of peyote cactus may cause serious toxicity requiring medical attention and may even cause fatality. Currently, there is no commercially available immunoassay for analysis of mescaline in body fluids and only chromatographic methods are available for its analysis. Although mescaline is metabolized into several different metabolites, a large amount of mescaline can be recovered unchanged in urine. Therefore, detection of mescaline in serum or urine can be used for establishing diagnosis of magic mushroom abuse. For death investigation, confirmation of the presence of mescaline in body fluid is essential in establishing the cause of death. Severe toxicity and even death may occur from mescaline overdose.

Conclusions

Various illicit drugs as well as prescription and nonprescription drugs are abused. On many occasions, abuse of drugs along with alcohol reduces the toxic level of many drugs and may cause fatality. However, deaths have also been reported from abuse of both illicit and prescription drugs. This issue is addressed in detail in Chapter 4, Combined Alcohol and Drug Abuse: A Potentially Deadly Mix.

References

[1] US Department of Health and Human Services. National survey on drug use and health. Washington, DC: US Department of Health and Human Services; 2014. (Office of Applied Studies). Published September 2015.
[2] Paulozzi LJ, Strickler GK, Kreiner PW, Koris CM, et al. Controlled substances prescribing patterns-prescription behavior surveillance system eight states, 2013. MMWR Surveill Summ 2015;64:1−14.
[3] Norn S, Kruse PR, Kruse E. History of opium poppy and morphine. Dan Medicinhist Arbog 2005;33:171−84.
[4] Vetulani J. Drug addiction. Part I. Psychoactive substances in the past and the presence. Pol J Pharmacol 2001;53:201−14.
[5] Zuardi AW. History of cannabis as a medicine: a review. Rev Bras Psiquiatr 2006;28:153−7.
[6] Courtwright DT. The controlled substances act: how a "big tent" reform became punitive drug law. Drug Alcohol Depend 2004;75:9−15.
[7] Sulzer D, Sonders MS, Poulsen NW, Galli A. Mechanisms of neurotransmitter release by amphetamines: a review. Prog Neurobiol 2005;75:406−33.
[8] Greene SL, Kerr F, Braitberg G. Review article: amphetamine and related drugs of abuse. Emerg Med Australas 2008;20:391−402.
[9] De Letter EA, Piette MH, Lambert WE, Cordonnier JA. Amphetamine as potential inducers of fatalities: a review in the district of Ghent from 1976−2004. Med Sci Law 2006;46:37−65.
[10] Logan BK, Fligner CL, Haddix T. Cause and manner of death in fatalities involving methamphetamine. J Forensic Sci 1998;43:28−34.
[11] Wollner K, Stockhausen S, Mubhoff F, Madea B. Death after intake of amphetamine/ecstasy: two case reports. Arch Kriminol 2015;235:53−61. [Article in German].

[12] Middleton RM, Kirkpatrick MB. Clinical use of cocaine: a review of the risks and benefits. Drug Saf 1993;9:212−17.

[13] Kloner RA, Hale S, Alker K, Rezkalla S. The effects of acute and chronic cocaine use on the heart. Circulation 1992;85:407−19.

[14] Buttner A. Neuropathological alterations in cocaine abuse. Curr Med Chem 2012;19:5598−600.

[15] Cressman AM, Natekar A, Kim E, Koren G, et al. Cocaine abuse during pregnancy. J Obstet Gynaecol Can 2014;36:628−31.

[16] Hamilton HE, Wallace JE, Shimek Jr EL, Land P, et al. Cocaine and benzoylecgonine excretion in humans. J Forensic Sci 1977;22:697−707.

[17] Jones AW, Holmgren A. Concentrations of cocaine and benzoylecgonine in femoral blood from cocaine related deaths compared with venous blood from impaired drivers. J Anal Toxicol 2014;38:46−51.

[18] Peretti FJ, Isenschmid DS, Levine B, Caplan Y. Cocaine fatality: an unexplained blood concentration in a fatal overdose. Forensic Sci Int 1990;48:135−8.

[19] Compton WM, Jones CM, Baldwin GT. Relationship between nonmedical prescription opioid use and heroin use. N Engl J Med 2016;374:154−63.

[20] Holden JE, Jeong Y, Forrest JM. The endogenous opioid system and clinical pain management. AACN Clin Issues 2005;16:291−301.

[21] Inturrisi CE. Clinical pharmacology of opioids for pain. Clin J Pain 2002;18(4 Suppl): S3−13.

[22] Yazdy MM, Desai RJ, Brogly SB. Prescription opioids in pregnancy and birth outcomes: a review of literature. J Pediatr Genet 2015;4:56−70.

[23] Hakkinen M, Launiainen T, Vuori E, Ojanpera I. Comparison of fatal poisoning by prescription opioids. Forensic Sci Int 2012;222:327−31.

[24] Madden ME, Shapiro SL. The methadone epidemic: methadone related deaths on the rise in Vermont. Am J Forensic Med Pathol 2011;32:131−5.

[25] Gambaro V, Agro A, Cippitelli M, Dell'Acqua L, et al. Unexpected variation of the codeine/morphine ration following fatal heroin overdose. J Anal Toxicol 2014;38:289−94.

[26] Algren DA, Monteilh CP, Punja M, Schier JG, et al. Fentanyl associated fatalities among illicit drug users in Wayne County Michigan (July 2005−May 2006). J Med Toxicol 2013;9:106−15.

[27] Dierksen J, Gonsoulin M, Walterscheid JP. Poor man's methadone: a case report of loperamide toxicity. Am J Forensic Med Pathol 2015;36:268−70.

[28] Eggleston W, Clark KH, Marraffa JM. Loperamide abuse associated with cardiac dysrhythmia and death. Ann Emerg Med 2016; April 26 [e-pub ahead of print].

[29] Bologini D, Ross RA. Medical cannabis vs synthetic cannabinoids: what does the future hold? Clin Pharmacol Ther 2015;97:568−70.

[30] Bui QM, Simpson S, Nordstrom K. Psychiatric and medical management of marijuana intoxication in the emergency department. West J Emerg Med 2015;16:414−17.

[31] Ashton CH. Pharmacology and effects of cannabis: a brief review. Br J Psychiatry 2001;178:101−6.

[32] Hemachandra D, McKetin R, Cherbuin N, Anstey KJ. Heavy cannabis users at elevated risk of stroke: evidence form a general population survey. Aust N Z J Public Health 2016;40:226−30.

[33] Hadener M, Weinmann W, Schurch S, Konig S. Development of a rapid column switching LC-MS/MS method for the quantification of THCCOOH and THCCOOH-glucuronide in whole blood for assessing cannabis consumption frequency. Anal Bioanal Chem 2016;408:1953−62.

[34] Bey T, Patel A. Phencyclidine intoxication and adverse effects: a clinical and pharmacological review of an illicit drug. Cal J Emerg Med 2007;8:9–14.

[35] McCarron MM, Schulze BW, Thompson GA, Conder MC, et al. Acute phencyclidine intoxication: incidence of clinical findings in 1,000 cases. Ann Emerg Med 1981;10:237–42.

[36] Boeckx RL. False positive EMIT DAU PCP assay as a result of an overdose dextromethorphan. Clin Chem 1987;33:974–5.

[37] Gao M, Rejaei D, Liu H. Ketamine use in current clinical practice. Acta Pharmacol Sin 2016;37:865–72. [e-pub ahead of print].

[38] Paltoniemi MA, Hagelberg NM, Olkkola KT, Saari T. Ketamine: a review of clinical pharmacokinetics and pharmacodynamics in anesthesia and pain therapy. Clin Pharamcokinet 2016; [e-pub ahead of print].

[39] Xy J, Leh H. Ketamine—an update on its clinical uses and abuses. CNS Neurosci Ther 2014;20:1015–20.

[40] Adamowicz P, Kala M. Urinary excretion rates of ketamine and norketamine following therapeutic ketamine administration: method and detection window consideration. J Anal Toxicol 2005;29:376–82.

[41] Johnson B. Risks associated with long term benzodiazepine use. Am Fam Physician 2013;88:225–6.

[42] Aljarallah S, Al-Hussain F. Acute fatal posthypoxic leukoencephalopathy following benzodiazepine overdose: a case report and review of literature. BMC Neurol 2015;15:69.

[43] Isbister G, O'Regan L, Sibbritt D, Whyte IM. Alprazolam is relatively more toxic than other benzodiazepines in overdose. Br J Clin Pharmacol 2004;58:88–95.

[44] Ambrozic J, Bunc M, Osredkar J, Brvar M. S100B protein in benzodiazepine overdose. Emerg Med J 2008;25:90–2.

[45] Nemeroff CB. The role of GABA in the pathophysiology and treatment of anxiety disorders. Psychopharmacol Bull 2003;37:133–46.

[46] Passie T, Halpern JH, Stichtenoth DO, Emrich HM, et al. The pharmacology of lysergic acid diethylamide: a review. CNS Neurosci Ther 2008;14:295–314.

[47] Klette KL, Anderson CJ, Poch GK, Nimrod AC, et al. Metabolism of lysergic acid diethylamide (LSD) in human liver microsomes and cryopreserved human hepatocytes. J Anal Toxicol 2000;24:550–6.

[48] Baselt RC, Cravey RC. Gamma-hydroxybutyrate. Disposition of toxic drugs and chemicals in man. Foster City, CA: Chemical Toxicology Institute; 1995. p. 348–9.

[49] Yeatmen DT, Reid K. A study of urinary endogenous gamma-hydroxybutyrate (GHB) level. J Anal Toxicol 2003;27:40–2.

[50] Caldicott DG, Chow FY, Burns BJ, Felgate PD, et al. Fatalities associated with the use of gamma-hydroxybutyrate and its analogs in Australia. Med J Aust 2004;181:310–13.

[51] Kintz P, Villain M, Pelissier AL, Cirimele V, et al. Unusually high concentrations in fatal GHB case. J Anal Toxicol 2005;29:582–5.

[52] Kintz P, Cirimele V, Jamey C, Ludes B. Testing for GHB in hair by GC/MS after single exposure. Application to document sexual assault. J Forensic Sci 2003;48:195–200.

[53] Gahlinger PM. Club drug: MDMA, gamma-hydroxybutyric acid (GHB), Rohypnol and ketamine. Am Fam Physician 2004;69:2619–26.

[54] Dekker AH. What is being done to address the new drug epidemic? J Am Osteopath Assoc 2007;107(9 Suppl. 5):E 21–26.

[55] Lessenger JE, Feinberg SD. Abuse of prescription and over the counter medications. J Am Board Fam Med 2008;21:45–54.

[56] Dasgupta A Pharmacology of commonly abused drugs Beating drug test and defending positive results: a toxicologist's perspective. Totowa, NJ: Humana Press, 2010.

[57] Gonomori K, Yoshioka N. The examination of mushroom poisonings at Akita University. Leg Med (Tokyo) 2003;5(Suppl. 1):S83−6.

[58] Halpern JH, Sherwood AR, Hudson JI, Yugerlum-Todd D, Pope Jr. HG. Psychological and cognitive effects of long term peyote use among Native Americans. Biol Psychiatry 2005;58:624−31.

[59] Nichols DE. Hallucinogens. Pharmacol Ther 2004;101:131−81.

Designer drugs including bath salts and spices

3

Introduction

Amphetamine-like designer drugs such as 3,4-methylenedioxy-methamphetamine (MDMA) along with 3,4-methylenedioxyamphetamine (MDA) have been widely abused for many years. Although other designer drugs such as piperazines and pyrrolidinophenones are already known for many years, more recently new classes of psychoactive substances have emerged in the underground market including bath salts (synthetic cathinone) and spices (synthetic cannabinoids). In general, abuse of designer drugs is a serious public health issue because many designer drugs are not detected during routine urine drug screening conducted in most hospital based clinical laboratories.

Designer drugs were initially synthesized by clandestine laboratories in order to bypass legal consequences of manufacturing and selling illicit drugs. Then in 1986, the United States Controlled Substances Act was amended in order to make manufacturing and marketing of designer drugs illegal. Abuse of designer drugs is most prevalent in males in their mid to late 20s but ranges from teen to adults of 40 years of age. People who abuse designer drugs tend to be single and have a lower level of education and income [1].

Designer drugs can be purchased through the Internet and from street drug sellers in a variety of forms including powders, crystals, tablets, liquids, prerolled joints, smoking blends, as well as herbal mixtures. Although many products are labeled with warnings "Not for Human Consumption" they are abused by humans. The active component may vary widely between products. There are many novel psychoactive substances. There were 236 new psychoactive substances reported to the European Monitoring Centers for Drugs and Drug Addiction from May 2005 to December 2012. According to the update provided by the same organization, there are more than 450 psychoactive substances currently monitored by this organization with 101 new substances reported in 2014 alone [2].

Designer drugs can be broadly classified as psychostimulants, synthetic cannabinoids, opioid-like designer drugs, and hallucinogens/dissociative agents. Psychostimulants in general mimic the pharmacological actions of other stimulants such as amphetamine, methamphetamine, 3,4-methylenedioxymethamphetamine (MDMA), and cocaine, to varying degrees. Bath salts are psychostimulants which are beta-keto derivatives of amphetamine.

Alcohol, Drugs, Genes and the Clinical Laboratory. DOI: http://dx.doi.org/10.1016/B978-0-12-805455-0.00003-8

Bath salts

Bath salts are synthetic cathinones which have recently emerged as popular drugs of abuse in United States. These drugs are often marketed as "Legal Highs" and sold as "Bath Salts" or "Plant Food" and in order to defy laws labeled as "not for human consumption." Cathinone, a beta-keto derivative of amphetamine, is a naturally occurring compound found in leaves and other parts of the khat plant (*Catha edulis*), a flowering evergreen shrub cultivated as a bush or small tree native to Ethiopia, East Africa, and the Southern Arabian Peninsula. The leaves of khat pants are chewed in African countries and the Middle East for stimulation and euphoria. Khat use is a part of Yemini culture where approximately 90% of males and 50% of females chew khat leaves on a regular basis. Even 15−20% of children below the age of 12 chew khat plants. Global distribution of khat has increased significantly in last three decades where khat is available in both European and US markets. However, most consumers of khat in Western countries are immigrants from East Africa or the Middle East while the mainstream population in Western countries does not use khat due to unfamiliarity with its use [3]. The World Health Organization considers khat as a drug of abuse. Khat is banned in European countries, the United States, and Canada, while it is lawful in Yemen, Somalia, and Ethiopia [4]. Other than the major active compound cathinone, khat leaves contain over 40 compounds including alkaloids, tannins, flavonoids, terpenoids, sterols, glycosides, amino acids, vitamins, and minerals. Cathinone is degraded with time to cathine (inactive metabolite) and norephedrine by enzymatic actions. The degradation of cathinone is accelerated due to exposure to sunlight and heat. As a result, after cultivation khat plants are wrapped with banana leaves to reduce degradation. Usually 100−200 g of fresh leaves wrapped in banana leaves are chewed for getting the stimulatory effects of cathinone present in khat leaves [5].

Synthetic cathinones

Although abuse of khat leaves is limited to immigrants from certain parts of Africa and the Middle East in the United Stated, abuse of synthetic cathinones is widespread among Americans. Synthesis of cathinone derivatives has been reported as early as 1920s with methcathinone synthesized in 1928 and mephedrone in 1929. Although few derivatives of cathinones entered clinical trial for potential use as drugs, only bupropion is used clinically as a smoking cessation-aid and also to treat depression. Since 2007, Internet-based drug forums described abuse of synthetic cathinone [6]. In Europe and United States, commonly abused bath salts include 4-methylmethcathinone (mephedrone), 4-methethcathinone, butylone, methylone (beta-keto-MDMA), ethylone (beta-keto-3,4-methylenedioxy-*N*-ethylamphetamine (MDEA)), 4-fluoromethcathinone, 4-methoxymethcathinone, and (3,4-methylenedioxypyrovalerone (MDPV)). Based on the structure, bath salts can be categorized either as a secondary amine or a tertiary amine (Table 3.1). Currently cathinone and most baths salts are Schedule I drugs with no known medical use. Death from abuse of bath salts has been reported. The common routes of administration of bath salts

Table 3.1 Classification of bath salts as secondary or tertiary amine

Type of amine	Example
Secondary amine	Mephedrone (4-methylmethcathinone)
	Methedrone (4-methoxymethcathinone)
	Methylone (beta, keto-MDMA)
	Flephedrone (4-FMC: 4-fluoromethcathinone)
	Methcathinone
	4-MEC (4-methylcathinone)
	4-EMC (4-ethylmethcathinone)
	Butylone (beta-keto-*N*-ethylbenzodioxolybutanamine)
	Ethylone (3,4-methylenedioxy-*N*-ethylcathinone)
	Ethcathinone
	Pentylone (alpha-methylaminovalerophenone)
	Pentedrone (beta-keto-methylbenzodioxolypentanamine)
Tertiary amine	MDPV (3,4-methylenedioxypyrovalerone)
	Pyrovalerone
	Naphyrone (napthylpyrovalerone)
	MPBP (4-methyl-alpha-pyrrolidinobutiopheone)
	MDPBP (3,4-methylenedioxy-alpha-pyrrolidinobutiopheone)

are snorting and oral ingestion. Smoking, intramuscular injection, and intravenous injection routes are less common. The desired effects of abusing bath salts are euphoria, alertness, sexual arousal, talkativeness, and overall positive feelings. The desired effects may be observed within 30−45 min after administration and effects may last 1−3 h. Chemical structures of amphetamine, cathinone, and commonly encountered synthetic cathinone are given in Fig. 3.1.

Synthetic cathinones (bath salts) in general mimic the psychostimulant properties of amphetamine, MDMA, or cocaine. These drugs act by increasing synaptic levels of monoamines (noradrenaline, dopamine, and serotonin) by interacting with plasma membranes of various monoamine transporters including noradrenaline, dopamine, and serotonin transporters thus inhibiting reuptake of respective neurotransmitters. However, their selectivity varies among various synthetic cathinones. Some drugs such as cathinone, mephedrone, methcathinone, can promote release of dopamine while other drugs such as mephedrone, methylone, ethylone, butylone, can release serotonin. Based on types of interactions with various transporters, synthetic cathinones can be broadly classified under four categories [7]:

- Cocaine-MDMA mixed synthetic cathinones
- Methamphetamine-like synthetic cathinones
- MDMA-like synthetic cathinones
- Selective catecholamine uptake inhibitors

Classification of synthetic cathinones based on interactions with various monoamine transporters are summarized in Table 3.2. Bath salts are very addictive and are a serious public health challenge [8,9].

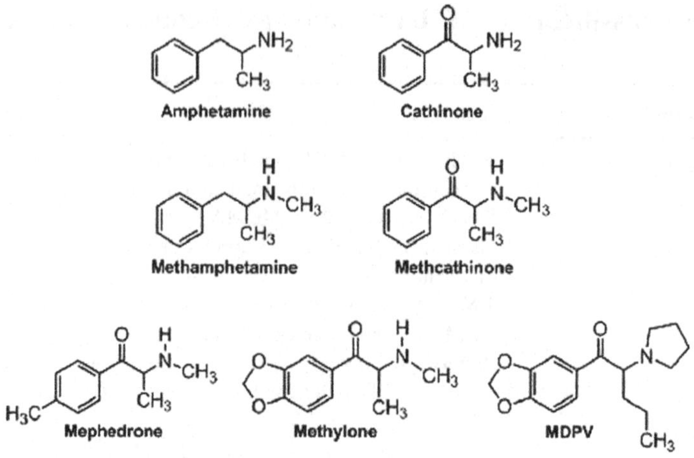

Figure 3.1 Chemical structures of amphetamine, cathinone, and commonly encountered synthetic cathinone.
Source: Adopted from Baumann MH, Partilla JS, Lehner K. Psychoactive "bath salts": not so soothing. Eur J Pharamcol 2013;698:1−5. Fig. 3.1, Elsevier, Reprinted with permission.

Table 3.2 Synthetic cathinones classified based on interaction with receptors

Type of synthetic cathinone	Mechanism of action	Examples
Cocaine-MDMA mixed synthetic cathinone	These drugs are nonselective monoamine uptake inhibitors like cocaine with five times higher affinity for dopamine transporters than serotonin transporters. These drugs also induce release of neurotransmitter serotonin similar to MDMA. Mephedrone also releases dopamine.	Mephedrone, methylone, ethylone, butylone
Methamphetamine-like synthetic cathinones	Similar to methamphetamine, these drugs act as preferential catecholamine (dopamine and noradrenaline) uptake inhibitors	Cathinone, methcathinone, flephedrone
MDMA-like synthetic cathinones	These drugs are potent noradrenaline and serotonin transporter inhibitors but have low potency towards dopamine transporters. These drugs release neurotransmitters serotonin and noradrenaline	Methedrone
Selective catecholamine uptake inhibitors	These drugs do not evoke release of monoamines. However, MDPV is 50 times more potent in interacting with dopamine transmitter compared to cocaine and 10 times more potent with noradrenaline transporter	MDPV and pyrovalerone

Metabolism of bath salts

Synthetic cathinone are extensively metabolized by the liver enzymes. Mephedrone is demethylated to a primary amine reduction of the ketone moiety to alcohol. Further oxidation may occur and some of the alcohols are conjugated via glucuronidation and sulfation and excreted in the urine. MDPV is first metabolized by opening of the methylenedioxy ring followed by demethylation leading to a catechol ring that is methylated by catechol-O-methyltransferase enzyme. Methylcatechol pyrovalerone and catechol pyrovalerone along with the parent drug has been identified in human urine. The most common metabolite of methylone is 4-hydroxy-3-methoxymethcathinones, although other metabolites have also been identified. Although the parent drug methylone was detected for 36 h, the metabolite was detected up to 48 h after exposure.

Toxicity and fatality associated with bath salts abuse

Patients abusing synthetic cathinone may present to the emergency department with agitation, psychosis, combative behavior, hyperthermia, and tachycardia. There is no antidote for treating poisoning from synthetic cathinones and the treatment is primarily supportive in nature. Belhadj-Tahar and Sadeg reported the case of a 29-year old woman who was admitted to the hospital with coma due to drug toxicity. Her blood alcohol level was 167 mg/dL and analysis of urine showed the presence of benzodiazepines and high levels of methcathinone; 17.24 mg/L, ephedrine; 11.60 mg/L, and methylephedrine; 11.10 mg/L. The analysis of serum also showed the presence of methcathinone (0.50 mg/L), methylephedrine (0.19 mg/L), and bromazepam (8.89 mg/L). The authors concluded that ingestion of alcohol and bromazepam altered the typical symptoms of methcathinone induced intoxication namely hypertension and convulsion. The authors further stated that the identification of methylephedrine, which is an impurity in the synthesis of methcathinone, can serve as a tag indicating fraudulent synthetic origin of methcathinone [10].

Fatality from bath salt abuse has been documented. The highest number of fatal intoxication has been reported with abuse of mephedrone. Kesha et al. reported fatal intoxication in a man due to consumption of MDPV where postmortem heart blood showed 0.7 mg/L of MDPV and peripheral blood showed 1.0 mg/L of MDPV [11]. In another report, the authors described fatality of a 36-year old man after the use of mephedrone, a bath salt. Postmortem analysis showed the presence of high amounts of mephedrone in the femoral blood and trace amounts of cocaine, MDMA, and oxazepam. The stomach content also showed the presence of an estimated 113 mg of mephedrone [12]. Busardo et al. reviewed 18 fatal cases involving mephedrone and concluded that 9 fatalities where mephedrone concentrations in postmortem blood ranged from 1.33 to 22 ng/mL were certainly due to mephedrone overdose. Other fatalities were related to multidrug abuse including mephedrone [13].

Liveri et al. reported a case of a 42-year old man who died due to myocardial infraction as a result of drug overdose. Postmortem analysis showed the presence of MDPV, pentedrone (2-methylamino-1-pehnylpentan-1-one), etizolam, olanzapine, mirtazapine, and ephedrine. The authors concluded that the death was related to use of new psychoactive substances [14]. Carbone et al. reported a case of a 19-year old healthy male who died suddenly due to methylone overdose. The postmortem blood showed methylone concentration of 0.07 mg/dL, a level below level of MDMA encountered in fatal cases [15]. Kudo et al. described fatality of a woman due to use of newer bath salts; 4-methoxy PV8, PV9, and 4-methoxy PV9. Various benzodiazepines (triazolam, flunitrazepam, and nitrazepam) and a dissociative agent diphenidine were also detected in blood and stomach content [16].

Although, synthetic cathinones are commonly used in date rape situations (commonly used drugs are gamma-hydroxy butyrate (GHB), ketamine, and flunitrazepam), there is a report of sexual assaults in 6 cases (out of 45 cases) where methylone, a synthetic cathinone, was identified in urine specimen. Following validation, in 2013, 45 victims were presented to the Rape Treatment Center in Miami-Dade and reported rape that required toxicology analysis of urine samples. The specimens were screened using immunoassays as well as using gas chromatography/mass spectrometry (GC/MS: screening for over 200 drugs). Synthetic cathinones along with methamphetamine, MDMA, and MDA were further confirmed also by using GC/MS after derivatization with heptafluorobutyric anhydride. The authors confirmed the presence of methylone in urine specimens of all six victims but ethanol, GHB, or ketamine were absent. The authors concluded that methylone might also be used in a drug-facilitated rape situation [17].

Bath salts if present in urine may not cause positive test results with amphetamine/methamphetamine immunoassays. However, a drug of abuse array V biochip array assay by Randox Corporation is capable of detecting synthetic cathinone if present in the urine specimen. This biochip assays have two antibodies specific for identification of various bath salts. Bath Salt I antibody is antimethcathinone antibody with 100% cross-reactivity to mephedrone. The Bath Salt II antibody is anti-MDPV antibody capable of detecting MDPV as well as 3,4-methylenedioxy-alpha-pyrrolidinobutiophenone. Other baths salts known to cross-react with these two antibodies include methylone, flephedrone, naphyrone, and pentedrone. The proposed manufacturer's cut-off is 5 ng/mL for Bath Salt I assay and 39 ng/mL for Bath Salt II assay.

The detection window of bath salts in urine is usually two days but metabolites may be detected for a longer time. Both GC/MS and liquid chromatography combined with tandem mass spectrometric (LC-MS/MS) methods are available for analysis of bath salts in various biological matrices. For GC/MS analysis usually derivatization using trifluoroacetic anhydride, pentafluoropropionic anhydride, heptafluorobutyric anhydride, or O-bis-trimethylsilyl-trifluoroacetamide is used. Hong et al. analyzed six synthetic cathinones (mephedrone, methylone, butylone, ethylone, pentylone, and MDPV) in urine using GC/MS after derivatization with heptafluorobutyric anhydride [18]. Concheiro et al. used liquid chromatography combined with high resolution mass spectrometry for analysis of 28 synthetic cathinones and metabolites in urine [19].

Other psychostimulant designer drugs

Amphetamine is a sympathomimetic amine which is structurally related to phenethylamine. Designer drugs structurally related to phenethylamine such as MDMA

(Ecstasy) and MDA are widely abused. In addition to MDMA other designer drugs structurally related to amphetamine such as para-methoxyamphetamine (PMA), para-methoxymethamphetamine (PMMA), and 4-methylthioamphetamine (4-MTA) have also been encountered at rave parties. MDMA associated deaths have been reported where a number of mechanisms including hyperpyrexia, cardiac arrhythmia, and liver failure have contributed in the death. In one report, the author reviewed 59 cases where deceased had MDMA in the postmortem blood and reported that in 13 cases where death was attributable to toxic effect of MDMA alone, the mean blood MDMA level was 8.43 mg/L (range: 0.478−53.9 mg/L; median 3.49 mg/L) [20].

PMA and PMMA are also commonly sold as "Ecstasy" but are more toxic than MDMA causing higher rate of morbidity and mortality than MDMA. Felgate et al. reported six fatalities involving abuse of PMA. Postmortem femoral blood PMA varied from 0.24 to 4.9 mg/L (mean: 2.3 mg/L). The authors concluded that PMA is more toxic than MDMA and blood levels exceeding 0.5 mg/L are associated with toxicity [21]. Johansen et al. also reported fatalities associated with abuse of both PMA and PMMA [22]. These compounds are associated with more severe hyperthermia than MDMA. 4-MTA is the methyl-thio analog of PMA, which produces MDMA-like effects and is also abused along with MDMA. The bath salt methedrone is a beta-keto-substituted analog of PMMA. Benzofurans and benzodifurans are also groups of designer drugs that are ring substituted amphetamines. These drugs are also structurally related to MDMA and similarly inhibit monoamine transporters. However, pharmacological action may be more intense than MDMA.

There are many designer drugs that are psychostimulant and have amphetamine-like action although many of these drugs are more potent than amphetamine and there are reports of fatalities associated with use of such drugs. The common examples of these designer drugs include MDEA, 2,5-dimethoxy-4-methylamphetamine, 2,5-dimethoxy-4-methylthioamphetamine, and 4-bromo-2,5-dimethoxyphenethylamine (2C-B) [23]. Classification of psychostimulant designer drugs based on structures is summarized in Table 3.3.

Metabolism

The designer drug 4-bromo-2,5-dimethoxyamohetamine (DOB) is metabolized by O-demethylation followed by oxidative deamination to the respective ketones as well as deamination followed by reduction to the corresponding alcohols. Other metabolic pathways involve O,O-bisdemethylation, or hydroxylation of the side chain followed by O-demethylation and deamination to the corresponding alcohol. All metabolites carrying the hydroxyl group were found to be in conjugated form in rat urine. The designer drug 4-iodo-2,5-dimethoxyamphetamine is also extensively metabolized by O-demethylation. The 2C (2,5-dimethoxy phenylamine) series of drugs are mainly metabolized by O-demethylation in positions two and five of the ring respectively, by deamination followed by oxidation to the corresponding alcohol. Further metabolic steps included side chain hydroxylation. Glucuronidation or sulfation of these metabolites has also been reported.

Table 3.3 Classification of designer psychostimulants based on structure type

Structure	Example
Beta-keto amphetamines	Synthetic cathinones (bath salts)
2,5-Dimethoxyamphetamine	DOB: 4-bromo-2,5-dimethoxyamphetamine
	DOC: 4-chloro-2,5-dimethoxyamphetamine
	DOI: 4-iodo-2,5-dimethoxyamphetamine
	DOM: 2,5-dimethoxy-4-methylamphetamine
	MDOB: 4-bromo-2,5-dimethoxymethamphetamine
	TMA-2: 2,4,5-trimethoxyamphetamine
2,5-Dimethoxy phenylamine (2C-series)	2C-B: 4-bromo-2,5-dimethoxyphenethylamine
	2C-I: 4-iodo-2,5-dimethoxyphenethylamine
	2C-D: 2,5-dimethoxy-4-methylphenethylamine
	2C-E: 4-ethyl-2,5-dimethoxyphenethylamine
	2C-T-2: 4-ethylthio-2,5-dimethoxyphenethylamine
	2C-T4: 4-isopropylthio-2,5-dimethoxyphenethylamine
	2C-T7: 2,5-dimethoxy-4-propylthiophenethylamine
Piperazines	BZP: 1-benzylpiperazine
	MeOPP: 1-(4-methoxyphenyl) piperazine
	TFMPP: trifluoromethyl-piperazine
	mCPP: 1-(4-chlorophenyl)piperazine
	pFPP:1, (4-fluorophenyl) piperazine
2-Aminoindanes	5-IAI: 5-iodo2-aminoindane
	MDAI: 5,6-methylenedioxy-2-aminoindane
Para-methoxy derivative	PMA: para-methoxyamphetamine
	PMMA: para-methoxymethamphetamine

Piperazine derivatives

Piperazine derivatives may be found in "Ecstasy" pills as a substitute for MDMA. Metachlorophenylpiperazine (mCPP) is an indirect serotonergic antagonist but another piperazine derivative trifluoromethyl-piperazine is a direct serotonergic antagonist but both drugs do not have any dopaminergic activity. Benzyl piperazine is an indirect dopamine and noradrenaline agonist without serotonergic properties. However, drug abusers report more unpleasant effects with this drug compared to MDMA. Aminoindanes such as 5,6-methylenedioxy-2-aminoindane and 5-iodoaminoindane are also abused but are less neurotoxic than MDMA [24].

Detection of designer drugs

Although recent abuse of MDMA or MDA can be detected by urine drug screen using amphetamine immunoassays, many designer drugs related to amphetamines cannot be detected by amphetamine immunoassays due to poor cross-reactivity with assay antibodies. A 39-year old African American woman presented to the emergency room after a night of partying. The urinary drug screen was positive for amphetamines. The LC-MS/MS analysis confirmed the presence of MDA (5.56 mg/L) and 4-iodo-2,5-dimethoxyphenethylamine (2C-I) (0.311 mg/L). Further investigation showed that 2C-I had no cross-reactivity (up to 100,000 ng/mL concentration tested) with the amphetamine screening assay (cloned enzyme donor immunoassay assay). Therefore, positive amphetamine screen was due to the presence of MDA in the urine [25].

Because of poor cross-reactivity of amphetamine-like designer drugs, chromatographic techniques including GC/MS or liquid chromatography combined with mass spectrometry or tandem mass spectrometry are most suitable for detection of these designer drugs. Pichini et al. described a LC-MS/MS determination of MDMA along with related designer drugs 2,5-diemethoxy-4-methylphenethylamine, 2C-B, 1-(8-bromo-2,3,6,7-tetrahydrobenzo [1,2-b:4,5-b'] difuran-4-yl)-2-aminoethane, 4-ethylthio-2,5-dimethoxyphenethylamine, 2C-I, 4-ethyl-2,5-dimethoxyphenethylamine, mCPP, 4-hydroxy-N,N'-disopropyltryptamine, and 4-acetoxy-N,N'-diisopropyltrypt amine in human urine. The authors used 3,4-methylenedioxypropylamphetamine as the internal standard. Extraction was performed using solid phase extraction and chromatographic separation was achieved by using a reverse phase C-18 column using a linear gradient of 10 mM ammonium bicarbonate, pH 7.3, and acetonitrile as a mobile phase. Separated analytes were identified by single ion monitoring using atmospheric pressure ionization-electrospray ionization interface [26].

Ewald et al. analyzed designer drugs DOB and 4-bromo-2,5-diemethoxymethamphetamine using GC/MS [27]. Takahashi et al. created a psychoactive drug data library by performing analysis using liquid chromatography with photodiode array spectrophotometry and GC//MS. This library has data of 104 drugs with the potential to abuse [28].

Abuse of synthetic cannabinoids (spices)

The abuse of synthetic cannabinoids was first reported in Europe in the early 2000s and in the United States around 2008. However, popularity of recreational use of synthetic cannabinoids are on rapid rise with synthetic cannabinoid related intoxication calls to poison control centers in United Stated increased by 240% between 2010 and 2011. In order to deal with severe health risks associated with use of synthetic cannabinoids, The Drug Enforcement Administration of United States passed Synthetic Drug Abuse Prevention Act in 2012 which classified many synthetic cannabinoids in Schedule I drug indicating no known medical use but high abuse potential. Unfortunately, to circumvent this classification many clandestine laboratories introduced newer versions of synthetic cannabinoids as evidenced by 330% increase in calls to poison control centers between January 2015 and May 2015. In 2014, 177 synthetic cannabinoids were reported to the United Nations Office on Drugs and Crime early warning advisory from 58 countries. Serious poisoning and even fatalities have been reported due to use of synthetic cannabinoids [29].

Synthetic cannabinoids were initially synthesized for research purposes. One of the first reported uses of synthetic cannabinoids, JW-018, was originally synthesized by John William Huffman, a chemist at Clemson University to evaluate therapeutic potential of synthetic cannabinoids. It has been speculated that a chemist in a clandestine laboratory copied his method and JWH-018 was introduced as a recreational drug in the underground market because JWH-018 like natural cannabinoid (tetrahydrocannabinol: THC) can interact with cannabinoid receptors in the brain.

Usually synthetic cannabinoids are sprayed on herbal mixtures and wrapped in foil packages with the warning label "Not for Human Consumption" (street names: spice, K2, K2 blond, etc.). These products, like cannabis, are often smoked via a joint or water pipe but also can be consumed orally or intranasally. Compared to natural THC, synthetic cannabinoids are more potent and may have a longer half-life. The effects may appear within 10 min after inhalation and may last 2−6 h after use [1]. Now there are many synthetic cannabinoids found through the Internet but most synthetic cannabinoids detected today can be broadly classified as aminoalkylindoles synthesized by John William Hoffman (JWH-018, JWH-122) or Alexander Makriyannis (AM-2201), cyclohexylphenols originally synthesized at Pfizer (CP 47,497 and its analogs), benzoylindoles produced by Research Chemical Suppliers (RCS-4), and classical synthetic cannabinoids such as HU-210 produced at the Hebrew University [30]. Commonly encountered synthetic cannabinoids are listed in Table 3.4 and Fig. 3.2.

Pharmacology and toxicology of synthetic cannabinoids

Similar to natural THC, synthetic cannabinoids bind with cannabinoid receptor 1 (CB1) and cannabinoid receptor 2 (CB2), which are found mostly in the central nervous system but also may be found in peripheral tissues including lungs, liver, and kidneys. However, within the brain, these receptors are mostly located in the cerebral cortex, hippocampus, basal ganglia, and cerebellum. In contrast to THC, which is a partial CB1 receptor agonist, synthetic cannabinoids are more potent full CB1 agonists thus rendering their pharmacological effects. Therefore, in general synthetic cannabinoids have much higher affinity for CB1 receptors than THC.

As well as stimulating CB1 receptors more than CB2 receptors, synthetic cannabinoids also nonspecifically bind to other receptor membranes including opioid and benzodiazepine receptors. These compounds are metabolized by the liver cytochrome P450 mixed function oxidase enzymes but unlike THC which is metabolized to inactive THC-COOH (major metabolite, but minor metabolite of THC; 11-OH-THC is active), metabolites of JWH-018, JWH-073, and AM-2201 have high affinity for CB1 receptors. Because of higher affinity for cannabinoids receptors, synthetic cannabinoids are associated with higher rates of toxicity and hospital admission compared to abusers of natural cannabis. The most commonly reported toxicities associated with synthetic cannabinoids include tachycardia, agitation and irritability, hallucination, delusion, hypertension, nausea, confusion, dizziness, vertigo, and chest pain. Acute kidney injury is also strongly associated with abuse of synthetic cannabinoids. Treatment is mostly supportive care [31].

Table 3.4 Common synthetic cannabinoids

Chemical class	Examples
Aminoalkylindoles	JWH-007, JWH-015, JWH-018, JWH-019, JWH-020, JWH-073, JWH-081, JWH-122, JWH-200, JWH-203, JWH-210, JWH-250, JWH-251, JWH-397, JWH-412, AM-1220
Cyclohexylphenols	CP 47,497 and its homologs, CP 55,940
Benzoylindoles	AM-694, AM-679, AM-2201, AM-2233, RCS-4
Synthetic cannabinoids analog	HU-210, HU-211, HU-239, HU-243, HU-308, HU-320
Others	UR-144, WN 55,212

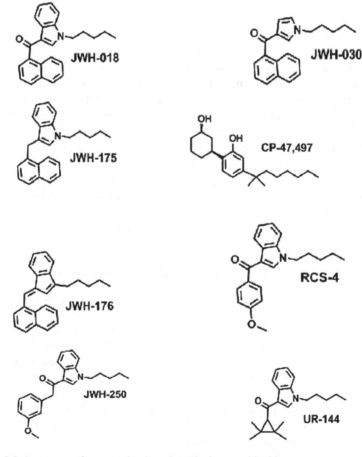

Figure 3.2 Structures of commonly abused synthetic cannabinoids.
Source: Adopted from Fantegrossi WE, Moran JH, Radominska-Pandya A, Prather PL. Distinct pharmacology and metabolism of K2 synthetic cannabinoid compared to Δ^9-THC: mechanism underlying greater toxicity. Life Sciences 2014;97:45–54. Fig. 3.1, Elsevier, Reprinted with permission.

Metabolism of synthetic cannabinoids

Detailed metabolic pathways of synthetic cannabinoids are still under investigation but there is contrast between metabolism of natural cannabinoids (marijuana; delta-9-tetrahydrocannabinol (Δ^9-THC)) and synthetic cannabinoids. The metabolism of Δ^9-THC via oxidation into 11-hydroxy-Δ^9-THC (active metabolite) involves CYP2C9 and CYP3A4 and then this metabolite is further metabolized 11-nor-9-carboxy-Δ^9-THC (THC-COOH; major metabolite) which is an inactive metabolite. THC-COOH is then conjugated and excreted in urine. In contrast to THC-COOH, which is inactive, many metabolites of synthetic cannabinoids retain some pharmacological activity. Synthetic cannabinoid JWH-1018, other aminoalkylindoles, cyclohexylphenols, and benzylindoles that show structural similarities are oxidized by cytochrome P450 enzymes and then are conjugated by the action of uridine 5'-diphospho (UDP)-glucuronosyltransferase enzyme present in the liver.

However, unlike metabolism of Δ^9-THC where CYP3A4 plays an important role, CYP3A4 plays a minor role in metabolism of synthetic cannabinoids. In vitro metabolism studies indicate that CYP2C9 and CYP1A2 are major isoenzymes involved in metabolism of synthetic cannabinoids. However, CYP2D6 may also play an important role in regulating brain concentrations of metabolites of synthetic cannabinoid for binding with cannabinoids receptors. CYP2D6 is expressed in the cerebral cortex, hippocampus, and cerebellum of the brain in vicinity to CB1 receptors. Then these metabolites are further conjugated and excreted as glucuronides. Two isoforms of UDP-glucuronosyltransferase (UGT2B7 and UGT1A2) play important role in glucuronidation of synthetic cannabinoid metabolites. As mentioned earlier, many metabolites of synthetic cannabinoids retain some pharmacological activities. In particular omega-hydroxyl metabolite of JWH-018 retains activity for CB1 receptor. Interestingly, even glucuronide derivative of this metabolite retains affinity for CB1 receptor but acts as a neutral antagonist [32].

Fatalities associated with synthetic cannabinoids use

Fatalities associated with synthetic cannabinoids abuse have been reported. Shanks et al. reported three cases where fatalities were associated with synthetic cannabinoid use. In case one, a 57-year old man died due to use of JWH-018. The cardiac blood showed 199 ng/mL of JWH-018 along with other prescription drugs. In the second case a 52-year old year man died who showed 19.6 ng/mL of JWH-018 and 68.3 ng/mL of JWH-073 in cardiac blood. In the third case a 29-year old man died who showed only the presence of JWH-018 (83.3 ng/mL) in the cardiac blood but no other drug [33]. Labay et al. recently reviewed cases where death was related to use of synthetic cannabinoids. The authors identified six deaths related to abuse of JWH-018 (postmortem blood levels: 0.11−0.65 ng/mL), six deaths related to abuse of JWH-122, six deaths related to abuse of JWH-210, one each associated with abuse of JWH-175 and JWH-250, respectively. In addition, two fatalities associated with abuse of XLR-11 and nine fatalities associated with abuse of AM-2201 (postmortem blood levels: 0.13–17.0 ng/mL) were also reported [34]. Patton et al. also reported death of a 23-year old man due to AM-2201 overdose. The metabolite of AM-2201 was detected in the postmortem blood [35].

Death due to use of synthetic cannabinoids (S)-methyl-2-(1-(5-fluoropentyl)-1H-indazole-3-carboxamido)-3-methylbutanoate (5F-AMB), a new synthetic cannabinoid first reported in Japan in early 2014, has also been reported. The concentration of 5F-AMB was only 0.3 ng/mL. However, the authors concluded that the death was accidental [36]. Shanks et al. described a death associated with use of a new synthetic cannabinoid ADB-4-fluorobenzyl-1H-indazole-3-carboxamide (FUBINACA). In this drug, 1-amino-3,3-deimethoxy-1-oxobutane-2yl (ABD) group is linked with FUBINACA base at the amide group. The concentration of this relatively new synthetic cannabinoid in the postmortem blood was 7.3 ng/mL. However, a small amount of THC (1.1 ng/mL) and its metabolite THC-COOH (4.7 ng/mL) was also detected in the postmortem blood using LC-MS/MS [37].

Detection of synthetic cannabinoids

Synthetic cannabinoids do not cross-react with marijuana immunoassay. Therefore, urine toxicology screen is usually negative in a person suspected to have synthetic cannabinoids overdose unless marijuana is also smoked along with synthetic cannabinoid. In this case urine screen for marijuana metabolite should be positive. However, recently enzyme-linked immunosorbent assay (ELISA assay) (National Medical Services JWH-018 direct assay targeting JWH-018 metabolite: JWH-018 N-(5-hydroxylpentyl)) for detecting certain synthetic cannabinoids in urine has been evaluated [38]. The drug of abuse array V biochip array assay by Randox Corporation is also capable of detecting certain synthetic cannabinoids if present in the urine specimen. In general, synthetic cannabinoids are not routinely analyzed in most hospital based clinical laboratories. Therefore, specimens should be shipped to a reference laboratory or a major academic medical center where such tests may be available.

Chromatographic methods for analysis of synthetic cannabinoids have been reported in the medical literature. Dresen et al. described a protocol for analysis of JWH-015, JWH-018, JWH-073, JWH-081, JWH-200, JWH-250, and related compounds, after liquid–liquid extraction from serum and quantification by LC-MS/MS. The authors analyzed 101 serum specimens from 80 subjects provided by hospitals, detoxification and therapy centers, forensic psychiatry centers, and police authorities and observed that 57 specimens were positive for at least 1 of these compounds [39]. In another report, the authors used LC-MS/MS for detection of JWH-018, JWH-019, JWH-073, JWH-122, JWH-200, JWH-210, JWH-250, JWH-398, RCS-4, AM-2201, MAM-2201, UR-144, CP 47,497-C7, and CP 47,497-C8 and their metabolites in urine [40].

Opioid related designer drugs

Heroin (diacetylmorphine), which was synthesized from morphine in 1874, can be considered as the first designer drug that belongs to opioid class. Heroin is a Class I scheduled drug in the United States with no known medical use but this drug is highly abused throughout the world. Heroin is metabolized to 6-monoacetylmorphine (also known as 6-acetylmorphine) and then finally to morphine. Fortunately a heroin abuser can be easily identified by opiate assay during urine drug screen.

Fentanyl is a widely used synthetic narcotic analgesic that is approximately 75—100 times more potent than morphine. Several analogs of fentanyl such as sufentanil, alfentanil, lofentanil, and remifentanil have been synthesized by pharmaceutical industries and are used clinically. Currently in the United States, fentanyl is a Schedule II drug which is used as an anesthetic. Fentanyl is also available as lozenges and transdermal patches (Duragesic) for pain management. Oral transmucosal fentanyl citrate (Actiq) is also available. Therapeutic range of fentanyl is considered as 1—3 ng/mL in serum and toxicity of fentanyl is similar to opiate toxicity [41]. Fentanyl is widely abused and many fentanyl related deaths have been reported. Martin et al. reported that 54 deaths in Ontario, Canada from 2002 to 2004 were related to fentanyl where postmortem fentanyl blood concentrations ranged from 3.0 to 383 ng/mL [42].

Fentanyl derivatives

Fentanyl analog designer drugs China White (α-methylfentanyl) appeared in the underground market of California in 1979 causing over 100 deaths. Gillespie et al. determined postmortem blood, bile, and liver concentrations of α-methylfentanyl in a drug overdose victim. The blood concentration of α-methylfentanyl was 3.1 ng/mL, bile concentration was 6.4 ng/mL while the level in liver was 78 ng/g of liver tissue [43]. In 1984, another illicit designer drug 3-methylfentanyl appeared as a street drug in California, which was also related to fatal drug overdose. Ojanpera et al. described three fatal poisoning cases involving 3-methylfentanyl. The mean blood level of 3-methylfentanyl was 0.5 ng/mL (range: 0.3—0.9 ng/ml). The blood fentanyl levels were measured using tandem mass spectrometric technique [44].

Recently, McIntyre et al. described a fatality associated with butyr-fentanyl. Using GC/MS, the authors demonstrated that butyr-fentanyl concentration in the peripheral blood was 58 ng/mL while the concentration in vitreous was 40 ng/mL. The liver concentration was 320 ng/g [45]. Death due to abuse of acetyl fentanyl has also been reported. The acetyl fentanyl peripheral blood concentration was 260 ng/mL while the liver concentration was 1000 ng/kg [46].

Fentanyl and its analogs are metabolized through N-dealkylation. The major metabolite of fentanyl is nor-fentanyl. The minor metabolites are hydroxyfentanyl and hydroxynorfentanyl. Similarly major metabolite of alpha-methyl fentanyl is nor-fentanyl but 3-methyl fentanyl is converted into nor-3-methyl fentanyl.

Neither fentanyl nor its analogs can be detected in routine urine drug testing by regular opiate screening assays because these compounds do cross-react with antibodies used in opiate assays, which are specific for morphine. However, there is a specific ELISA assay for determination of fentanyl in urine. The concentrations of fentanyl and its analogs can be measured in serum, urine, and other biological matrices using GC/MS.

Meperidine derivatives

Meperidine (Demerol) is a synthetic opioid which is used as a narcotic analgesic. It is available both as an injectable form and for oral use supplied as hydrochloride salt. Both meperidine and several of its analogs are abused. A common designer drug which is a meperidine analog is 1-methyl-4-phenyl-4-propionoxypiperdine (MPPP). An impurity found in some illicitly synthesized MPPP preparations which is identified as 1-methyl-4-phenyl-1,2,3,6-tetrahydropyridine caused permanent Parkinsonism in a number of intravenous drug abusers [47]. Meperidine and its analogs have negligible cross-reactivity with the opiate screening assay for drugs of abuse. However, specific enzyme immunoassay is available for detection of meperidine and its metabolites in urine. Chromatographic techniques are also available for analysis of meperidine and its analog.

Designer drugs which are phencyclidine analogs

Phencyclidine (PCP) was introduced in the 1950s as a human anesthetic but was discontinued due to significant side effects. PCP undergoes extensive metabolism by liver cytochrome P450 enzymes (especially CYP3A4) into several hydroxy metabolites.

There are a number of designer drugs that are analogs of phencyclidine. These drugs include N-(1-phenylcyclohexyl)-propanamine, N-(1-phenylcyclohexyl)-3-methoxypropanamine, N-(1-phenylcyclohexyl)-2-methoxyethanamine, and N-(1-phenylcyclohexyl)-2-ethoxyethanamine. These drugs are extensively metabolized by liver enzymes [48].

Drugs related to GHB

GHB is an endogenous constituent of the mammalian brain that is present in nanomolar concentration and acts as a neurotransmitter. GHB was sold in the 1990s in health food stores but following reports of toxicity Federal Food and Drug Administration (FDA) banned the sale of GHB. However, GHB can be obtained illegally and is often used in date rape situations (see chapter: Drugs of Abuse: an Overview). Absorption of GHB from the gastrointestinal tract is rapid, with onset of effects within 15 min. The elimination half-life is 27 min but clinical effects may last 6–10 h after use.

Several GHB analogs such as gamma-butyrolactone (GBL), 1,4-butanediol (1,4-BD), gamma-hydroxy valeric acid (GHV), and gamma-valerolactone (GVL) are abused. Wood et al. reported that in 2006, only eight patients reported to the emergency department of the authors' hospital with GBL toxicity but 150 patients reported to the emergency department with GHB toxicity. In contrast, out of 418 specimens seized 85 specimens contained GHB but 140 contained GBL. None of the samples seized contained 1,4-BD [49]. Street names and common features of GHB and related compounds are summarized in Table 3.5.

Table 3.5 Abused drugs related to GHB

Drug	Street names	Comments
Gamma-hydroxybutyric acid	G, liquid ecstasy, liquid, liquid E, easy lay, Cherry Meth, natural sleep 500, woman Viagra, etc.	GHB is an endogenous inhibitory neurotransmitter. It is synthesized from gamma-aminobutyric acid endogenously. Used in date rape situations due to rapid onset of action as 2–3 g dosage may cause deep sleep. Usually detected in urine up to 12 h after abuse. Fatality has been reported
Gamma-butyrolactone (GBL)	Blue nitro, midnight blue, cleaner, magic stripper gamma, GH revitalizer, etc.	GBL is converted into GHB by the action of enzyme lactonase present in peripheral tissues. Usually GBL is not detected in humans after abuse and toxicity is mainly due to GHB
1,4-Butanediol (1,4-BD)	Weight belt, serenity, review, etc.	1,4-BD is first converted into gamma-hydroxybutyraldehyde by the action of alcohol dehydrogenase. Then it is finally converted into GHB by the action of aldehyde dehydrogenase. Effect of 1,4-BD may last longer than GHB abuse alone. Abuse of 1,4-BD may be fatal
GHV (gamma-hydroxy valeric acid)		GVL is a precursor of GHV
Gama valerolactone (GVL)		Metabolized by lactonase enzyme into gamma-hydroxyvaleric acid (GHV) also known as 4-methyl-GHB. After GVL abuse GHV is detected in blood and urine

Both GBL and 1,4-BD are precursors of GHB and can be viewed as prodrugs of GHB. Because GBL is widely used in industry, it is readily available from commercial chemical supply companies. In 1999, FDA issued a warning regarding the danger of consuming GBL containing supplements and asked manufacturers to voluntarily recall such products. As GBL containing products were recalled, some manufacturers substituted GBL with 1,4-BD. However, 1,4-BD is also toxic.

After ingestion, GBL is rapidly converted into GHB by the action of lactonase enzyme present in peripheral tissues. However, 1,4-BD is first metabolized into gamma-hydroxybutyraldehyde by the action of alcohol dehydrogenase enzyme. Then gamma-hydroxybutyraldehyde is converted into GHB by the action of another enzyme aldehyde dehydrogenase. The toxicity is prolonged if 1,4-BD and alcohol is consumed at the same time because alcohol is a preferred substrate for alcohol dehydrogenase. Thai et al. studied the pharmacology of 1,4-BD in human and observed that 1,4-BD is quickly absorbed and cleared with a maximum plasma concentration achieved at an average of 24 min after ingestion and the elimination half-life was 39.3 min on average. 1,4-DB is also extensively converted into GHB endogenously and the average half-life of GHB was 32.3 min [50].

In one case report, the authors observed serious toxicity in an adolescent female who consumed a soft drink containing two teaspoons of a health food called "Serenity." She had a Glasgow Coma Scale score of 5 although her urine toxicology screen was negative. Two acquaintances brought in the bottle of herbal supplement which listed 1,4-BD as a component. She was discharged next morning after psychiatric evaluation [51]. The health risks of 1,4-BD is similar to abuse of GHB and GBL and death from abuse of 1,4-BD has also been reported. Zvosec et al. reported toxic events in eight patients who ingested 1,4-BD and two patients died from such overdose. The blood GHB in the first deceased was 432 mg/L while the corresponding urine concentration was 5430 mg/L. In addition, 1,4-BD (845 mg/L) was detected in the urine. In the second deceased the blood and urine GHB concentrations were 837 and 1161 mg/L, respectively. The concentration of 1,4-BD in blood and urine were 220 and 1756 mg/L, respectively. However, in nonfatal cases no 1,4-buitanediol was detected in blood or urine. The amount of 1,4-BD ingested by the two who died ranged from 5.4 to 20 g while in nonfatal cases the amount ingested varied from 1 to 14 g [52]. Ortman reported a case of a 20-month old child after ingesting a plastic toy containing 1,4-BD which is used in manufacturing of plastic. Fortunately the child recovered [53].

Neither GBL nor 1,4-BD directly binds to GHB receptors but GHV binds directly to GHB receptors but with less affinity than GHB. Although, both GBL and 1,4-BD are endogenously converted into GHB, GVL does not metabolize to GHB but into gamma-hydroxyvaleric acid (GVH also known as 4-methyl-GHB). Anderson-Streichert et al. reported a case of a woman who was sexually assaulted under the influence of GVL. Her urine showed the presence of GHV at a concentration of 3.0 mg/L. In the blood ethanol was detected but no GHV [54].

There is no antidote for treating overdose due to GHB as well as drugs related to GHB and management is mostly supportive with emphasis on airway management. For suspected overdose with GVL and 1,4-BD, analysis of GHB in blood or urine is also recommended because both agents are rapidly converted into GHB. Unfortunately, GHB cannot be detected by routine drugs of abuse testing protocol. In the case of suspected overdose of GHB, a more sophisticated analytical technique such as GC/MS should be employed for confirming the presence of GHB in blood or urine.

GHB in blood can be determined using GC/MS after liquid–liquid extraction and di-trimethylsilyl-derivatization [55]. Couper and Logan also used a simple liquid–liquid extraction for extraction of GHB from biological fluid and GC/MS analysis after forming di-trimethylsilyl-derivatization. Using the technique the authors determined GHB concentration of 3.2 mg/L in the blood of a sexual assault victim. In addition GHB levels of two drivers who were accused of DUI were 33 and 34 mg/L [56]. GHB in human serum or urine can also be determined by liquid chromatography combined with mass spectrometry. Kaufmann and Alt have reported analysis of GHB in human serum and urine using this technique after conversion of GHB to its respective n-butyl ester derivative. The authors used hexadeutero GHB as the internal standard [57].

Conclusions

Abuse of synthetic cathinones (bath salts) and synthetic cannabinoids (spice, K2, etc.) are on rise most commonly among the young male population. GHB and related drugs are also abused, including in date rape situations. There are also other designer drugs which are psychostimulants. Except for MDMA and MDA, designer drugs including synthetic cathinones and synthetic cannabinoids cannot be detected in routine toxicology analysis. Although specialized immunoassays are available for analysis of cathinone, synthetic cathinones, and synthetic cannabinoids, such assays may not be readily available in many small to medium sized hospital based clinical laboratories. However, using chromatographic methods (GC/MS and liquid chromatography combined with mass spectrometry or tandem mass spectrometry) these designer drugs can be readily analyzed, but only reference laboratories and large academic medical centers have such capabilities.

References

[1] Weaver MF, Hopper JA, Gunderson EW. Designer drugs 2015: assessment and management. Addict Sci Clin Pract 2015;10:8.
[2] New psychoactive substance sin Europe: European Monitoring Centre for Drugs and Drug Abuse. March 2015 report.
[3] Anderson D, Beckerleg S, Hailu D, Klein A. The khat controversy: stimulating the debate on drug. Oxford: Berg; 2006.
[4] El-Menyar A, Mekkodathil A, Al-Thani H, Al-Motarreb A. Khat use: history and heart failure. Oman Med J 2015;30:77–82.
[5] Yousef G, Huq Z, Lambert T. Khat chewing a cause of psychosis. Br J Hosp Med 1995;54:322–6.

[6] Prosser JM, Nelson LS. The toxicology of bath salts: a review of synthetic cathinones. J Med Toxicol 2012;8:33–42.

[7] Zawilska JN. Legal highs-an emerging epidemic of novel psychoactive substances. Int Rev Neurobiol 2015;120:273–300.

[8] Iversen L, White M, Treble R. Designer psychostimulants: pharmacology and differences. Neuropharmacology 2014;87:59–65.

[9] Baumann MH, Partilla JS, Lehner K. Psychoactive "bath salts": not so soothing. Eur J Pharamcol 2013;698:1–5.

[10] Belhadj-Tahar H, Sadeg N. Methcathinone: a new postindustrial drug. Forensic Sci Int 2005;153:99–101.

[11] Kesha K, Boggs CL, Ripple MG, Allan CH, Levine B, Jufer-Phipps R, et al. Methylenedioxypyrovalerone (bath salts) related death: case report and review of the literature. J Forensic Sci 2013;58:1654–9.

[12] Lusthof KJ, Ooxting R, Maes A, Verschaagen M, et al. A case of extreme agitation and death after use of mephedrone in the Netherland. Forensic Sci Int 2011;206: e93–5.

[13] Busardo FP, Kyriakou C, Napoletano S, Marinelli E, et al. Mephedrone related fatalities: a review. Eur Rev Med Pharmacol Sci 2015;19L:3777–90.

[14] Liveri K, Constatinoua MA, Afxentiou M, Kanari P. A fatal intoxication related to MDPV and pentedrone combined with antipsychotic and antidepressant substances in Cyprus. Forensic Sci Int 2016;265:160–5.

[15] Carbone PN, Carbone DL, Carstairs SD, Luzi SA. Sudden cardiac death associated with methylone use. Am J Forensic Med Pathol 2013;34:26–8.

[16] Kudo K, Usumoto K, Kikura-Hanajiri R, Sameshima N, et al. A fatal case of poisoning related to new cathinone designer drugs, 4-methoxy PV8, PV9 and 4-methoxy PV9 and a dissociative agent. Leg Med (Tokyo) 2015;17:421–6.

[17] Hagan KS, Reidy L. Detection of synthetic cathinones in victims of sexual assault. Forensic Sci Int 2015;257:71–5.

[18] Hong WY, Ko YC, Lin MC, Wang PY, et al. Determination of synthetic cathinones in urine using gas chromatography-mass spectrometry technique. J Anal Toxicol 2016;40: 12–16.

[19] Concheiro M, Anizan S, Ellefsen K, Huestis MA. Simultaneous quantification of 28 synthetic cathinones and metabolites in urine by liquid chromatography-high resolution mass spectrometry. Anal Bioanal Chem 2013;405:9437–48.

[20] Milroy CM. Ecstasy associated deaths: what is fatal concentration? Analysis of a case series. Forensic Sci Med Pathol 2011;7:248–52.

[21] Felgate HE, Felgate PD, James PA, Sims DN, et al. Recent paramethoxyamphetamine deaths. J Anal Toxicol 1998;22:169–72.

[22] Johansen SS, Hansen AC, Muller IB, Lundemose JB, et al. Three fetal cases of PMA and PMMA poisoning in Denmark. J Anal Toxicol 2003;27:253–6.

[23] Christophersen AS. Amphetamine designer drugs-an overview and epidemiology. Toxicol Lett 2000;112–113:127–31.

[24] Liechti M. Novel psychoactive substances (designer drugs): overview and pharmacology of modulation of monoamine signaling. Swiss Med Wkly 2015;145:W14043.

[25] Dress JC, Stone JA, Wu AH. Morbidity involving the hallucinogenic designer amines MDA and 2CI. J Forensic Sci 2009;54:1485–7.

[26] Pichini S, Pujadas M, Marchei E, Pellegrini M, et al. Liquid chromatography-atmospheric pressure ionization electrospray mass spectrometric of hallucinogenic designer drugs in urine of consumers. J Pharm Biomed Appl 2008;47:335–42.

[27] Ewald AH, Fritschi G, Bork WR, Maurer HH. Designer drugs 2,5-dimethoxy-4-bromo-amphetamine (DOB) and 2,5-diemthoxy-4-bromo-methamaphetamine (MDOB): studies of their metabolite and toxicological detection in rat urine using gas chromatography/mass spectrometric techniques. J Mass Spectrom 2006;41:487—98.

[28] Takahashi M, Nagashima M, Suzuki J, Seto T, et al. Creation and application of psychoactive designer drugs data library using liquid chromatography with photodiode array spectrometry detector and gas chromatography-mass spectrometry. Talanta 2009; 77:1245—72.

[29] Cooper ZD. Adverse effects of synthetic cannabinoids: management of acute toxicity and withdrawal. Curr Psychiatry Rep 2016;18:52.

[30] Seely CA, Lapoint J, Moran JH, Fattore L. Spice drugs are more than harmless herbal blends: a review of the pharmacology and toxicology of synthetic cannabinoids. Prog Neuropsychopharmacol Biol Psychiatry 2012;39:234—343.

[31] Mills B, Yepes A, Nugent K. Synthetic cannabinoids. Am J Med Sci 2015;350:59—62.

[32] Su MK, Seely KA, Moran JH, Hoffman RS. Metabolism of classical cannabinoids and synthetic cannabinoids. Clin Pharmacol Ther 2015;97:562—4.

[33] Shanks KG, Dahn T, Terrell AR. Detection of JWH-018 and JWH-073 by UPLC-MS-MS in postmortem whole blood. J Anal Toxicol 2012;36:145—52.

[34] Labay LM, Caruso JL, Gilson TP, Phipps RJ, et al. Synthetic cannabinoid drug use as a cause or contributory cause of death. Forensic Sci Int 2016;260:31—9.

[35] Patton AL, Chimalakonda KC, Moran CL, McCain KR, et al. K2 toxicity: fatal case of psychiatric complications following AM2201 exposure. J Forensic Sci 2013;58: 1676—80.

[36] Shanks KG, Behonick GS. Death after use of the synthetic cannabinoids 5F-AMB. Forensic Sci Int 2016;262:e21—4.

[37] Shanks KG, Clark W, Behonick G. Death associated with the use of the synthetic cannabinoids ADB-FUBINACA. J Anal Toxicol 2016;40:236—9.

[38] Barnes AJ, Spinelli E, Young S, Martin TM, et al. Validation of an ELISA synthetic cannabinoids urine assay. Ther Drug Monit 2015;37:661—9.

[39] Dresen S, Kneisel S, Weinmann W, Zimmermann R, et al. Development and validation of a liquid chromatography-tandem mass spectrometry method for the quantitation of synthetic cannabinoids of the aminoalkylindole type and methanandamide in serum and its application to forensic samples. J Mass Spectrom 2011;46:163—71.

[40] Scheidweiler KB, Huestis MA. Simultaneous quantification of 20 synthetic cannabinoids and 21 metabolites and semi-quantitative quantification of 12 alkyl hydroxy metabolites in human urine by liquid chromatography-tandem mass spectrometry. J Chromatogr A 2014;1327:105—17.

[41] Mystakidou K, Katsouda E, Parpa E, Vlahos L, et al. Oral transmucosal fentanyl citrate: overview of pharmacological and clinical characteristics. Drug Deliv 2006;13: 269—76.

[42] Martin TL, Woodall KL, McLellan BA. Fentanyl related deaths in Ontario, Canada: toxicological findings and circumstances of death in 112 cases (2002—2004). J Anal Toxicol 2006;30:603—10.

[43] Gillespie TJ, Gandolfi AUJ, Davis TP, Morano RA. Identification and quantification of alpha-methylfentanyl in post mortem specimens. J Anal Toxicol 1982;6:139—42.

[44] Ojanpera I, Gergov M, Rasanen I, Lunetta P, et al. Blood levels of 3-methylfentanyl in 3 fetal poisoning cases. Am J Forensic Sci 2006;27:328—31.

[45] McIntyre IM, Trochta A, Gary RD, Wright J, et al. An acute butyr-fentanyl fatality: a case report with postmortem concentrations. J Anal Toxicol 2016;40:162—6.

[46] McIntyre IM, Trochta A, Gary RD, Malamatos M, et al. An acute acetyl fentanyl fatality: a case report with postmortem concentrations. J Anal Toxicol 2015;39:490−4.

[47] Johannessen JN, Markey SP. Assessment of the opiate properties of two constituents of a toxic illicit drug mixture. Drug Alcohol Depend 1984;13:367−74.

[48] Maurer HH. Chemistry, pharmacology, and metabolism of emerging designer drugs. Ther Drug Monit 2010;32:544−9.

[49] Wood DM, Warren-Gash C, Ashraf T, Greene SL, et al. Medical and legal confusion surrounding gamma-hydroxybutyrate (GHB) and its precursors gamma-butyrolactone (GBL) and 1,4-butanediol (1,4-BD). QJM 2008;101:23−9.

[50] Thai D, Dyer JE, Jacob P, Haller CA. Clinical pharmacology of 1,4-butanediol and gamma-hydroxybutyrate after oral 1,4-butanediol administration to healthy volunteers. Clin Pharmacol Ther 2007;81:178−84.

[51] Micahel S, Quang L. Gamma hydroxybutyrate, gamma-butyrolactone and 1,4-butanediol: a case report and review of literature. Pediatric Emerg Care 2000;16:435−40.

[52] Zvosec DL, Smith SW, McCutcheon JR, Spillance J, et al. Adverse events including death associated with the use of 1,4-butanediol. N Eng J Med 2001;344:87−94.

[53] Ortmann LA, Jaeger MW, James LP, Schexnayder S. Coma in a 20 month old child from ingestion of a toy containing 1,4-butanediol, a precursor of gamma-hydroxybutyrate. Pediatr Emerg Care 2009;25:758−60.

[54] Andersen-Streichert H, Jungen H, Gehl A, Muller A, et al. Uptake of gamma-valerolactone detection of gamma-hydroxyvaleric acid in human urine samples. J Anal Toxicol 2013;37:250−4.

[55] Elian AA. GC-MS determination of gamma-hydroxybutyric acid (GHB) in blood. Forensic Sci Int 2001;122:43−7.

[56] Couper FJ, Logan BK. Determination of gamma-hydroxybutyrate (GHB) in biological specimens by gas chromatography-mass spectrometry. J Anal Toxicol 2000;24:1−7.

[57] Kaufmann E, Alt A. Determination of GHB in urine and serum by LC/MS using a simple one-step derivative. Forensic Sci Int 2007;168:133−77.

Combined alcohol and drug abuse: a potentially deadly mix

Introduction

Illicit drug use is a major public health issue not only in the United States but globally, because it has been estimated that 230 million people worldwide (approximately 5% of world population) had abused an illicit drug at least once in their life. The number of regular illicit drug users worldwide is approximately 27 million (roughly 0.6% of world population). Approximately 15.9 million people worldwide may inject illicit drugs and among them an estimated 3 million people may be positive for HIV. Sharing needles is a major cause of spreading HIV virus [1]. According to the World Health Organization's report, approximately half of the total world population drinks alcohol. The proportion of users varies widely among countries from 18% to 90% among males and from 1% to 81% among females [2].

In United States, data from combined surveys from 2008 to 2012 indicate that 8.7% full time workers aged 18−64 used alcohol heavily, 8.6% used illicit drugs, while 9.5% suffered from substance use disorder. The highest rates of heavy alcohol use were found in mining (17.5%), and construction industries (16.5%). The highest rates of illicit drug use were observed in accommodations and food service industries (19.1%). In addition highest percentage of people with substance use disorder (16.9%) was also found in the accommodations and food industries. The lowest percentage of people who abused illicit drugs worked for educational services (4.8%) [3].

Many drug abusers abuse both alcohol and drugs at the same time in order to enhance the buzz. Unfortunately, alcohol interacts with many drugs in a clinically significant way enhancing the toxicity of a drug. Abusing drugs and alcohol at the same time is a deadly combination because alcohol may lower the threshold of toxic concentration of a specific illicit or prescription drug, thus causing life threatening toxicity or even fatality. In general, illicit drugs such as cocaine, opioids (heroin as well as prescription opioids such as morphine, methadone, codeine, and oxycodone) are more commonly encountered in drug overdose situations. Fentanyl, an opioid receptor agonist that is used as filler for street heroin, is 80 times more potent than morphine and as a result a slight change of dosage may cause fatality [4].

Data collected from drivers killed in road traffic crashes in Sweden between 2003 and 2007 showed alcohol was the substance most commonly found in blood of drivers killed in roadside accidents. Out of 1403 cases studies, 835 cases (60%) showed no presence of illicit drugs or alcohol. Alcohol alone was detected in 242 victims while another 73 cases had both alcohol and illicit drugs. There were

Alcohol, Drugs, Genes and the Clinical Laboratory. DOI: http://dx.doi.org/10.1016/B978-0-12-805455-0.00004-X

253 cases where both prescription and illicit drugs were present [5]. Drug poisoning deaths in Sweden also showed a predominance of alcohol. Moreover, mono-intoxication deaths were mostly alcohol related. Interestingly, the number of drugs found in postmortem blood varied from only 1−12 drugs (median 3−4 drugs) indicating that polydrug abuse is also common. In alcohol related mono-intoxication cases mean and median blood alcohol levels were 3.06 g/L (306 mg/dL) and 3.10 g/L (310 mg/dL), respectively. However, lower concentration of alcohol was observed where alcohol was found along with a prescription or illicit drug, indicating adverse drug−alcohol interaction. Interestingly, when alcohol and one drug were detected, the mean alcohol level reduced from 306 into 215 mg/dL but with two drugs, mean alcohol level was further reduced to 178 mg/dL. When three, four, five, and more drugs were detected along with alcohol, the corresponding mean alcohol blood levels were 155, 149, 137, and 125 mg/dL respectively. The occurrence of a single drug along with alcohol was also a common finding. The mean blood alcohol concentration was lowest with morphine (150 mg/dL) and highest with diazepam (320 mg/dL). The mean concentrations of some of the drugs observed in mono-intoxication in blood were 0.5 mg/L for (500 ng/mL) for morphine, 2.0 mg/L (2000 ng/mL) for amphetamine, 3.9 mg/L (3900 ng/mL) for propoxyphene, 0.4 mg/L (400 ng/mL) for 7-aminoflunitrazepam (metabolite of flunitrazepam). Elevated morphine levels found in those poisoned patients were related to morphine abuse as verified by detecting 6-monocaetyl morphine, the marker of heroin abuse in the blood of those deceased [6]. In Chapter 2, Drugs of Abuse: an Overview an overview of abused drugs is provided. This chapter focuses on interactions between alcohol and illicit drugs with an emphasis on toxicity and fatality associated with combined abuse of alcohol and illicit drugs or abuse of prescription drugs.

Alcohol drug interaction

Alcohol interacts with many drugs (prescription, over the counter, and illicit drugs) and such interactions are often clinically significant. Alcohol−medication interactions can be broadly classified as pharmacokinetic interactions or pharmacodynamic interactions. For certain drugs, for example diazepam, both pharmacokinetic and pharmacodynamic interactions have been reported. However, pharmacodynamic interactions between alcohol and drugs are more common that pharmacokinetic interactions.

After ingestion, alcohol passes into the stomach where a small amount is metabolized and some part is absorbed into the portal system. Alcohol is absorbed slowly from the stomach but rapidly from the upper small intestine and as a result gastric emptying time has influence on blood alcohol levels. Alcohol in the circulation is metabolized by alcohol dehydrogenase into acetaldehyde. Then acetaldehyde is further metabolized into acetate by the action of aldehyde dehydrogenase. In heavy drinkers, cytochrome P-450 pathway of alcohol metabolism is activated and mainly CYP2E1 is responsible for the conversion of alcohol into acetaldehyde. However, CYP3A4 and CYP1A2 also have minor roles in alcohol metabolism. Therefore, alcohol consumption may affect metabolism of drugs which are metabolized via CYP3A4 and CYP1A2.

Drugs that slow gastric emptying generally reduce blood alcohol level whereas drugs that increase gastric emptying time may potentially elevate blood alcohol level. Cimetidine and ranitidine increase the gastric emptying time and also inhibit alcohol dehydrogenase present in stomach mucosa. Therefore, if alcohol is consumed with cimetidine or ranitidine, higher blood alcohol level is observed. Aspirin also increases gastric emptying and may inhibit alcohol dehydrogenase enzyme. Therefore, elevated blood alcohol may be observed (depending on dosage of aspirin) in people taking aspirin and consuming alcohol. Erythromycin also increases blood alcohol level by increasing gastric emptying time. If nonsteroidal antiinflammatory drugs such as ibuprofen, naproxen, diclofenac, ketoprofen, and fenoprofen are taken with alcohol, risk of gastrointestinal bleeding may be increased [7]. Acetaminophen is metabolized by CYP2E1 and CYP3A4. Alcohol increases hepatoxicity of acetaminophen by inducing CYP2E1, which is responsible for formation of hepatotoxic metabolite of acetaminophen (N-acetyl-p-benzoquinone amine). Therefore, acute ingestion of a large amount of alcohol may increase risk of acetaminophen-induced hepatotoxicity [8].

Drugs that inhibit alcohol dehydrogenase usually prolong elimination half-life of alcohol while drugs that inhibit aldehyde dehydrogenase result in an increased concentration of acetaldehyde, which is associated with unpleasant reactions after intake of alcohol. Fomepizole, which is used in treating ethylene glycol and methanol poisoning, inhibits alcohol dehydrogenase. Disulfiram, which is used in patients enrolled in alcohol rehabilitation programs, acts by inhibiting aldehyde dehydrogenase. Unpleasant reactions after consuming alcohol in patients taking disulfiram deter them from consuming alcohol. The antibacterial drug metronidazole may inhibit aldehyde dehydrogenase thus increasing alcohol blood level. Moreover metronidazole may cause disulfiram-like reactions possibly by also inhibiting aldehyde dehydrogenase [9]. Other antibiotics such as sulfonamides, nitrofurantoin, and chloramphenicol are known to cause disulfiram-like reactions. Ornidazole, a broad spectrum antibiotic, has been also reported to cause disulfiram-like reactions [10].

At this time there is insufficient evidence that indicates warfarin−alcohol interaction. Havrda et al. described a case report where international normalized ratio (INR) of a 58-year old man was increased from 2.18 to 8.0 after he started consuming a low amount of alcohol (one-half can of light beer every other day). After discontinuing beer, his INR returned to the baseline value [11]. Major drug (excluding prescription drugs that are abused and illicit drugs)−alcohol interactions are summarized in Table 4.1.

Table 4.1 Examples of some drug (excluding prescription drugs which are also abused)—alcohol interaction

Drug/drug class	Drug—alcohol interaction
Aspirin	Higher alcohol level due to faster absorption of alcohol and inhibition of alcohol dehydrogenase
Acetaminophen	Alcohol increases toxicity of acetaminophen due to faster formation of toxic metabolite
Antihistamines	Alcohol enhances sedative effects of antihistamines such as diphenhydramine (Benadryl), chlorpheniramine, clemastine, hydroxyzine, promethazine, and cyproheptadine but alcohol has no effect on nonsedative antihistamines, e.g., cetirizine and loratadine
Antibiotics	Erythromycin may increase blood alcohol level by increasing gastric emptying time. Antibiotics such as metronidazole, sulfonamides, nitrofurantoin, chloramphenicol, and ornidazole are known to cause disulfiram-like reaction. Isoniazid induced liver toxicity may be enhanced with chronic alcohol consumption
Antidiabetic	In general, chronic consumption of alcohol along with taking antidiabetic medications may increase the risk of hypoglycemia. Chlorpropamide, glyburide, and tolbutamide may cause disulfiram-like reaction. Metformin if consumed with alcohol may increase lactic acid levels in blood
Anticancer	Methotrexate (also used as a disease modifying agent in treating rheumatoid arthritis) induced risk of liver damage is increased with alcohol consumption
Antihypertensive agents	Alcohol appears to have a pharmacodynamic interaction with felodipine as subjects experienced lightheadedness when felodipine was consumed with alcohol. This may be due to more profound reduction in diastolic blood pressure with a resultant increase in heart rate and cardiac index. Although blood pressure did not change due to nifedipine—alcohol interaction, increased heart rate was observed. Norverapamil, a metabolite of verapamil may accumulate due to administration of alcohol because unlike verapamil, which is metabolized by CYP3A4, norverapamil is metabolized by CYP2E1. Verapamil may also increase the subject's perception of alcohol intoxication
Antiulcer (H_2 receptor antagonists)	Increased blood alcohol level because of cimetidine, nizatidine, and ranitidine inhibits stomach alcohol dehydrogenase (thus reducing first pass metabolism) and also increases alcohol absorption by increasing gastric emptying time

(Continued)

Table 4.1 **(Continued)**

Drug/drug class	Drug–alcohol interaction
Gabapentin	Gabapentin, an antiepileptic drug which is also used in treating neurological pain, enhances tachycardia associated with alcohol in a dose-dependent manner
Monoamine oxidase (MAO) inhibitors	MAO inhibitors such as phenelzine and tranylcypromine, if consumed with red wine, may cause sever high blood pressure due to presence of tyramine in red wine
Nonsteroidal antiinflammatory drugs	Ibuprofen, fenoprofen, ketoprofen, naproxen and diclofenac if consumed with alcohol may increase risk of gastrointestinal bleeding
Procainamide	Ethanol consumption can increase elimination of procainamide, an antiarrhythmic drug, because alcohol consumption increases formation of acetyl-CoA, which is an important cosubstrate for conversion of procainamide to N-acetyl procainamide by N-acetyl transferase enzyme
Tricyclic antidepressants	Amitriptyline, clomipramine, desipramine, doxepin, imipramine, nortriptyline, and trimipramine may increase drowsiness and orthostatic hypotension if consumed with alcohol. Atypical antidepressants such as nefazodone and trazodone may cause enhanced sedation when consumed with alcohol
Warfarin	A case report indicated that when a person started consuming alcohol, his INR increased from 2.18 to 8.0

Interactions between abused drugs and alcohol

Many prescription drugs which are abused (mostly amphetamines, benzodiazepines, barbiturates, and opioids) as well as illicit drugs such as cocaine (on some occasions cocaine is used as a topical anesthetic in ENT surgeries), heroin, and marijuana (synthetic marijuana Marinol has therapeutic use) interact with alcohol. Again, such interactions are mostly pharmacodynamic in nature but pharmacokinetic reactions have also been documented. There are conflicting results regarding pharmacokinetic interactions between alcohol and some abused drugs. However, pharmacodynamic interactions between alcohol and drugs are well established. Interactions between alcohol and illicit drugs and well as prescription drugs that are abused are summarized in Table 4.2.

Interactions between barbiturates and alcohol

Barbiturates are sedatives while phenobarbital is used for treating seizure. In general, alcohol increases sedative effects of barbiturates including the sedative effect of phenobarbital. Therefore, patients taking barbiturates should be warned not to perform tasks requiring alertness such as driving or operating heavy

Table 4.2 **Interaction between abused drugs as well as certain prescription drugs which are abused and alcohol**

Drug/drug class	Drug–alcohol interaction
Barbiturates	The effect is mostly pharmacodynamic because both barbiturates and alcohol are CNS depressants. Therefore, alcohol enhances sedative and hypnotic effects of barbiturates. Severe respiratory depression may occur from combined use of barbiturate and alcohol, and overdose fatalities have also been reported
Benzodiazepines	Both benzodiazepines and alcohol are CNS depressant and as a result alcohol enhances the effects of benzodiazepines causing increased sedation, increased drowsiness, but significantly decreased motor skill (causing severe driving impairment). Some pharmacokinetic interactions between alcohol and specific drugs in this family have also been reported
Cannabinoid (marijuana: THC; Δ^9-tetrahydrocannabinoid)	Alcohol has additive effect on impairment of cognitive function by THC. Combination of alcohol and THC is associated with severe driving impairment. Alcohol also prolongs duration of euphoria induced by THC
Cocaine	Mixing cocaine with alcohol is a potentially deadly combination due to formation of cocaethylene, a very potent active metabolite of cocaine
MDMA	Alcohol prolongs euphoria induced by MDMA and perception of well-being. Some pharmacokinetic interaction between MDMA and ethanol has also been reported
Methamphetamine	Although there is no pharmacokinetic interaction between alcohol and methamphetamine, methamphetamine may decrease subjective perception of alcohol intoxication. Moreover, combination of alcohol and methamphetamine is associated with lower systolic blood pressure and increased heart rate thus increasing harmful cardiovascular effects
Opioids	In general, alcohol enhances sedation and drowsiness effects of opioids and also causes further impairment of motor skills. All patients taking prescription opioids should be warned regarding additive effects of alcohol on opioid-induced drowsiness and significantly impaired driving skills associated with mixing opioid prescription drugs with alcohol. Combined overdose of alcohol and opioids may be life threatening because such a combination significantly reduces breathing and cough functions. As a result a person may be at high risk getting food or fluid stuck in the airways, thus impairing the breathing ability of a person. Moreover, a person overdosed with both opioid and alcohol may be unable to breath and may die from such combined overdose although death from opioid overdose without involvement of alcohol has also been reported. Pharmacokinetic interaction between alcohol and heroin as well as between alcohol and morphine has also been reported

machinery after drinking and simultaneously taking a medication belonging to barbiturate class [7]. Barbiturate use in conjunction with alcohol can result in severe respiratory depression and significant incidence of overdose deaths. Both barbiturates and alcohol enhance gamma aminobutyric acid (GABA) mediated chloride current, which is the primary source of inhibitory signal within central nervous system (CNS). Ethanol and pentobarbital together may cause severe respiratory depression including lethal apnea [12].

Combined effect of alcohol and secobarbital showed differences between people with a family history of alcohol abuse and people with no family history of alcohol abuse. Subjects with a family history of alcohol abuse showed more extended intoxication and greater withdrawal effect after simultaneous administration of secobarbital and alcohol [13].

Okamoto studied the interaction between alcohol and pentobarbital and compared such effects with alcohol and chlordiazepoxide interaction using mice model. The authors reported that interaction between alcohol and pentobarbital produced greater effect because at a dosage of 4 g/kg of ethanol, the lethal dose of pentobarbital (LD_{50}) was reduced by 41% while LD_{50} of chlordiazepoxide was reduced by only 2%. The authors commented that this data supports the clinical observation that accidental benzodiazepine intake in conjunction with alcohol is less likely to cause death whereas high a incident of deaths has been reported with barbiturate−ethanol combination. The authors further demonstrated that alcohol increased pentobarbital elimination half-life by 1.39 times and also caused increased peak pentobarbital concentration. Therefore, duration of pentobarbital effect was increased by administration of alcohol. Alcohol also inhibited metabolism of chlordiazepoxide [14]. Kinoshita et al. described a case of fatal poisoning due to combined effect of alcohol, phenobarbital, and amoxapine. The postmortem femoral blood concentration of alcohol, phenobarbital, and amoxapine were 286 mg/dL, 6.80 μg/mL, and 0.41 μg/mL, respectively. It is important to note than phenobarbital is metabolized by CYP2E1 [15].

Interactions between benzodiazepines and alcohol

Benzodiazepines have been associated with road traffic accidents and such incidence is increased due to combined use of benzodiazepine and alcohol. Alcohol and benzodiazepine have an additive effect (pharmacodynamic interaction) that causes further reduction in psychomotor skills needed for safe driving. In general, short acting benzodiazepines cause lesser impairment than long acting benzodiazepines. Moreover, both barbiturates and benzodiazepines like alcohol can impair memory. Therefore, consumption of alcohol along with ingestion of barbiturates or benzodiazepines may exacerbate memory-impairing effects. This effect is exploited in drug assisted date rape situations where alcoholic beverages are mixed with flunitrazepam, a rapid acting benzodiazepine [7]. Flunitrazepam is not Federal Food and Drug Administration approved for clinical use in United States.

There are also pharmacokinetic interactions between alcohol and some benzodiazepines. Alcohol ingestion may increase absorption of some benzodiazepines [16]. Some benzodiazepines are metabolized by CYP3A4 through hydroxylation (triazolam, midazolam, diazepam, alprazolam), demethylation (diazepam), and also through nitro-reduction (clonazepam). Diazepam is also metabolized by CYP2C19. Acute alcohol ingestion may increase blood concentrations of benzodiazepines which are metabolized by cytochrome P-450 enzymes (CYP) but have minimal or no effect for oxazepam and lorazepam which are conjugated by uridine 5'-diphospho-glucuronosyltransferase enzyme. The inhibition of some benzodiazepines' metabolism due to acute alcohol ingestion is responsible for increased benzodiazepine concentrations. Studies have shown that area under the curve (AUC) of N-desmethyldiazepam (also known as nor-diazepam, an active metabolite) may be decreased by up to 50% due to administration of alcohol, suggesting that metabolism of diazepam via CYP2C19 was reduced due to inhibition of this enzyme as a result of acute alcohol administration. However, chronic alcohol ingestion may induce CYP enzymes and as a result clearance of diazepam may be increased. This may be due to induction of CYP enzymes due to chronic alcohol administration. However, overall interaction between alcohol and benzodiazepines are pharmacodynamic in nature [7]. The frequency and quantity of alcohol consumption is a major consideration in patients who may need therapy with benzodiazepines. Alcohol affects GABA−benzodiazepine−chloride ionophore complex and has an agonist-like effect that is responsible for the addictive effects of alcohol and benzodiazepine, causing more CNS depression associated with increased drowsiness, increased sedation, and significant impairment of motor skills. Moreover, alcohol also has anxiolytic effect, and as a result, many patients taking prescription benzodiazepines may also consume alcohol [17].

It appears that fatal poisoning (suicidal and nonsuicidal) occurs more often when alcohol is consumed with multiple benzodiazepines rather than ingestion of alcohol and a single benzodiazepine. Many of these fatalities involved triazolam probably due to lower therapeutic concentration of triazolam (2−20 ng/mL) compared to other benzodiazepines [18]. Drummer et al. investigated eight deaths involving flunitrazepam and observed very high concentrations of 7-aminoflunitrazepam, a metabolite of flunitrazepam in all cases. In four cases no other drug was detected but in another four cases alcohol (mean concentration 160 mg/dL) was also present. The mean 7-aminoflunitrazepam concentration was 0.45 mg/L in four cases where no alcohol was involved but the mean 7-aminoflunitrazepam concentration was significantly lower (0.16 mg/L) in four other cases where alcohol was also present. Because only moderate amounts of flunitrazepam were detected in postmortem blood, the authors speculated that 7-aminoflunitrazepam was produced postmortem and may be a marker for flunitrazepam use. The authors also concluded that the presence of alcohol reduces the amount of flunitrazepam needed to cause death [19]. Alcohol may also increase the absorption of marijuana, resulting in an increase in positive subjective mood effects of smoked marijuana. This may contribute to popularity of combined use of alcohol and marijuana [20].

Interactions between cannabinoid and alcohol

The interaction between cannabinoid (marijuana: Δ^9-tetrahydrocannabinoid (THC)) and alcohol is mostly pharmacodynamic in nature because studies on potential pharmacokinetic interactions between THC and alcohol produced conflicting results with some studies reporting no significant interaction, whereas other studies reported decreased blood ethanol concentration due to administration of THC. In general, THC has been shown to cause impairment in cognitive function and when combined with alcohol more impairment may be observed because effects are additive, possibly synergistic. Studies evaluating THC and ethanol using driving stimulators showed that the effect of THC on driving impairment was small to moderate (up to 300 μg/kg dose) when taken alone but the combination of a moderate dosage of THC with even a low dose of alcohol resulted in severe impairment in driving ability [7].

Dubois et al. studied association between combined effect of alcohol and THC and fatal crash risk. The authors reported that over the past two decades, the prevalence of THC and alcohol in car drivers involved in fatal crashes has increased approximately fivefold (below 2% in 1991 to above 10% in 2008). The authors calculated that drivers who were positive for THC alone had a 16% increased risk of potentially unsafe driving actions. The odds of potentially unsafe driving, when alcohol and THC were combined, increased by 8−10% for each of 0.01% (10 mg/dL) blood alcohol level increase [20]. Hartman et al., based on a study of 18 subjects, reported that cannabis and alcohol increased weaving within the lane (using National Advanced Driving Simulator) when drivers had either THC or alcohol in blood. Increase of blood THC levels from 8.2 to 13.1 ng/mL caused similar impairment as observed with increasing blood alcohol levels (breath alcohol was actually measured) from 0.05% to 0.08% (80 mg/dL, the legal limit of driving). THC and alcohol had additive effects on driving impairment as THC concentrations of 5 ng/mL combined with blood alcohol of 0.05% (50 mg/dL) caused the same degree of impairment as observed with 0.08% blood alcohol (80 mg/dL). The authors also observed that even low amounts of alcohol significantly increased peak THC concentration in blood [21]. Lukas and Orozco reported that alcohol might increase absorption of THC resulting in an increase in the positive mood effects of smoked marijuana [22]. This may contribute to the popularity of drinking alcohol and smoking marijuana simultaneously in order to prolong euphoria.

Cocaine and alcohol: a deadly mix

Cocaethylene is a toxicologically important compound formed due to coadministration of cocaine and ethanol. The hepatic carboxyltransferase enzyme is responsible for formation of cocaethylene. Unlike benzoylecgonine, which is the inactive metabolite of cocaine formed in the absence of alcohol, cocaethylene is an active metabolite of cocaine. Moreover, cocaethylene has a plasma half-life of three to five times the half-life of cocaine and is associated with seizure, liver damage, and compromised immune function. Moreover, LD50 of cocaethylene is significantly lower than cocaine and as a result carries an 18−25 fold increase over cocaine alone in risk of immediate death [23].

In the presence of alcohol, peak concentration of cocaine is also increased by approximately 20%, possibly due to higher rates of absorption of cocaine in the presence of alcohol. The higher cocaine blood concentration due to coadministration of alcohol is also associated with higher cardiotoxicity induced by cocaine. However, alcohol does not affect half-life or other pharmacokinetic parameters of cocaine. The combined presence of cocaine and cocaethylene in blood is responsible for increased euphoria and other cocaine related pleasurable effects. However, such a combination also increases the heart rate and higher plasma cortisol concentration. It has been suggested that the enhanced effect of cocaine when abused along with alcohol may be due to initial higher concentration of cocaine in blood as well as additive effects of cocaethylene, but a pharmacodynamic interaction between cocaine and alcohol cannot be ruled out [7]. Bailey reported that cocaethylene was always found (except in one case) along with benzoylecgonine and cocaine in urine, but in urine specimens where no cocaethylene was present, benzoylecgonine may or may not be present without simultaneous presence of cocaine. The mean alcohol concentration in blood was also higher (132 mg/dL) in patients where cocaethylene was detected compared to blood alcohol level (63 mg/dL) where no cocaethylene was detected [24].

Interactions between methamphetamine, amphetamine, MDMA, and alcohol

Although there is no significant pharmacokinetic interaction between methamphetamine and alcohol, addition of alcohol to methamphetamine was associated with higher heart rate and higher blood pressure, thus increasing harmful cardiovascular toxicity of methamphetamine. Interestingly, methamphetamine users who were nondrinkers or light drinkers developed a tendency to dislike alcohol after methamphetamine abuse but no such effect was observed in heavy drinkers. Coadministration of methamphetamine with alcohol results in long acting and more complicated changes in the brain's neurotransmitter functions. Alcohol also plays an important role in the fatal effect of methamphetamine, especially from small dosage [25]. Alcohol enhances driving impairment caused by amphetamine [26].

3,4-Methylenedioxymethamphetamine (MDMA) is often abused along with alcohol. In one study using human volunteers to investigate interaction between MDMA and alcohol, the authors reported that plasma concentration of MDMA showed a 13% increase after use of alcohol whereas plasma concentration of alcohol showed 9−15% decrease after MDMA administration. The MDMA−alcohol combination induced longer-lasting euphoria and subjective feelings of well-being compared to when alcohol or MDMA was administered alone. Overall MDMA reduced the subjective feeling of sedation induced by alcohol but MDMA did not reverse alcohol induced psychomotor impairment. Therefore, persons drinking alcohol and at the same time abusing MDMA may feel that they are driving better when actual performance may be severely impaired [27]. Veldstra et al. studied effect of MDMA and alcohol on stimulated driving performance and concluded that the dissociation between subjective perceptions and objective performance in individuals taking MDMA and alcohol is an important notion for traffic safety because this may affect a driver's judgment of whether or not it is safe to drive. For example, an intoxicated individual may decide to drive because of feelings of alertness caused by MDMA that may cloud the impairing effects of other drugs such as alcohol thus creating a potentially serious risk for traffic safety [28].

Interactions between opioids and alcohol

Heroin is a widely abused drug which interacts pharmacokinetically with alcohol. Heroin is first metabolized into 6-monoacetylmorphine (6-MAM) and then 6-MAM further breaks down into morphine. Based on their study of forensic autopsy cases all containing 6-MAM, Thaulow et al. showed that the concentration ratios of morphine/6-MAM, morphine-3-glucuronide/morphine, and morphine-6-glucuronide/ morphine in blood samples were all significantly lower in alcohol positive cases compared to alcohol negative cases. For subgroup of cases revealing a very recent intake of heroin ($n = 645$), only the morphine/6-MAM ratio was significantly lower in ethanol positive cases than ethanol negative cases. For subgroup of cases with a less recent heroin intake ($n = 817$), lower morphine-3-glucuronide/ morphine and morphine-6-glucuronide/morphine ratios were found in alcohol positive subjects. The authors concluded that alcohol interacts pharmacokinetically with heroin and inhibits two steps in heroin metabolism; the hydrolysis of 6-MAM to morphine and glucuronidation of morphine into morphine-3-glucronide or morphine-6-glucuronide [29].

Hoiseth et al. reported morphine-3-glucuronide/morphine ratio was lower in alcohol positive cases compared to cases where no alcohol was involved (4.9 with alcohol and 6.7 without alcohol). The ratio of morphine-6-glucuronide to morphine was also lower in alcohol positive cases compared to alcohol negative cases (0.62 vs 0.96). The authors concluded that less metabolite is formed from morphine in the presence of alcohol due to inhibition of glucuronidation of morphine and such pharmacokinetic interaction could lead to increased terminal half-life of morphine and also more accumulation after repeated dosage [30]. Although there was no pharmacokinetic effect of alcohol on oxycodone, studies have shown that oxycodone significantly reduced breath alcohol concentrations at 15 and 30 min after low dose of alcohol and 15, 20, and 60 min after use of high dose of alcohol. However, there was no effect of other opioids such as propoxyphene, morphine, and hydromorphone on breath alcohol concentrations in similar situations [7].

Another major concern for combining opioid prescription drugs with alcohol is due to the possibility of dose dumping which is defined as unintended rapid release (over a short period of time) of the entire amount or major fraction which is originally intended for extended release. In vitro studies with Avinza (morphine sulfate extended release capsules) showed accelerated release of morphine that was dependent on alcohol concentration. This is the reason why box warnings of Avinza as well as other extended release opioid formulations advise patients not to drink alcoholic beverages or nonprescription medications containing alcohol during therapy. Moreover, combination of alcohol and opioid use increases the risk of fatal overdose from opioids due to a combination of CNS and respiratory depressant effects of such a combination. Fatal poisoning involving prescription opioids are frequently associated with alcohol use. Opioids also significantly decrease the ventilatory response to hypercapnia when administered with alcohol. Increased pleasurable subjective effects have been reported by health volunteers after administration of a combination of oxycodone and alcohol, compared to when such volunteers took oxycodone or alcohol alone [31].

Hickman et al. commented that epidemiological evidence shows that opiate overdose deaths rarely involve a single drug. The most common agent found along with opioid in such cases is alcohol. Moreover, heroin abusers who also drink may require a lesser quantity of heroin for overdose than heroin abusers who do not consume alcohol. Moreover, postmortem morphine levels are usually below the levels expected of highly tolerant individuals [32]. Levine et al. also commented that an even small amount of alcohol is clearly a risk factor in deaths due to heroin [33].

Conclusions

The interaction between a drug and alcohol can be pharmacokinetic or pharmacodynamic or both in nature although pharmacodynamic interactions are more common than pharmacokinetic interaction. Alcohol should be avoided when using certain medication such as benzodiazepines and extended release opioid formulations. Alcohol potentiates sedative effects of benzodiazepines that result in significant impairment while driving or operating heavy machinery. Abuse of MDMA along with alcohol may confuse a person and the person may underestimate sedation due to use of alcohol. Therefore, the person may think that he or she is capable of driving when in reality the driving skills of that person may be severely impaired. This may significantly increase the risk of an accident. The combination of cocaine and alcohol is deadly due to formation of cocaethylene, an active metabolite of cocaine that is only formed in the presence of alcohol. Concurrent use of alcohol also increases the risk of death from heroin abuse.

References

[1] Khazaei S, Poorolajai J, Mahjub H, Esmailnasab N, et al. Estimation of the frequency of intravenous drug users in Hamadan City, Iran using the capture-recapture method. Epidemiol Health 2012;34:e2012006.
[2] Huu Bich T, Thi Quynh Nga P, Ngoc Quang L, Van Minh H, et al. Pattern of alcohol consumption in diverse rural populations in the Asian region. Glob Health Action 2009;28:2. Available from: http://dx.doi.org/10.3402/gha.v2io.2017.
[3] Bush DM, Lipari RN. Substance abuse and substance abuse disorder by industry. The CBHSQ Report. Rockville (MD): Substance Abuse and Mental Health Services Administration (US); 2013–2015 Apr 16.
[4] Martins SS, Sampson L, Cerda M, Galea S. Worldwide prevalence and trends in unintentional drug overdose: a systematic review. Am J Public Health 2015;105:e29–46.

[5] Jones AW, Kugelberg FC, Holmgren A, Ahlner J. Five year update on the occurrence of alcohol and other drugs in blood samples from drivers killed in road traffic crashes in Sweden. Forensic Sci Int 2009;186:56−62.

[6] Jones AW, Kugelberg FC, Holmgren A, Ahlner J. Drug poisoning deaths in Sweden show a predominance of ethanol in mono-intoxications, adverse drug-alcohol interactions and poly-drug use. Forensic Sci Int 2011;206:43−51.

[7] Weathermon R, Crabb DW. Alcohol and medication interactions. Alcohol Res Health 1999;23:40−51.

[8] Chan LN, Anderson GD. Pharmacokinetic and pharmacodynamic drug interactions with ethanol (alcohol). Clin Pharmacokinet 2014;53:1115−36.

[9] Langford NJ, Ferner RE. The medico-legal significance of pharmacokinetic interactions with ethanol. Med Sci Law 2013;53:1−5.

[10] Guler S, Aytar H, Soyuduru M, Ramadan H. Disulfiram like reaction with ornidazole. Am J Emerg Med 2015;33:1330.e7−8.

[11] Havrda DE, Mai T, Chonlahan J. Enhanced antithrombotic effect of warfarin associated with low-dose alcohol consumption. Pharmacotherapy 2005;25:303−7.

[12] Ren J, Ding X, Geer JJ. Respiratory depression in rats induced by alcohol and barbiturates and rescue by ampakine CX717. J Appl Physiol 2012;113:1004−11.

[13] McCaul ME, Turkhan JS, Svikis DS, Bigelow GE. Alcohol and secobarbital effects as function of familial alcoholism: extended intoxication and increased withdrawal effects. Alcohol Clin Exp Res 1991;15:94−101.

[14] Okamoto M, Rao SN, Aaronson LM, Walewski JL. Ethanol drug interaction with chlordiazepoxide and pentobarbital. Alcohol Clin Exp Res 1986;9:516−21.

[15] Konoshita H, Nishiguchi M, Kasuda S, Ouchi H, et al. An autopsy case of poisoning with ethanol and psychotropic drugs. Soud Lek 2008;53:16−17.

[16] Fraser AG. Pharmacokinetic interactions between alcohol and other drugs. Clin Pharmacokinet 1997;33:79−90.

[17] Linnoila MI. Benzodiazepines and alcohol. J Psychiatr Res 1990;24(Suppl. 2):121−7.

[18] Tanaka E. Toxicological interactions between alcohol and benzodiazepines. J Toxicol Clin Toxicol 2002;40:69−75.

[19] Drummer OH, Syrjanen ML, Cordner SM. Deaths involving benzodiazepine flunitrazepam. Am J Forensic Med Pathol 1993;14:238−43.

[20] Bubois S, Mullen N, Weaver B, Bedard M. The combined effects of alcohol and cannabis on driving: impact on crash risk. Forensic Sci Int 2015;248:94−100.

[21] Hartman RL, Brwon TL, Milavetz G, Spurgin A, et al. Cannabis effects on driving lateral control with and without alcohol. Drug Alcohol Depend 2015;154:25−37.

[22] Lukas SE, Orozco S. Ethanol increases delta (9)-tetrahydrocannabinol (THC) levels and subjective effects after marijuana smoking in human volunteers. Drug Alcohol Depend 2001;64:143−9.

[23] Andrews P. Cocaethylene toxicity. J Addict Dis 1997;16:75−84.

[24] Bailey DN. Cocaethylene (ethylcocaine) detection during toxicological screening of a university medical center patient population. J Anal Toxicol 1995;19:247−50.

[25] Yamamura T, Hisida S, Hatake K. Alcohol addiction of methamphetamine abusers in japan. J Forensic Sci 1991;36:754−64.

[26] Perez-Reyes M, White WR, McDonald SA, Hicks RE. Interaction between ethanol and dextroamphetamine: effects on psychomotor performance. Alcohol Clin Exp Res 1992;16:75−81.

[27] Hernandez-Lopez C, Farre M, Roset PN, Menoyo E, et al. 3,4-methylenedioxymethamphetamine (ecstasy) and alcohol interaction in human: psychomotor performance, subjective effects and pharmacokinetics. J Pharmacol Exp Ther 2002;300:236−44.

[28] Veldstra JL, Brookhuis KA, de Eaard D, Molmans BH, et al. Effects of alcohol (BAC 0.5%) and ecstasy (MDMA) on stimulated driving performance and traffic safety. Psychopharmacology (Berl) 2012;222:377−90.

[29] Thaulow CH, Hoiseth G, Anderson JM, Handal M. Pharmacokinetic interactions between ethanol and heroin: a study on post-mortem cases. Forensic Sci Int 2014;242:127−34.

[30] Hoiseth G, Andersen JM, Morland J. Less glucuronidation of morphine in the presence of ethanol in vivo. Eur J Clin Pharmacol 2013;69:1683−7.

[31] Guidin JA, Mogali S, Jones JD, Comer SD. Risks, management and monitoring of combination opioid, benzodiazepines and/or alcohol. Postgrad Med 2013;125:115−30.

[32] Hickman M, Lingford-Hughes A, Bailey C, Macleod J, et al. Does alcohol increases the risk of overdose death: the need for a translational research. Addiction 2008;103:1060−2.

[33] Levine B, Green D, Smialek JE. The role of ethanol in heroin deaths. J Forensic Sci 1995;40:808−10.

Link between environmental factors, personality factors, and addiction

Introduction

Behavioral addiction is defined as an intense desire to repeat some action that is pleasurable, or perceived to improve well-being, or capable of alleviating some personal distress, despite the awareness that such an action may have negative consequences. From a psychological, neurological, and social standpoint such repeated patterns of actions which are characterized as "addictive behavior" include drug as well as alcohol addiction. In the new "Diagnostics and Statistical Manual of Mental Disorders" (DSM-5; 5th edition, published by American Psychiatric Association), gambling disorder is included in the "Substance Related and Addictive Disorder" chapter because such behavior produces similar activations in the brain as seen with alcohol or substance use disorder [1].

Clinicians used DSM-IV criteria, through a structured interview, for many years for diagnosis of psychiatric illnesses including alcohol and substance use disorders—which are themselves psychiatric illnesses. There are significant overlaps between DSM-5 and DSM-IV criteria, except DSM-IV describes two distinct disorders: alcohol abuse and alcohol dependence, with specific criteria for each disorder. However, in DSM-5, both disorders are integrated into one disorder termed as alcohol use disorder (AUD) with subclassification of mild, moderate, and severe disorder. There are 11 symptoms in DSM-5 and using this guideline, the presence of at least 2 of the 11 criteria in past 12 months in a patient indicates the patient is suffering from AUD. If only two to three criteria are present the diagnosis is mild, if four to five criteria are present then it is moderate AUD and if six or more criteria are present then the diagnosis is severe AUD. In one study using DSM-5 criteria, the prevalence of AUD was 10.8% among 34,653 surveyed participants. According to DSM-IV criteria, 9.7% in the same population would have AUD diagnosis [2]. DSM-5 is also used for diagnosis of substance use disorder (cannabis, hallucinogens, inhalants, opioids, sedative/hypnotic, stimulants, and tobacco). In contrast to DSM-IV which has two criteria: substance abuse and substance dependence, DSM-5 guidelines combine them into one criterion: substance abuse disorder. There are other guidelines for diagnosis of alcohol and/or substance abuse disorder. For example, an Alcohol Use Disorder Identification Test score can also be used to establish diagnosis of alcohol dependence.

Grant et al. recently reported that based on DSM-5 criteria, prevalence of lifetime drug use disorders in United States was 9.9%. Drug use disorders included

Alcohol, Drugs, Genes and the Clinical Laboratory. DOI: http://dx.doi.org/10.1016/B978-0-12-805455-0.00005-1

use of sedatives/tranquilizers, cannabis, amphetamine, cocaine, heroin, and other opioids, hallucinogens, club drugs (3,4-methylenedioxymethamphetamine, ketamine, etc.), as well as solvent/inhalant use. The most prevalent drugs were cannabis, opioids, and cocaine. The odds of drug use were generally greater among men, younger individuals who were unmarried or previously married, individuals on a lower income, and those with high school and lower education. Moreover, white men and Native American individuals had a higher probability of drug abuse than men belonging to other ethnic groups. The drug use disorder was highly associated with AUD and nicotine use disorder. The authors also observed significant association between a history of the past 12 months drug use and major depressive disorder, dysthymia, bipolar disorder, posttraumatic stress syndrome, borderline personality disorder, antisocial personality disorder (ASPD), and schizotypal personality disorder. Similar associations were observed among lifetime drug abusers. However, in addition to these disorders associations between generalized anxiety disorders, panic disorders, social phobia, and drug use were only observed in lifetime drug users. A previous 12-month history of drug abuse was also associated with disability. Only 13.5% of respondents with a history of the past 12 months drug use and only 24.6% respondents with lifetime drug use received treatment indicating that DSM-5 drug use disorder is a common highly comorbid and disabling disorder which is largely untreated in the United States [3].

Many factors are associated with susceptibility of a person to alcohol and/or drug addiction. Certain environmental factors and personality traits may precipitate risk of alcohol and/or drug addiction in certain individuals. In many instances an individual may abuse both alcohol and drugs. In general, more men than women abuse alcohol and/or drugs. Women typically initiate drug abuse later than men and their drug abuse is often influenced by boyfriends or spouses. Moreover, woman and men use drugs for different reasons but women often enter treatment earlier than men. However, women also have higher prevalence of comorbid psychiatric disorders such as depression and anxiety than men and such mood disorders are often associated with substance abuse. Although such factors may appear to complicate treatment in women, research indicates that men and women are equally responsive to drug rehabilitation treatment [4].

Environmental factors and addiction

Scientists have determined that certain personality traits such as novelty-seeking behavior and low harm-avoidance increase the risk of alcohol and drug abuse. On the other hand, a person with a good social network has much lower risk of alcohol dependence. It has been speculated that environmental factors are more important in making an individual susceptible to alcohol and drug abuse. Childhood neglect or abuse is a major risk factor for drug and alcohol abuse. Peer pressure experienced by teenagers contributes significantly to their first underage experiments with alcohol. The attitudes of parents and adult relatives towards alcohol play an important role in determining the risk of underage drinking behavior. A pregnant mother should not drink alcohol at all, in order to avoid fetal alcohol spectrum of disorders as well as fetal alcohol syndrome. During pregnancy no amount of alcohol regardless of the type of alcoholic beverage (beer, wine, or liquor) is safe, and there is no trimester when drinking may be less harmful [5]. Prenatal exposure of alcohol is associated with higher likelihood of the child abusing alcohol or other substances during adolescent years compared to individuals where fetuses were not exposed to alcohol. Hannigan et al. reported that young adults with detailed histories of prenatal exposure to alcohol showed higher ratings of perceptions of pleasantness of alcohol odors. Moreover, when the prenatal exposure to alcohol was higher the young adult reported greater pleasure from alcohol odor [6].

Risks for adolescent alcohol/drug abuse

Family studies have shown that the risk for alcohol dependence is 4–10 fold higher in the offspring of an alcoholic parent (see also chapter: Pharmacogenomics of Abused Drugs). In addition, many other household factors are linked with risk of substance abuse in adolescent years. Jurich et al. concluded that nine family factors which have an impact on drug abuse include parental absence, less discipline, scapegoating, hypocritical morality, parent–child communication gap, parental divorce, mother–father conflicts, family breakups, and the use of "psychological crutches" to cope with stress [7]. Tomcikova et al., based on a study sample of 3882 individuals, concluded that living with 1 parent is associated with increased risk of frequent drinking and drunkenness among adolescents. Moreover, low quality of communication between mother and child is associated with increased risk of adolescent drinking [8]. Melotti et al. commented that although alcohol drinking was more common among young people coming from higher-income families, binge drinking, and alcohol consumption was less common with higher levels of maternal education. However, tobacco abuse was lower among young people from higher income families [9]. Having strict parental rules is associated with postponement of drinking by adolescents. In general, parents who impose strict drinking rules also consume less alcohol. However, parents who drink alcohol may consider themselves less credible to impose strict drinking rules. Therefore, parent's permissiveness towards drinking is associated with higher frequency of heavy alcohol consumption [10].

The Federal Child Abuse Prevention and Treatment Act defines maltreatment as a child abuse or neglect which encompasses any act or lack of act by a child's caretaker that results in physical or emotional harm. Studies have shown that childhood maltreatment including physical abuse and neglect is linked to increased risk of adolescent substance use, with one study reporting that 29% of children who experienced maltreatment participated in some form of substance abuse while another study reported that 16% of maltreated children later abused drugs [11]. Physical abuse during childhood is associated with higher risk of adolescent alcohol or drug abuse. In most states the definition of physical child abuse is any act that causes a child physical harm, and such harm is not accidental. Although boys are more likely to be physically abused, girls often experience sexual abuse. Many studies have shown that physical abuse and sexual abuse predicted later substance abuse. In one study based on a clinical samples of 655 adolescents divided into 2 groups (polydrug users and nonpolydrug users), the authors observed that polydrug abusers had a greater prevalence of all types of maltreatments (physical abuse, sexual abuse, emotional abuse, physical neglect, and emotional neglect) although most associated with this group were sexual abuse and emotional neglect. Other relevant variables to adolescent drug abuse were diagnosis of depressive disorder, the presence of an anxiety trait, and a family history of alcohol dependence [12]. Skinner et al. followed 332 participants from childhood (18 months to 6 years of age) to adulthood (31−41 years of age) and observed that childhood sexual abuse was fully mediated by adolescent alcohol use and depression. Children exposed to severe emotional abuse are at high risk of comorbid substance abuse, depression, and anxiety in their adolescent years and also mid-30s [13].

UNICEF has estimated that between 133 million to 275 million children around the world witness frequent parental intimate partner conflict or violence. Studies have shown that one in four women and one in seven men in United States has experienced intimate partner violence in their lifetime. Schiff reported that women who experienced intimate partner conflict were 4.43 times more likely to develop depression later in life and those who experienced intimate partner violence were 7.64 times more likely to develop depression. Young males who were exposed to parental intimate partner violence at 14 years of age were more likely to develop anxiety, nicotine, alcohol, and cannabis use disorder later in life, but in general female offspring were more affected than males. However, intimate partner conflicts had much less effect on offspring with almost no effects on males but some impact on females [14]. Smith et al. concluded that exposure to sever intimate partner violence as an adolescent significantly increased the odds of alcohol use problems in early adulthood for young women but not for young men [15].

Studies have shown that parental supervision and monitoring resulted in lower alcohol or substance abuse among 8th and 10th graders. However, one developmental transition characteristic of adolescence is moving from home after finishing high school, and increasing involvement with peers. Studies have indicated that peer use of alcohol and/or drugs is a strong predictor of alcohol and/or substance abuse by young adults. In one study, the authors concluded that predictors of drinking and heavy episodic drinking during the first year after high school included being white, living on campus, a previous drinking history, lower parental expectations, and having peers who drink [16]. Guo et al. reported that on average, being randomly assigned to a drinking peer as opposed to no drinking peer increased college binge drinking by 20−40% per month. However, such an effect was observed among youths with medium levels of genetic propensity for alcohol use indicating that gene−environment analyses can uncover social−contextual effects likely to be missed by traditional sociological approaches [17]. Studies have shown that misbehavior and peer encouragement of misbehavior were positively associated with substance abuse. Moreover, school disengagement, failure in school, or skipping school also increase risk of substance abuse. In contrast, good grades, education expectations, and school bonding protect from alcohol or substance abuse. Studies have shown that religiosity protects adolescents from alcohol and substance abuse. Good self-esteem also protects adolescents from alcohol or substance abuse [18].

All adolescents who participate in bullying, whether they are the perpetrators, victims, or a combination of both roles, have been shown to have higher risk of psychological problems later in life compared to those who do not participate in bullying nor are victims of bullying. Research has shown that females are more likely to be bulled via verbal attacks whereas males are physically bullied. Studies indicated that playing the role of bully has been positively associated with increased alcohol use [11]. Stone and Carlisle, based on review of a data of 7585 subjects, observed that racial bully perpetrators were most likely to have used cigarettes, alcohol, and marijuana followed by youths in mixed victim/perpetrator groups [19]. Gang affiliation is also associated with higher risk of alcohol and substance use. Specifically, higher rates of alcohol and marijuana have been reported among gang members than among those affiliated with a group of deviant peers [11]. Alcohol advertisements are also associated with higher alcohol use by young adults. Ross et al. concluded that there is a robust relationship between underage youth's brand-specific exposure to alcohol advertisements on television and their consumption of those same alcohol brands during the past 30 days [20]. Various risk factors for adolescent alcohol or drug abuse, except personality trait/disorders, are summarized in Table 5.1.

However, there are environmental factors that may protect an adolescent from alcohol or drug abuse. Good performance in school, good communication with parents, coming from an intact family, parental supervision, and participation of adolescents in religious activities, all have protective effects. Many studies have shown that higher levels of religiosity have been associated with lower rates of alcohol abuse, marijuana abuse, and cigarette smoking among adolescents. Rostosky et al. also observed protective effect of religiosity on alcohol and substance abuse in adolescents, but such protection was only observed in heterosexual adolescents [21].

Stressful life events and susceptibility to alcohol/drug abuse

The body responds to stress with self-regulating processes that contain both physiological and behavioral components. In response to stress, neurons in the paraventricular nucleus release two hormones, corticotropin releasing factor (CRF) and arginine vasopressin, into the blood vessels connecting to the hypothalamus and pituitary. Both hormones stimulate anterior pituitary and as a result adrenocorticotropic hormone is secreted into the blood, which eventually results in secretion of adrenocorticoid hormones, mainly cortisol, in humans. In summary, the stress hormone cortisol is produced due to activation of hypothalamic-pituitary-adrenal axis (HPA-axis).

Table 5.1 Various risk factors (other than personality trait/disorders) for adolescent alcohol or drug abuse

Risk factor	Comments
Maternal abuse of alcohol	Fetal alcohol syndrome or fetal alcohol spectrum of disorders may result due to maternal alcohol use. Offspring of mothers who drank during pregnancy have higher risk of alcohol or substance abuse during adolescent years. Moreover, such offspring may experience pleasure from even alcoholic odor.
Familial risk factors	Alcohol or substance abuse by parents increases risk of alcohol/substance abuse in offspring. Young adults living with one parent have higher risk of substance abuse. However, strict parental rules deter adolescents from alcohol use.
Childhood maltreatment/ physical and sexual abuse	Increased incidences of alcohol or substance abuse during adolescent years. Childhood maltreatment also increases risk of adolescence substance abuse.
Emotional abuse	Emotional abuse of child is associated with incidences of substance abuse during adolescent years. Witnessing violence also increases the risk of substance abuse disorder (alcohol, nicotine, marijuana, or hard drugs) during adolescent years.
Intimate partner conflict/violence	Exposure of adolescents to parental conflict/violence is associated with anxiety disorder in males, but alcohol and substance abuse in females, indicating that females are more affected than males.
Peer pressure	Sometimes peer pressure or desire to be popular may increase the risk of substance abuse especially if an individual believes that substance abuse may make him or her more popular with the group
Bullying	Males are involved in bullying more than females. Playing the role of a bully is associated with higher risk of alcohol abuse.
Gang affiliation	Gang affiliation results in significantly increased risk of substance abuse.
Availability of alcohol	If alcohol is easily available it may increase the risk of alcohol use by adolescents.
Advertisement	Advertisements for alcohol may increase the risk of alcohol use.

Cortisol can bind with two types of receptors; Type I receptors (mineralo-corticoid receptors with high affinity for cortisol) and Type-II (glucocorticoid receptors with low affinity for cortisol). During normal activity cortisol usually binds with Type I receptors thus maintaining the required basal level of cortisol needed for daily activity, but when cortisol level is high in response to stress, it binds with Type II receptors and such binding also terminates the stress signal (negative feedback) which is essential to maintain blood cortisol to a predetermined set point. A healthy acute stress response is characterized by a quick rise in blood cortisol level followed by decline of cortisol level to the basal level with the termination of stressful event. However, when a person is exposed to chronic stress, it may deregulate the normal activity of HPA-axis, which may result in metabolic and/or neuropsychiatric problems including susceptibility to alcohol or drug abuse.

Three factors, including genetic makeup of a person, early life environment, and current life stress, determine the function of HPA-axis. Maternal use of alcohol may impair HPA-axis responsivity in adulthood. Maternal stress during gestation may also modify HPA-axis responsivity during childhood as well as adulthood. Childhood traumas including physical abuse or sexual abuse adversely affect the developing brain and may permanently alter the normal stress response capacity of HPA-axis. This may explain why childhood adverse events may increase the risk of alcohol and drug abuse in adulthood. Independent of prenatal and childhood stressors, periods of severe stress in adults such as family and work related problems, neighborhood violence, combat exposure, chronic illness, etc., may also alter HPA-axis dynamics and may increase cortisol burden of the body. This alteration in function of HPA-axis causes higher cortisol exposure or greater cortisol burden following each stressful event [22].

Acute alcohol consumption activates HPA-axis. In social drinkers acute alcohol intake is associated with increased cortisol levels in blood particularly if the blood alcohol level exceeds 100 mg/dL. Chronic consumption of alcohol results in hypercortisolism and shift to alcohol dependence may be accompanied by allostatic shift in HPA-functioning resulting in low cortisol responsivity. Cortisol may also interact with brain's dopaminergic rewards pathway thus contributing to its reinforcing effects. Cortisol may play a role in the regions of the brain that are important for cognitive learning, and memory retrieval. Therefore, perturbation in HPA-axis may consolidate the habit base learning that sustains the maladaptive behaviors related to alcohol abuse [19].

Abnormalities in the HPA-axis are well documented in men using illicit drugs. Wisniewski et al. demonstrated higher concentrations of cortisol in blood in both men and woman using heroin and cocaine compared to controls [23]. Moreover, a higher salivary cortisol level in response to stress is associated with an inability to remain in a substance abuse treatment program [24]. Although cocaine affects the HPA-axis, and the brain nuclei responsible for movements and rewarding effects, several neurobiological systems have been implicated with cocaine addiction, including dopamine, serotonin, and glutamate systems, opioid receptors and opioid neuropeptide gene systems, stress responsive systems including CRF, vasopressin, and/orexin [25].

Extensive research both clinical and preclinical demonstrated that exposure to stress has significant impact on drug addiction. Animal experiments have shown acquisition to amphetamine and cocaine were enhanced when rats were subjected to stress such as social isolation or tail pinch or born to female rats restrained during pregnancy or male rats exposed to attack by an aggressive male rat. Therefore, activation of HPA-axis by stress may be linked to susceptibility to substance abuse. One explanation for the high concordance between stress related disorders and drug addiction is the self-medication hypothesis, which suggests that a person may use alcohol or drugs to cope with the tension associated with life stressors or to relieve symptoms of anxiety and depression resulting from a traumatic life event. Another characteristic of self-administration of drugs or alcohol is that the person has direct control on how much substance to abuse and its subsequent effect on the HPA-axis activation. This controlled activation of HPA-axis may result in the production of an internal state of arousal or stimulation that is intended by that individual (sensation seeking hypothesis). During abstinence, exposure to a stressor again or drug/alcohol associated cue may stimulate the HPA-axis to remind the individual regarding pleasurable effects of drugs or alcohol in the past, which eventually may lead to craving or relapse [26].

Various life stressors may promote susceptibility of an individual to alcohol use. In the 2001–02 National epidemiological survey on alcohol and related conditions, respondents reported on common general life stressors such as changing job or moving, trouble with a boss or coworker, trouble with a neighbor or family member, poor health, being a victim of a crime, being fired or unemployed, and divorce or breakup. The data demonstrated that the number of past year stressors experienced was related to any current drinking, binge drinking, or AUDs. For men the relationship with each stressor and alcohol use steadily increased from 0 to approximately 6 stressors and then tapered off or tended to decrease at 10 or more stressors but for women the relationship of alcohol use and stressor was linear with each stressor with increased prevalence at each increase in the past year. Moreover, stress such as problems at work, trouble with the police, or breakup of romantic relationships may be influenced by an AUD.

Terrorist attack may also increase alcohol use among people as studies have shown that following the terrorist attack that destroyed the World Trade Center in New York in 2001, alcohol consumption was increased in New York City and elsewhere for a short term after the attack. Longer-term studies showed increased alcohol consumption 1 and 2 years later among New Yorkers who had greater exposure to the attack [27]. Stressful life events may also increase the risk of substance abuse. In addition, substance abuse and alcohol use is associated with domestic partner abuse, violence, and crime. Many investigators reported a close link between violent behavior, homicide, and alcohol intoxication. Studies conducted on convicted murders suggest that about half of them were under heavy influence of alcohol at the time of murder [28]. Various life stressors that may increase susceptibility to alcohol or drug abuse are listed in Table 5.2.

Marriage has a protective effect on alcohol or substance abuse. Kendler et al. based on a population study involving 3,220,628 individuals concluded that first marriage to a spouse with no lifetime AUD is associated with a large reduction in risk of AUD. These observations are consistent with the hypothesis that the psychological and social aspects of marriage and in particular health-monitoring spousal interactions, strongly protect against the development of AUD [29]. Close ties with family members, a good social network, having peers and friends

Table 5.2 Life stressors that may increase risk of alcohol or substance abuse

• Being fired from job
• Prolonged unemployment
• Health related issues/health related issues of spouse
• Serious or life threating illness in family member/close friend
• Serious financial trouble
• Divorce or separation
• Living alone/social isolation
• Victim of violence/crime
• Changing job or moving
• Difficulty with coworker/boss
• Difficulty with spouse/family member
• Problem with children
• Difficulty with neighbors
• Living in a neighborhood with a high crime rate
• Legal trouble

who do not abuse alcohol or drugs, and religiosity/spirituality are protective factors against the development of alcohol or drug use. Practice of yoga and meditation may have protective effect against alcohol or drug abuse. Reddy et al. concluded that a specialized yoga therapy may play a role in attenuating the symptoms of posttraumatic stress disorder (PTSD), reducing risk of alcohol, and drug use [30]. Haaga et al. observed that instructions in transcendental meditation lowered drinking risks among male university students but not female students [31].

Personality factors and alcohol/drug use

The five factor model of personality developed by McCreae and John is one of the most commonly used models in psychology. The model was derived initially from studies in English language with an aim of identifying essential domains of personality. Later studies in other languages found agreement with the initial five factor model developed from research in English language. The model consists of five personality factors which can be evaluated using revised NEO Personality Inventory Facet Scale [32].

- Openness (Various facets: Fantasy, Aesthetics, Feelings, Actions, Ideas, and Values)
- Conscientiousness (Various facets: Competence, Order, Dutifulness, Achievement Striving, Self-Discipline, and Deliberation)
- Extraversion (Various facets: Warmth, Gregariousness, Assertiveness, Activity, Excitement-Seeking, and Positive Emotions)
- Agreeableness (Various facets: Trust, Straightforwardness, Altruism, Modesty, and Tender-Mildness)
- Neuroticism (Various facets: Anxiety, Angry Hostility, Depression, Self-Consciousness, Impulsivity, and Vulnerability)

Gore and Widiger commented that the DSM-5 maladaptive trait dimensional model proposal which included 25 traits organized within 5 broad domains (i.e., negative affectivity, detachment, antagonism, disinhibition, and psychoticism) may align with the five factor model. For example, negative affectivity would align with neuroticism of the five factor model while disinhibition would align with low conscientiousness. The authors, based on a study of 445 undergraduates along with the personality inventory of DSM-5, concluded that the results provided support for the hypothesis that all 5 domains of the DSM-5 dimensional trait model are maladaptive variants of the five factor model general personality structure [33]. A substantial body of research also indicates that the personality disorders included within the DSM-5 can be understood as extreme and/or maladaptive variants of the five factor model [34].

Martin and Sher, based on a study of 468 young adults, observed that AUD was positively associated with neuroticism and negatively associated with agreeableness and conscientiousness [35]. Terracciano et al. observed that compared to never users, current marijuana abusers scored higher on openness, average on neuroticism, and lower on agreeableness as well as conscientiousness. Compared to never users, current cocaine users scored higher on neuroticism and lower on conscientiousness. The authors concluded that high levels of negative affect and impulsive traits were associated with substance abuse. Moreover, there was also a link between low score on conscientiousness and substance use [36]. Users of drugs are more prone to negative emotions (neuroticism) and tend to be distrustful, manipulative, unreliable, and undisciplined. Sutin et al. also observed the same pattern of elevated neuroticism, decreased agreeableness, and decreased conscientiousness among current users of cocaine/heroin. Interestingly, low conscientiousness was a risk factor for drug use only among those with relatively more financial resources. Individuals who are high on neuroticism, low on agreeableness, or low on conscientiousness tend to act on impulse when faced with high level of emotional distress. Constellations of these traits have also been observed in alcohol dependence, smoking, gambling, and risky sexual behavior [37].

Impulsivity is related to risk taking, quick decision making, and lack of planning. Such behavior is often committed in a spur of the moment without paying attention to consequences, including negative effects. The five factor model can be used to clarify the multifaceted nature of impulsivity [38]. However, impulsivity is commonly determined by using Barratt Impulsivity Scale (BIS-11), which is a psychometric measure. Temperament consists of four traits including novelty seeking, harm avoidance, reward dependence, and persistence. Character consists of three dimensions; self-directedness, cooperativeness, and self-transcendence. Cloninger defines impulsive behavior as the coexistence of four heritable temperament traits; high novelty seeking, low harm avoidance, low persistence and rarely, high reward dependence [39]. Impulsivity is closely linked to alcohol and substance abuse, both as a contributor to use and as consequences of use. Bozkurt et al., based on a study of alcohol dependent patients ($n = 94$) and healthy controls ($n = 63$), observed that the mean impulsivity score was higher in alcohol dependent subjects than control (BIS-11 score; 69.34 in alcohol dependent subjects vs 58.81 in health controls) [40].

Mudler suggested that the most vulnerable individuals to substance dependency might be those with high impulsivity and/or high novelty-seeking behavior [41]. Novelty seeking is positively associated with extraversion and negatively with conscientiousness in the five factor model. Individuals with high novelty-seeking behavior tend to be quick tempered, excitable, curious, exploratory, easily bored, impulsive, and disorderly [42]. Wingo et al. commented that the novelty-seeking trait, which is affected by both genetic and environmental factors, is positively associated with drug addiction in humans [43].

Interestingly, there are similar relationships between five factor model of personality and behavioral addiction. Andreassen et al. showed positive associations between neuroticism with Internet addiction, exercise addiction, compulsive buying, and study addiction. Extraversion was positively associated with Facebook addiction, exercise addiction, mobile phone addiction, and compulsive buying. Openness to experience was negatively associated with Facebook addiction, and mobile phone addiction. Agreeableness was negatively associated with Internet addiction, exercise addiction, mobile phone addiction, and compulsive buying. Conscientiousness was negatively associated with Facebook addiction, video game addiction, Internet addiction, and compulsive buying. However, conscientiousness was positively associated with exercise addiction and study addiction [44].

Comorbid substance use disorder and personality disorder

When two disorders occur simultaneously in the same person it is referred to as comorbid (Table 5.3). Many individuals with substance use disorder have comorbid

Table 5.3 Common mental disorders and personality disorders where prevalence of substance abuse/comorbid substance abuse disorders is significant

Anxiety disorder (generalized anxiety disorder, panic disorder, and social anxiety/phobia)
Antisocial personality disorder
Avoidant personality disorder
Bipolar disorder
Borderline personality disorder
Delusional disorder
Dysthymia
Histrionic personality disorder
Major depressive disorder
Narcissistic personality disorder
Obsessive compulsive disorder
Paranoid personality disorder
Schizophrenia
Schizotypal
Schizoid disorder
Posttraumatic stress disorder

mental illness, and vice-versa. Comorbid mental illness and substance use disorder may occur through any of the three mechanisms [45]:

- Alcohol or drug abuse may cause a mental problem, e.g., alcohol induced depressive disorder, cocaine induced psychotic disorder, and stimulant induced anxiety disorder. This is the most common situation.
- Substance abuse may be secondary to mental illness. For example a person may drink alcohol to alleviate symptoms of an anxiety disorder such as social phobia.
- Substance abuse and mental disorder are may be coincidental and not related to each other.

There are several personality disorders and psychiatric disorders which are associated with higher prevalence of substance use disorders. Smith et al. also observed higher prevalence of substance abuse among people with ASPD. This type of personality disorder is characterized by a pervasive pattern of disregard for and violation of the rights of others, occurring since age 15 in persons of at least 18 years of age. In general, fulfilling three of the seven criteria (failure to follow social norms, deceitfulness, impulsivity, irritability, and aggressiveness, reckless disregard for safety of the individual person and others, consistent irresponsibility and lack of remorse after illicit behavior) can establish that the person has ASPD. It has been estimated that 1−3% of the general population (3.0−6.8% among male and 0.8−1% in females) may have ASPD but in the prison population the prevalence is estimated to be 35−47% and prevalence is 18−40% among substance-dependent individuals. In one study involving rural populations using nonmedical prescription opioids, the authors observed that 31% had ASPD. In multivariate analyses, the authors observed that distrust and conflict within an individual's social network, as well as past 30 days use of heroin and crack cocaine, male gender, younger age, lesser education, heterosexual orientation, and comorbid major depressive disorder were associated with meeting diagnostic criteria of ASPD [46].

Decades of research have shown that anxiety disorders and substance abuse disorders co-occur at greater rates than expected by chance alone. Anxiety disorders are more strongly associated with substance dependence than substance abuse. Generalized anxiety disorders and panic disorders with or without agoraphobia showed the highest association with substance use disorders. There are also associations between obsessive compulsive disorder (OCD) and alcohol use [47]. Clinical data clearly established an association between PTSDs with alcohol or drug use. PSTD is due to direct experience of a traumatic stressor or witnessing such stressors which may cause serious harm to an individual, including death. Such traumatic stressors include military combat, sexual assault, severe violence, serious accidents, natural disasters such as earthquakes or man-made disasters, e.g., terrorist attack. The association between PTSD and alcohol/drug use disorders is well established, particularly among veterans, adolescents, and patients enrolling in substance abuse programs. Individuals who meet the criteria of PTSD have up to 4.5 times higher likelihood of having alcohol or substance abuse disorder compared to the normal population. It has been postulated that individuals exposed to PTSD are at risk of substance abuse because they may wish to manage symptoms of PSTD by substance or alcohol intake. PTSD symptoms such as elevated hyperarousal symptoms (hypervigilance, irritability, etc.) are associated with drug use while avoidance and numbing symptoms are associated with alcohol use [48].

Driessen et al. investigated the prevalence of PTSD among 459 treatment-seeking subjects with substance dependence and observed that 25.3% of all subjects had PSTD. However, among subjects using both alcohol and drugs the prevalence was 34.1%, among subjects using only drugs it was 29.9%, but the prevalence of PTSD among subjects abusing alcohol only was significantly lower at 15.4%, indicating that prevalence of PTSD was much higher among subjects abusing drugs compared to subjects abusing only alcohol. The comorbidity of substance use disorder with PTSD resulted in lower levels of social functioning and more psychological distress as well as poor outcome from treatment for substance abuse [49]. Smith et al. concluded that PTSD is more strongly associated with substance use for women than men [50].

The presentation of major depression disorder is often complicated by co-occurance of substance abuse disorder such as alcohol or illicit drug abuse or dependence. Nearly one-third of patients with a major depressive disorder also have substance abuse disorder and the comorbidity is associated with higher rates of suicide and greater social or personal impairment [51]. Dysthymic disorder is defined as a low-grade chronic depression that lasts for 2 years for adults. This disorder has a prevalence of 6% in the general population. There is an elevated comorbidity rate between various mood disorders including dysthymia and substance abuse. Cassidy et al. concluded that substance abuse is a major comorbidity in bipolar patients with nearly 60% reporting a history of some lifetime substance abuse [52].

Toftdahl et al., based on a survey of 463,003 psychiatric patients in the Danish Register, observed that the out of that patient population 140,811 (30.4%) patients were also enrolled in different registers with diagnosis of substance abuse. Out of 463,003 patients, 114,359 (24.7%) used alcohol, 17,563 used opioids (3.8%), 20,964 used cannabis (4.5%), 21,520 used sedatives (4.7%), 3368 used cocaine (0.7%), 6182 used psycho-stimulants (1.35%), and 1514 used hallucinogens (0.3%). Additional substance abuses included solvent (426 patients), multiple drugs, or other psychoactive substances (15,994 patients). The authors observed that prevalence of any lifetime substance abuse disorder was 37% for schizophrenia, 35% schizotypal disorder, 28% for other psychoses, 32% for bipolar disorder, 25% for depression, 25% for anxiety, 11% for OCD, 17% for PTSD, and 46% for personality disorders. These personality disorders included paranoid, schizoid, dissocial, emotionally unstable, histrionic, anankastic, anxious, dependent, unspecified, and mixed disorders [53]. Mauri et al. also reported that 34.7% of first episode schizophrenia patients had a lifetime history substance abuse. The age of onset of schizophrenia was significantly lower for drug abusers than patients without any type of abuse and for alcohol abusers. In multidrug users, cannabis was used more frequently (49%), followed by alcohol (13%), and cocaine (4%) [54]. Noorbakhsh et al. observed a significant correlation between stimulant use and histrionic personality disorder, ASPD, and narcissistic personality disorder. In addition, correlation between avoidant, histrionic, narcissistic, depressed, antisocial, and borderline personality disorder and narcotic use was significant [55].

Cooccurrence of substance use with other addictions

Many illicit drug users are also nicotine dependent. Evidence suggest that tobacco use contributes to an increased likelihood of becoming cannabis dependent and similarly cannabis use promotes more intense use of tobacco (nicotine dependence) [56]. Studies have shown high comorbidity of gambling disorders with substance abuse disorders with rates of nicotine dependence approaching 70%, alcohol abuse or dependence approaching 50−75%, and other drug use problems nearing 40%. Moreover, individuals with substance use disorders are very likely to also have pathological gambling disorder. Similarly studies have found high rates of substance abuse disorders among individuals with kleptomania (23−50%) and compulsive buying (30−46%) [57]. Fisoun et al. reported that Internet addiction in adolescents was associated with increased chance of drug abuse [58]. Yen et al. based on a study of 2453 college students concluded that Internet addiction is associated with harmful alcohol use [59].

Conclusions

Many environmental factors are associated with alcohol or substance abuse among adolescents, which is a serious public health issue. Life stressors may also make an individual vulnerable to alcohol or drug abuse and such vulnerability increases significantly if a person has poor coping skills. Moreover, substance abuse disorders are comorbid with many personality disorders and psychiatric disorders. It is important to recognize environmental issues and mental health issues in treating a patient for substance abuse and/or mental health disorder.

References

[1] Munno D, Saroldi M, Bechon E, Sterpone SC, et al. Addictive behavior and personality traits in adolescents. CNS Spect 2016;21:207−31.
[2] Agrawal A, Heath AC, Lynskey M. DSM-IV to DSM-5: the impact of proposed revisions on diagnosis of alcohol use disorder. Addiction 2011;106:1935−43.
[3] Grant BF, Saha TD, Ruan WJ, Goldstein RB, et al. Epidemiology of DSM-5 drug use disorder: results from the national epidemiologic survey on alcohol and related conditions-III. JAMA Psychiatry 2016;73:39−47.
[4] Brady KT, Randall CL. Gender differences in substance use disorders. Psychiatr Clin North Am 1999;22:241−52.
[5] Williams JF, Smith VC. Committee on Substance Abuse. Fetal alcohol spectrum of disorders. Pediatrics 2015;136:e1395−1406.
[6] Hannigan JH, Chiodo LM, Sokol RJ, Janisse J, et al. Prenatal alcohol exposures selectively enhances young adult perceived pleasantness of alcohol odors. Physiol Behav 2015;148:71−7.

[7] Jurich AP, Polson CJ, Jurich JA, Bates RA. Family factors in the lives of drug users and abusers. Adolescence 1985;20:143—59.

[8] Tomcikova Z, Veselska ZD, Geckova AM, van Dijk JP, et al. Adolescents drinking and drunkenness more likely in one parent families and due to poor communication with mother. Cent Eur J Public Health 2015;23:54—8.

[9] Melotti R, Heron J, Hickman M, Macleod J, et al. Adolescent alcohol and tobacco use and early socioeconomic position: the ALSPAC birth cohort. Pediatrics 2011;127: e948—55.

[10] Van der Vorst H, Engles RC, Meeus W, Dekovic M. The impact of alcohol-specific rules, parental norms about early drinking and parental alcohol use on adolescent's drinking behavior. J Child Psychol Psychiatry 2006;47:1299—306.

[11] Whitesell M, Bachand A, Peel J, Brown M. Familial, social, and individual factors contributing to risk for adolescent substance use. J Addict 2013;579310.

[12] Alvarez-Alonso MJ, Jurado-Barba R, Martinez-Martin N, Espin-Martin N, et al. Association between maltreatment and polydrug use among adolescents. Child Abuse Negl 2016;51:379—89.

[13] Skinner ML, Hong S, Herrenkohl TI, Brown EC. Longitudinal effects of early childhood maltreatment on the co-occurring substance misuse and mental health problems in adulthood: the role of adolescent alcohol use and depression. J Stud Alcohol Drugs 2016;77:464—72.

[14] Schiff M, Plotnikova M, Dingle K, Williams GM. Does adolescent's exposure to parental intimate partner conflict and violence predict psychological distress and substance use in young adulthood? A longitudinal study. Child Abuse Negl 2014;38:1945—54.

[15] Smitah CA, Elwyn LK, Ireland TO, Thornberry TP. Impact of adolescent exposure to intimate partner violence on substance use in early adulthood. J Stud Alcohol Drugs 2010;71:2190230.

[16] Simons-Mortyon B, Haynie D, Liu D, Chaurasia A, et al. The effect of residence, school status, work status, and social influence on the prevalence of alcohol use among emerging adults. J Stud Alcohol Drugs 2016;77:121—32.

[17] Guo G, Li Y, Wang H, Cai T. Peer influence, genetic propensity, and binge drinking: a natural experiment and a replication. AJS 2015;121:914—54.

[18] Patrick ME, Schulenberg JE. Prevalence and predictions of adolescent alcohol use and binge drinking in the United States. Alcohol Res 2013;35:193—200.

[19] Stone AL, Carlisle SK. Racial bulling and adolescent substance use: an examination of school-attending young adolescents in the United States. J Ethn Subst Abuse 2015;21:1—20.

[20] Ross CS, Maple E, Siegel M, DeJong W, et al. The relationship between brand specific alcohol advertisement on television and brand specific consumption among underage youth. Alcohol Clin Exp Res 2014;38:2234—42.

[21] Rostosky SS, Danner F, Riggle ED. Is religiosity a protective factor against substance abuse in young adulthood? Only if you're straight. J Adolesc Health 2007;40:440—7.

[22] Stephens MA, Wand G. Stress and the HPA axis: role of glucocorticoids in alcohol dependance. Alcohol Res 2012;34:468—83.

[23] Wisniewski AB, Brown TT, John M, Cofranceso J, Golub ET, et al. Cortisol levels and depression in men and woman using heroin and cocaine. Psychoneuroendocrinology 2006;31:250—5.

[24] Daughters SB, Richards JM, Gorka SM, Sinha R. HPA axis response to psychological stress and treatment retention in residential substance abuse treatment: a prospective study. Drug Alcohol Depend 2009;105:201—8.

[25] Picetti R, Schlussman SD, Zhou Y, ray B, et al. Addiction and stress: clues for cocaine pharmacotherapies. Curr Pharm Des 2013;19:7065−80.
[26] Goeders NE. The impact of stress on addiction. Eur Neuropsychopharmacol 2003; 13:435−6.
[27] Keyes KM, Hatzenbuehler ML, Grant BF, Hasin DS. Stress and alcohol: epidemiological evidence. Alcohol Res 2012;34:391−400.
[28] Palijan TZ, Kovacevic D, Radeljak S, Kovac M, et al. Forensic aspects of alcohol abuse and homicide. Coll Anthropol 2009;33:893−7.
[29] Kendler KS, Lonn SL, Salvatore J, Sundquist J, et al. Effect of marriage on risk of onset of alcohol use disorder: a longitudinal and co-relative analysis in a Swedish national sample. Am J Psychiatry 2016; May 16 [e-pub ahead of print].
[30] Reddy S, Dick AM, Geber MR, Mitchell K. The effect of a yoga intervention on alcohol and drug abuse risk in veteran and civilian women in posttraumatic stress syndrome. J Altern Complement Med 2014;20:750−6.
[31] Haaga DA, Grosswald S, Gaylord-King C, Rainforth M, et al. Effects of the transcendental meditation program on substance abuse among university students. Cardiol Res Pract 2011;2011:537101.
[32] McCree RR, John OP. An introduction to five factor model and its applications. J Pers 1992;60:175−215.
[33] Gore WL, Widiger TA. The DSM-5 dimensional trait model and five factor model of general personality. J Abnorm Psychol 2013;122:816−21.
[34] Widiger TA, Presnall JR. Clinical application of the five-factor model. J Pers 2013;81:515−27.
[35] Martin ED, Sher KJ. Family history of alcoholism, alcohol use disorders and five factor model of personality. J Stud Alcohol 1994;55:81−90.
[36] Terracciano A, Lockenhoff CE, Crum RM, Bienvenu OJ, et al. Five factor model personality profiles of drug abusers. BMC Psychiatry 2008;8:22.
[37] Sutin AR, Evans MK, Zonderman AB. Personality traits and illicit substances: the moderating role of poverty. Drug Alcohol Depend 2013;131:247−51.
[38] Whiteside SP, Lynam DR. The five factor model and impulsivity: using a structural model of personality to understand impulsivity. Pers Ind Differ 2001;30:669−89.
[39] Cloninger CR. Assessment of the impulsive compulsive spectrum of behavior by seven factor model of temperament and character. In: Oldham JM, Hollander E, Skodol AE, editors. Impulsivity and compulsivity. Washington, DC: American Psychiatric Press; 1996. p. 59−95.
[40] Bozkurt M, Evren C, Cay Y, Evren B, et al. Relationship of personality dimension with impulsivity in alcohol dependent inpatients men. Nord J Psychiatry 2014;68:316−22.
[41] Mudler RT. Alcoholism and personality. Aust N Z Psychiatry 2002;36:(1):44−52.
[42] Prisciandaro JJ, McRae-Clark AL, Moran-Santa Maria M. Psychoticism and neuroticism predict cocaine and future use via different mechanism. Drug Alcohol Depend 2011;116:80−5.
[43] Wingo T, Nesil T, Choi JS, Li MD. Novelty seeking and drug addiction in humans and animals: from behavior to molecule. J Neuroimmune Pharmacol 2015;11:456−70.
[44] Andreassen CS, Griffiths MD, Gjertsen SR, Krossbakken E, et al. The relationship between behavioral addictions and the five factor model of personality. J Behav Addict 2013;2:90−9.
[45] Miele GM, Dietz Trautman KD, Hasin DS. Assessing comorbid mental and substance use disorders: a guide to clinical practice. J Pract Psychiatry Behav Health 1996;4:272−82.

[46] Smith RV, Young AM, Mullins UL, Havens JR. Individual and network correlates of antisocial personality disorder among rural nonmedical prescription opioid users. J Rural Health 2016; May 12 [e-pub ahead of print].

[47] Smith JP, Book SW. Anxiety and substance use disorders: a review. Psychiatr Times 2008;25:19−23.

[48] Ramoz Z, Fortuna LR, Porche MV, Wang Y, et al. Posttraumatic stress syndrome and their relationship to drug alcohol use in international sample of Latino immigrants. J Immigr Minor Health 2010; May 6 [e-pub ahead of print].

[49] Driessen M, Schulte S, Luedecke C, Schaefer I, et al. Trauma and PTSD in patients with alcohol, drug or dual dependance: a multi-center study. Alcohol Clin Exp Res 2008;32:481488.

[50] Smith KZ, Smith PH, Cercone SA, McKee SA. Past year non-medical opioid use and abuse and PTSD diagnosis: interactions with sex and associations with symptom cluster. Addict Behav 2016;58:167−74.

[51] Davis L, Uezato A, Newell JM, Fraizer E. Major depression and comorbid substance use disorder. Curr Opin Psychiatry 2008;21:14−18.

[52] Cassidy F, Ahearn EP, Carroll BJ. Substance abuse in bipolar disorder. Bipolar Disord 2001;3:181−4.

[53] Toftdahl NG, Nordentoft M, Hjorthoj C. Prevalence of substance abuse disorders in psychiatric patients, a nationwide Danish population based study. Soc Psychiatry Psychiatr Epidemiol 2016;51:129−40.

[54] Mauri MC, Volonteri LS, De Gaspari IF, Colasanti A, et al. Substance abuse in first episode schizophrenia patients: a retrospective study. Clin Pract Epidemiol Health 2006;23:4.

[55] Noorbakhsh S, Zeinodini Z, Khanjani Z, Poorshrifi H, et al. Personality disorders, narcotics, and stimulants; relationship in Iranian male substance dependent population. Iran Red Crescent Med J 2015;17:e23038.

[56] Rabin RA, George TP. A review of co-morbid tobacco and cannabis use disorder: possible mechanisms to explain high rates of co-use. Am J Addict 2015;24:105−16.

[57] Grant JE, Brewer JA, Potenza MN. The neurobiology of substance and behavioral addictions. CNS Spectr 2006;11:924−30.

[58] Fisoun V, Flores G, Siomos K, Geroukalis D, et al. Internet addiction as an important predictor in early detection of adolescent drug use experiment-implications for research and practice. J Addict Med 2012;6:77−84.

[59] Yen JY, Ko CH, Yen CF, Chen CS, et al. The association between harmful alcohol use and Internet addiction among college students: comparison of personality. Psychiatry Clin Neurosci 2009;63:218−24.

Genetic polymorphisms of alcohol metabolizing enzymes associated with protection from or increased risk of alcohol abuse

6

Introduction

Ethanol, commonly referred as "alcohol," is a small water-soluble polar molecule which is rapidly absorbed from the gastrointestinal tract. However, peak blood alcohol level is reached later if alcohol is consumed with food. Moreover, food can also result in lower blood alcohol levels for the same amount of alcohol consumed without food. A very small amount of alcohol is subjected to first pass metabolism. The majority of alcohol is metabolized via oxidative pathways mainly involving two enzymes: alcohol dehydrogenase (ADH) and aldehyde dehydrogenase (ALDH). Nicotinamide adenine dinucleotide (NAD^+) is a required cofactor for both enzymatic reactions and in this reaction NAD^+ is converted into NADH.

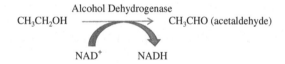

$$CH_3CH_2OH \xrightarrow[\;NAD^+ \quad NADH\;]{\text{Alcohol Dehydrogenase}} CH_3CHO \text{ (acetaldehyde)}$$

Then acetaldehyde is further metabolized by ALDH into acetate (CH_3COO^-).

$$CH_3CHO \xrightarrow[\;NAD \quad NADH\;]{\text{Aldehyde Dehydrogenase 2}} CH_3COO^-$$

However, alcohol may also be metabolized by liver cytochrome P450 enzyme systems, most commonly CYP2E1, especially in the presence of high blood alcohol level. Other enzymes such as catalase may also be capable of metabolizing alcohol, but this is a minor pathway. Polymorphisms of genes coding both ADH and ALDH enzymes affect blood alcohol metabolism. While some polymorphisms may protect an individual from alcohol abuse, others may increase the risk of alcohol abuse. Minor nonoxidative metabolic pathways for alcohol involve conjugation with glucuronic acid yielding ethyl glucuronide and conjugation with sulfate to produce ethyl sulfate. Various metabolic pathways of alcohol are summarized in Table 6.1.

Alcohol, Drugs, Genes and the Clinical Laboratory. DOI: http://dx.doi.org/10.1016/B978-0-12-805455-0.00006-3

Table 6.1 Metabolic pathways of alcohol metabolism

Major pathway of alcohol metabolism	• Alcohol dehydrogenase enzyme metabolizes alcohol into acetaldehyde and then aldehyde dehydrogenase further metabolizes acetaldehyde into acetate
Minor pathways of alcohol metabolism	• In alcohol abusers, in addition to alcohol dehydrogenase, CYP2E1 may also convert alcohol into acetaldehyde • Catalase can also convert alcohol in acetaldehyde • Regardless of pathway by which acetaldehyde is produced; it is finally converted into acetate by aldehyde dehydrogenase • A very small amount of alcohol is converted into ethyl glucuronide by the action of live enzyme uridine diphosphate-glucuronosyltransferase • Ethyl sulfate is also another minor metabolite of alcohol formed due to action of liver enzyme sulfotransferase. In general ethyl sulfate concentration in urine is lower than ethyl glucuronide • Fatty acid ethyl ester and phosphatidylethanol may also be considered as very minor metabolites of alcohol

Genes and alcohol abuse

In addition to polymorphisms of genes that encode ADH and ALDH, other polymorphisms of genes that encode different receptors and transporters also play some role in the genetic basis of alcohol addiction. However, the role of polymorphisms of genes that encode ADH and ALDH in either protecting an individual from alcohol abuse, or increasing the risk of alcohol abuse, is well characterized. Alcohol also interacts with dopamine receptors, dopamine transporters, serotonin receptors, gamma aminobutyric acid receptors, and cholinergic receptors. Polymorphisms of genes encoding such receptors may also determine susceptibility of an individual to alcohol abuse. Many such polymorphisms also increase risk of drug abuse and there are some common genetic links between alcohol abuse and drug abuse because individuals who are prone to alcohol abuse also have a higher risk of drug abuse. However, environmental factors also play important role in making a person susceptible to alcohol abuse. In this chapter, polymorphisms of genes that encode ADH and ALDH, and their effects on protecting an individual from alcohol abuse or making a person more susceptible to alcohol abuse, is discussed. In Chapter 8, Association Between Polymorphisms in Genes Encoding Various Receptors, Transporters and Enzymes and Alcohol/Drug Addiction the role of polymorphisms of genes that encode various brain receptors and transporters in making an individual more susceptible to alcohol and drug abuse is addressed.

Genes encoding alcohol dehydrogenase enzyme

ADH is zinc containing cytosolic enzyme consisting of two protein subunits. ADH— found mostly in the liver, followed by gastrointestinal tract, kidney, nasal mucosa, testes, and uterus—has broad substrate specificity and can metabolize not only ethyl alcohol (alcohol, the preferred substrate) but also methanol, propanol, and ethylene glycol [1]. Humans have seven genes (genes are usually written in italics) that encode ADH enzymes and all of these genes are clustered in a small region of chromosome 4 (4q21−24). The Class I ADH enzymes which can be either homodimer or heterodimer are responsible for approximately 70% metabolism of alcohol. These enzymes are encoded by *ADH1A*, *ADH1B*, and *ADH1C* genes. The *ADH4* gene encodes Class II ADH enzyme, which is a homodimer and is found in the liver and to a lesser extent in the kidney. The *ADH5* gene encodes Class III ADH which is usually a homodimer. This enzyme is a ubiquitously expressed form ALDH with a very low affinity for ethanol. The major function of this enzyme is to oxidize formaldehyde to formic acid and to terminate nitric oxide signaling. The Class III ADH is the only enzyme detected in the brain and plays little role in the overall metabolism of ethanol. The Class IV ADH is encoded by *ADH7* gene that produces sigma subunit. This ADH enzyme is capable of converting retinol to retinal as well as ethanol to acetaldehyde. The *ADH6* gene produces mRNA, which can be detected in both the fetal and the adult liver, but the enzyme has not been isolated [2].

Gene encoding aldehyde dehydrogenase enzyme

ALDHs are a group of NAD dependent enzymes that metabolize a wide variety of aliphatic and aromatic aldehydes [3]. Unlike *ADH* genes, which are located on a single chromosome (chromosome 4), *ALDH* genes are not localized in a single chromosome. Humans have 19 genes and 3 pseudogenes that encode the ALDH superfamily of isoenzymes but only 3 of these genes; *ALDH1A1*, *ALDH1B1*, and *ALDH2* are relevant to acetaldehyde metabolism. ALDH1A enzyme is usually found in cytosol while ALDH1B1 and ALDH2 enzymes exert their function in mitochondria. ALDH2 plays the most important role in oxidation of acetaldehyde [4].

The ALDH1A enzyme is encoded by the *ALDH1A1* gene which is located in chromosome 9 (9q21.13) and extending over 52 kb region. The ALDH2 enzyme is encoded by *ALDH2* gene which is located on chromosome 12 (12q24.2) and extending over 43 kb. ALDH2 enzyme is responsible for metabolism of acetaldehyde generated due to oxidation of alcohol into acetaldehyde by ADH enzyme. The medication disulfiram (Antabuse), which is used in treating alcohol detoxification, inhibits this key enzyme. In ALDH2 enzyme encoded by wild type gene (*ALDH2*1*), glutamic acid is present in position 504 of amino acid sequence. Polymorphism of *ALDH2* gene has been described and *ALDH2*2* allele is relatively common in East Asians. This allele (Glu504Lys; rs671 G>A) encodes a defective ALDH2 enzyme where lysine replaces glutamic acid at 504 (this substitution corresponds to substitution at position 487 in the mature ALDH2 enzyme) and as a result the enzyme is virtually inactive. Acetaldehyde level increases in individuals carrying this allele resulting in an unpleasant reaction to drinking. Therefore, this polymorphism may deter these individuals from drinking, thus protecting these individuals from alcohol abuse [4].

When ALDH2 enzyme is not functional due to the presence of *ALDH2*2* allele, ALDH1A enzyme present in liver cytosol plays an important role in metabolism of acetaldehyde. The wild type *ALDH1A1* gene is *ALDH1A1*1* which is observed among the population worldwide. Two polymorphisms in the promoter region of *ALDH1A1* gene have been described. The *ALDH1A1*2* allele is 17 bp deletion (from position -416 to position -432) and *ALDH1A1*3* allele is a 3 bp insertion (-524). The ALDH1B enzyme, which is a mitochondrial enzyme, is encoded by *ALDH1B1* gene located on chromosome 9. This gene does not contain introns in the coding sequence. However, effects of these variants on alcohol related issues have been poorly investigated.

Genetic polymorphisms that protect from alcohol abuse

People drink alcohol for its pleasurable effects but if drinking causes unpleasant reactions such as flushing (alcohol flush reaction or Asian flush), severe nausea, asthma attack, rapid heartbeat, and psychological distress due to aldehyde build up in blood, it may deter a person from drinking. In general, two types of polymorphisms may have protective effect on alcohol abuse:

- Polymorphism in *ADH* genes that lead to super active ADH enzyme
- Polymorphism in *ALDH2* gene causing poor activity of ALDH enzyme

Acetaldehyde may build up in blood due to super active ADH enzyme causing rapid conversion of alcohol to acetaldehyde. Alternatively, poorly functioning ALDH enzyme may cause acetaldehyde build up due to slow conversion of acetaldehyde into acetate. For normally-functioning ADH and ALDH enzyme, acetaldehyde concentration in blood is very small after consumption of reasonable amount of alcohol, and mostly undetected.

Gene polymorphism causing super active alcohol dehydrogenase enzyme

Most of the variants of *ADH* genes involve a single nucleotide polymorphism (SNP). Some of these variations occur in the part of the gene that is responsible for coding the protein and such SNPs are called "coding variations," that may result in the generation of ADH enzymes with altered activities. However, some variations may also occur in noncoding areas of the gene and such alterations are called "noncoding variations" but such variations may also affect the expression of the gene. The reference allele for *ADH1B* gene is *ADH1B*1* (wild type) which encodes beta-1 subunit of ADH enzyme with an arginine at amino acid position 48 (Arg48) and 370 (Arg370). This allele is the predominant allele observed worldwide among Caucasians, Native Americans, and people of African descent but it is less common among East Asians. The ADH enzyme encoded by the wild type gene has normal enzymatic activity.

There are two super active ADH enzymes due to polymorphisms of genes encoding ADH enzyme. One such polymorphism is *ADH1B*2* gene (Arg48His, rs1229984) which is found commonly among East Asians (Han Chinese, Japanese, Koreans, Filipinos, Malays, etc., and aborigines of Australia and New Zealand) and also among approximately 25% of people of Jewish origin. This allele is also encountered in a low frequency among Caucasians. Although *ADH1B*2* is more prevalent in Asians, if this allele is present in Caucasians it also provides protection from alcohol use disorders [5]. Toth et al. reported that Hungarians who carry *ADH1B*2* allele showed reduced risk of developing alcoholism [6]. Carr et al. reported that men in the *ADH1B*2* allele group reported more unpleasant reactions to alcohol compared to men carrying wild type *ADH1B*1* gene and conclude that carriers of *ADH1B*2* allele consumed alcohol less frequently than men who were homozygous for *ADH1B*1* [7].

Another polymorphism *ADH1B*3* (Arg370Cys, rs2066702) is found primarily in people of African descent and Native Americans. ADH isoenzymes encoded by *ADH1B*2* or *ADH1B*3* alleles are super active ADH enzymes (due to significantly higher turnover rate of these enzymes) that results in a 30−40 fold increase in metabolism of ethanol compared to normally-functioning enzymes encoded by the wild type *ADH1B*1* gene. As a result acetaldehyde may build up in blood causing facial flushing and adverse side effects after alcohol use thus discouraging people carrying such alleles from drinking [8]. McCarthy et al., using 91 African American young adults, observed that one-third of the participants had *ADH1B*3* allele and these individuals showed increased pulse rate (compared to individuals with wild type gene) and other uncomfortable effects of alcohol consumption due to acetaldehyde burst. The authors concluded that lower rates of alcohol dependence in individuals carrying *ADH1B*3* allele may be related to adverse response to alcohol [9].

Polymorphism causing less active aldehyde dehydrogenase

Acetaldehyde build up may also be related to poor activity of ALDH enzyme. Most common polymorphism is *ALDH2*2* allele that encodes poorly active ALDH2 enzyme thus protecting an individual from alcohol abuse due to acetaldehyde build up (slow degradation of acetaldehyde). The *ALDH2*2* allele is found among 45% of East Asians including Han Chinese, Japanese, and Koreans, but found rarely in other ethnic groups. It has been estimated that 540 million people worldwide (8% of world population) carry this allele. Although individuals who are *ALDH2*2* homozygotes (*ALDH2*2/*2*) show essentially inactive ALDH2 enzyme but heterozygotes (*ALDH2*1/*2*) may show partial ALDH2 activity. Genetic and epidemiological studies have shown *ALDH2*2* homozygous individuals are almost fully protected from developing alcohol use disorder but heterozygous individuals have partial protection (approximately 60%) [10]. Yamamoto et al., using 93 Asian subjects, showed that none of the subjects with homozygous for the *ALDH2*1* allele showed any detectable blood acetaldehyde level or facial flushing but all homozygous and heterozygous for *ALDH2*2* allele exhibited facial flushing and

Table 6.2 Polymorphism of alcohol dehydrogenase and aldehyde dehydrogenase genes that protects from alcohol abuse

Enzyme involved	Allele	Comments
Alcohol dehydrogenase	ADH1B*2	This polymorphism leads to super active ADH enzyme and rapid conversion of alcohol to acetaldehyde. Because of acetaldehyde build up and unpleasant reactions associated with acetaldehyde after consuming alcohol, this allele, if present, deters a person from drinking
Alcohol dehydrogenase	ADH1B*3	This polymorphism also leads to super active ADH enzyme and deters a person from drinking
Aldehyde dehydrogenase	ALDH2*2	This gene encodes inactive ALDH2 enzyme in homozygotes (ALDH2*2/*2) and significantly reduced enzyme activity in heterozygotes (ALDH2*1/*2). Asians carrying two alleles (homozygotes) have almost complete protection from developing alcoholism. Carriers of one allele also get significant protection from developing alcoholism

detectable blood acetaldehyde levels. As expected, blood acetaldehyde levels were significantly more elevated in individuals who were homozygous (ALDH2*2/*2) than heterozygous (ALDH2*1/*2) [11]. Genetic polymorphisms that protect against alcohol abuse are listed in Table 6.2.

Combination of super active alcohol dehydrogenase and less active aldehyde dehydrogenase enzyme: further protection from alcohol abuse

The combination of ALDH2*2 and ADH1B*2 alleles may provide further protection from alcohol abuse. Whitfield reported that the protective effect of ADH1B*2 in Caucasians was approximately half of the protective effect observed in Asians, suggesting that ALDH2*2 and ADH1B*2 each contribute to unique protective effect from developing alcohol dependence [12]. An individual possessing both ADH1B*2 and ALDH2*2 alleles may experience further build up of acetaldehyde in blood due to faster conversion of alcohol into acetaldehyde by ADH1B*2 as well as slower removal of acetaldehyde from blood due to ALDH2*2 allele. Luczak et al., using 784 Asian American students (Chinese and Korean descent), reported the effect of ADH1B*2 allele may be felt more strongly in Asians who already had heightened sensitivity to alcohol from possessing one ALDH2*2 allele [13].

Genetic polymorphisms that may increase risk of alcohol abuse

Wild type *ADH1B*1* allele and wild type *ALDH2*1* may increase the risk of alcohol use disorder because no acetaldehyde build up is associated with normally-functioning ADH and ALDH enzymes. Several studies have shown association of *ADH1B*1* and *ALDH2*1* with alcoholism, especially in the Asian population. Kim et al. studied 1032 Korean subjects and concluded alcohol dependence in 86.5% alcoholic subjects could be attributed to *ADH1B*1* and or *ALDH2*1* [14]. Tolstrup et al., in a large study involving genotyping of 9080 white men and women from the general population and using the brief Michigan Alcoholism Screening test, concluded that men with *ADH1B*1/*1* genotype (wild type homozygous) had a two to fourfold higher risk of developing alcoholism compared to men with *ADH1B*2/*1* or *ADH1B*2/*2* genotype. The authors further commented that because *ADH1B*1* allele is found in more than 90% Caucasians and less than 10% East Asians, the population attributable risk of alcoholism by *ADHB*1/*1* homozygous genotype was 62% among Caucasians compared with 24% among the East Asian population [15].

Polymorphism of *ADH4* gene may be associated with alcohol and drug dependence in European-Americans. Luo et al. genotyped 7 SNPs spanning *ADH4* gene in 365 healthy controls and 561 subjects affected with alcohol and or drug dependence and observed that SNP2 (rs1042363) at axon 9 or SNP6 (rs1800759) at the promoter region showed the greatest degree of Hardy−Weinberg disequilibrium with either alcohol dependence or drug dependence [16]. In addition to these polymorphisms, other rarely encountered polymorphisms of ADH genes may lead to alcohol dependence. Zuo et al., using 49,353 subjects, observed that a rare variant constellation across the entire *ADH* gene cluster (*AD7−ADH1C−ADH1B−ADH1A−ADH6−ADH4−ADH5*) was associated with alcohol dependence in European-Americans, European-Australians, and African Americans [17]. Van Deek et al. reported an association between age of onset of regular alcohol use and a SNP just upstream of *ADH7* (rs2654849) in the Dutch population. Significant association was also found between reactions to alcohol and polymorphism in *ADH5* (rs6827292) [18]. However, more research is needed to establish link between these genetic polymorphisms and alcohol abuse. Genetic polymorphisms that increase risk of alcohol abuse are listed in Table 6.3.

Polymorphism of CYP2E1 gene and alcoholism

With higher consumption of alcohol especially in individuals with alcohol use disorder, liver CYP2E1 enzyme is activated and contributes significantly to oxidation of ethanol into acetaldehyde in chronic alcohol abusers. The CYP2E1 enzyme is encoded by *CYP2E1* gene located on the chromosome 10 (10q26.3). Effect of polymorphism of *CYP2E1* gene on ethanol metabolism has also been studied. Although several *CYP2E1* polymorphisms have been reported, four polymorphisms, *CYP2E1*5B*

**Table 6.3 Polymorphism of alcohol dehydrogenase and aldehyde dehydrogenase genes that may increase the risk of alcohol abuse*__

Enzyme involved	Allele	Comment
Alcohol dehydrogenase	*ADH1B*1*	Wild type gene may increase the risk of alcohol abuse because no acetaldehyde is detected in blood
Aldehyde dehydrogenase	*ALDH2*1*	Wild type gene encoding normally active aldehyde dehydrogenase enzyme, which prevents aldehyde build up in blood
Alcohol dehydrogenase	Some polymorphisms of *ADH4, ADH6*, and *ADH7* genes	Currently results are inconclusive in establishing an association between these genetic polymorphisms and risk of alcoholism
CYP2E1	Various polymorphisms	Currently results are inconclusive in establishing an association between these genetic polymorphisms and risk of alcoholism

(c2 allele), *CYP2E1*6* (C allele), *CYP2E1*1B* (A1alelle), and *CYP2E1*1D* (IC allele), may have an association with alcoholism and related disorders. Carriers of c2 allele (CYP2E1*5B) have often been found to have increased risk for alcoholic liver disease possibly due to increased tendency to consume excessive amounts of alcohol. The C allele (*CYP2E1*6*) has been associated with predisposition of alcoholism in Japanese men [19]. However, other studies have found no association between *CYP2E1* gene polymorphism and alcohol use disorder. Cichoz-Lach et al. determined allele and genotype frequency of *ADH1B, ADH1C*, and *CYP2E1* in 204 alcohol dependent Polish men and 172 healthy volunteers who did not drink alcohol (control). The authors observed no statistical difference between distribution of *CYP2E1* allele and genotype between alcohol dependent subjects and controls [20].

Conclusions

Alcohol metabolism mainly takes place in the liver by cytosolic ADH enzyme and mitochondrial ALDH2 enzymes. In general it is assumed that carriers of *ADH1B*2* and *ADH1B*3* (which encodes super active ADH isoenzymes) alleles are protected from alcohol use disorder because these individuals may refrain from drinking due to acetaldehyde build up in blood following drinking. Similarly *ALDH2*2* allele results in an inactive ALDH2 enzyme and individuals with homozygotes (*ALDH2*2/*2*) (observed mostly in the East Asian population) are highly protected from alcohol use disorders. However, carriers of both *ALDH2*2* and *ADH1B*2* alleles (mostly found among the Asian population) are most protected from developing alcoholism regardless of sex [21].

References

[1] Cederbaum AI. Alcohol metabolism. Clin Liver Dis 2012;16:667−85.
[2] Meier P, Seitz HK. Age, alcohol metabolism and liver disease. Curr Opin Clin Nutr Metab Care 2008;11:21−6.
[3] Edenberg HJ. The genetics of alcohol metabolism: role of alcohol dehydrogenase and aldehyde dehydrogenase variants. Alcohol Res Health 2007;30:5−13.
[4] Hurley TD, Edenberg HJ, Li TK. The pharmacogenomics of alcoholism. In: Licinio J, Wong ML, editors. Pharmacogenomics: the search for individualized therapeutics. Weinheim, Germany: Wiley-VCH; 2002. p. 417−41.
[5] Wall TL, Shea SH, Luczak SE, Cook TA, Carr LG. Genetic association of alcohol dehydrogenase with alcohol use disorders and endo phenotypes in white college students. J Abnorm Psychol 2005;114:456−65.
[6] Toth R, Pocsai Z, Fiatal S, Szeles G, Kardos L, Petrovski L, et al. ADH1B*2 allele is protective against alcoholism but not chronic liver disease in Hungarian population. Addiction 2010;105:891−6.
[7] Carr LG, Foroud T, Stewart T, Castelluccio P, Edenberg HJ, Li TK. Influence of ADH1B polymorphism on alcohol use and its subjective effects in Jewish population. Am J Med Genet 2002;112:138−43.
[8] Jones AW. Evidence based survey of the literature of the elimination rates of ethanol from blood with applications in forensic casework. Forensic Sci Int 2010;200:1−20.
[9] McCarthy DM, Pedersen SL, Lobos EA, Todd RD, Wall TL. ADH1B*3 and response to alcohol in African Americans. Alcohol Clin Exp Res 2010;34:1274−81.
[10] Lai CL, Yao CT, Chau GY, Yang LF, Kuo TY, Chiang CP, et al. Dominance of the inactive Asian variant over activity and protein contents of mitochondrial aldehyde dehydrogenase 2 in human liver. Alcohol Clin Exp Res 2014;38:44−50.
[11] Yamamoto K, Ueno Y, Mizoi Y, Tatsuno Y. Genetic polymorphism of alcohol and aldehyde dehydrogenase and the effects on alcohol metabolism. Arukoru Kenkyuto Yakubutsu Ison 1993;28:13−25.
[12] Whitfield B. Alcohol dehydrogenase and alcohol dependence: variation in genotype-associated risk between populations. Am J Hum Genet 2002;71:1247−50.
[13] Luczak SE, Pandika D, Shea SH, Eng MY, Liang T, Wall TL. ALDH2 and ADH1B interactions in retrospective reports of low dose reactions and initial sensitivity to alcohol in Asian American college students. Alcohol Clin Exp Res 2011;35:1238−45.
[14] Kim DJ, Choi IG, Park BL, Lee BC, et al. Major genetic components underlying alcoholism in Korean population. Hum Mol Genet 2008;17:854−8.
[15] Tolstrup JS, Nordestgaard BG, Rasmussen S, Tybjaerg-Hansen A, Gronbaek M. Alcoholism and alcohol drinking habits predicted from alcohol dehydrogenase genes. Pharmacogenomics J 2008;8:220−7.
[16] Luo X, Kranzler HR, Zuo L, Lappalainen J, Yang BZ, Gelernter J. ADH4 gene variation is associated with alcohol dependence and drug dependence in European Americans: results from HWD tests and case control association study. Neuropsychopharmacology 2006;31:1085−95.

[17] Zuo L, Zhang H, Malison RT, Li CS, Zhang XY, Wang F, et al. Rare ADH variant constellations are specific for alcohol dependence. Alcohol Alcohol 2013;48:9–14.

[18] Van Beek JH, Willemsen G, de Moor MH, Hottenga JJ, Boomsma DI. Association between ADH gene variants and alcohol phenotypes in Dutch adults. Twin Res Hum Genet 2010;13:30–42.

[19] Webb A, Lind PA, Kalmijn J, Feiler HS, Smith TL, Schuckit MA, et al. The investigation of CYP2E1 in relation to the level of response to alcohol through a combination of linkage and association analysis. Alcohol Clin Exp Res 2011;35:10–18.

[20] Cichoz-Lach H, Celinski K, Wojcierowski J, Slomka M, Lis E. Genetic polymorphism of alcohol metabolizing enzyme and alcohol dependence in Polish men. Braz J Med Biol Res 2010;43:257–61.

[21] Chiang CP, Lai CL, Lee SP, Hsu WL, et al. Ethanol-metabolizing activities and isoenzyme protein contents of alcohol and aldehyde dehydrogenase enzymes in human liver: phenotypic traits of the ADH1B*2 and ALDH2*2 variant gene alleles. Pharmacogenetic Genomics 2016; Feb 9 [e-pub ahead of print].

Pharmacogenomics of abused drugs

7

Introduction

Drug abuse is a major public health problem not only in the United States but also worldwide. It has been estimated that up to 324 million individuals globally, aged between 15 and 65 years, have used illicit drugs. Many mental health problems such as depression, bipolar disorder, mood and anxiety disorders, antisocial personality disorder, and suicide attempts, are also associated with drug abuse [1].

Genetic makeup of a person may play some role in drug and alcohol abuse but there is no single gene which is associated with alcohol and drug abuse. Drug abuse is the result of a complex interplay between the genetic makeup of an individual and social, biochemical, and environmental factors. It is usually assumed that the vulnerability of an individual to drug abuse is roughly 50% determined by genetic factors while another 50% is nongenetic factors. As a result, many genes involved in modification of neurotransmitter balance collectively play some role in making an individual susceptible to alcohol and drug abuse. Since a number of genes are involved, the effect of an individual gene in making a person vulnerable to alcohol or drug abuse may be modest. Moreover, repeated exposure of a drug to the human brain may also cause epigenetic changes such as histone modification (acetylation and methylation), DNA methylation, and modification of noncoding RNA [2].

Like many drugs, drugs of abuse are also metabolized by various liver enzymes. Polymorphisms of genes causing modification of enzymatic activities of these enzymes are also linked to addiction as well as susceptibility of toxicity of certain abused drugs. In this chapter polymorphisms of genes encoding various liver enzymes that are responsible for metabolism of abused drugs are discussed along with their effects on making an individual more susceptible to drug toxicity. The role of various genes that encode dopamine receptors, transporters, serotonin receptors, and other receptors with which abused drugs interact are discussed in Chapter 8, Association between Polymorphisms in Genes Encoding Various Receptors, Transporters and Enzymes and Alcohol/Drug Addiction along with the links between various polymorphisms and alcohol/drug addiction.

Enzymes responsible for drug metabolism

The liver is the organ primarily responsible for biotransforming endogenous compounds and exogenous lipophilic chemicals into water-soluble substances that are more easily eliminated from the body. The process of drug biotransformation

Alcohol, Drugs, Genes and the Clinical Laboratory. DOI: http://dx.doi.org/10.1016/B978-0-12-805455-0.00007-5

is accomplished by two categories of reactions: Phase I and Phase II. Phase I reactions involve oxidation, reduction, or hydrolysis. Phase II biosynthetic conjugation reactions include glucuronidation, sulfation, acetylation, methylation, glutathione conjugation, or amino acid conjugation to endogenous substrates or Phase I metabolic products. Collectively both Phase I and Phase II reactions result in increased metabolite polarity and hydrophilicity resulting in enhanced renal elimination from the body. In addition to enzymes responsible for drug metabolism, drug transporters also play an important role in pharmacology of certain drugs. The best characterized drug transporter is the multidrug resistance protein MDR1 (also called *P*-glycoprotein). MDR1 is a glycosylated membrane-bound protein expressed mainly in intestines, liver, kidneys, and brain. A large number of structurally unrelated drugs are substrates for MDR1, which regulates their intestinal absorption, hepatobiliary secretion, renal secretion, and brain transport.

Phenotype demonstrating variation in individual response to certain drugs was first recognized in early 1950s where antimalarial drugs were found to cause in vivo hemolysis in patients with glucose-6-phosphate deficiency. Later, the pharmacogenetic differences in a number of Phase I and Phase II enzymes were reported, explaining many interindividual responses to metabolism of various drugs. Polymorphisms of genes encoding various enzymes including cytochrome P450 (CYP) isoenzymes, alcohol dehydrogenase, aldehyde dehydrogenase, dihydropyrimidine dehydrogenase, and esterases involved in Phase I metabolism have been well documented in the literature. In addition, polymorphism of genes encoding Phase II enzymes such as uridine diphosphate glucuronosyltransferase (UGT), *N*-acetyl transferase, and others have also been reported. However, various CYP isoenzymes play an important role in metabolism of various abused drugs. Therefore, only polymorphisms of genes encoding CYP isoform are discussed in detail in the chapter.

CYP family of enzymes

The CYP family of enzymes has many isoenzymes which play a very important role in the Phase I metabolism of many drugs. The CYP proteins comprise a superfamily of heme-containing proteins found in many organisms, with over 7700 known members across all species studied. The human CYP super family of enzymes is encoded by 57 functional genes and 58 pseudogenes producing over 50 isoenzymes (3 families) in humans. The name of the isoenzymes is derived from the characteristic maximum spectral absorption at 450 nm. While CYP3A4 is the most abundant enzyme (30%), other enzymes such as CYP1A2 (13%), CYP2A6 (4%), CYP2C (20%), CYP2D6 (2%), and CYP2E1 (7%) are also important members of CYP family of isoenzymes. In general CYP3A4 is responsible for metabolism of approximately 50% of drugs while CYP1A2, CYP2A6, CYP2C, CYP2D6, and CYP2E1 are responsible for 13%, 4%, 25%, 2%, and 7% metabolism of all drugs. Overall CYP families of enzymes are responsible for metabolism of approximately 80% of all drugs. Polymorphisms in the CYP family also have a large impact on metabolism of drugs. Polymorphisms of genes encoding CYP2D6, CYP2C9, and CYP2C19 account for most the frequent variation of Phase I metabolism of drugs. Approximately 5−14% Caucasians, 0−5% Africans, and 0−1% Asians lack CYP2D6 enzyme activity and are poor metabolizers (PMs) of drugs involving this enzyme. Polymorphisms also occur in genes encoding CYP1A1, CYP1A2, CYP1B1, CYP2C8, CYP2E1, CYP3A4, and CYP3A5 enzymes [3].

Important polymorphisms of CYP enzymes

Polymorphisms of genes encoding CYP isoenzymes may result in wide interindividual variation in drug metabolism. Based on metabolism, individuals are classified into four groups:

- Extensive metabolizers (EMs): These individuals belong to "normal population" and have two functional alleles. As a result these individuals metabolize the drug at expected normal rate.
- Poor metabolizers (PMs): These individuals carry two defective alleles and as a result have enzymes with poor or no activity. These individuals metabolize a particular drug slowly or not at all.
- Intermediate metabolizers (IMs): These individuals are heterozygous for a defective allele or carrying two alleles encoding enzymes with reduced activity. These individuals metabolize a particular drug at a rate in between EM and PM.
- Ultrarapid metabolizers (UMs): These individuals carry more than two active gene copies in the same allele and as a result produce enzymes with much higher activity than normal individuals.

Some of the genes encoding CYP isoenzymes are highly polymorphic while others show less polymorphisms or without important functional polymorphisms with respect to drug metabolism. While CYP isoenzymes encoded by *CYP2D6*, *CYP2C9*, *CYP2C19*, *CYP2A6*, and *CYP2B6* genes are highly polymorphic, other CYP isoenzymes such as CYP1A1, CYP1A2, CYP2E1, and CYP3A4 do not show widely different metabolic activities due to functional polymorphism [4].

Despite low hepatic content (2%), CYP2D6 enzyme is very important in drug metabolism because approximately 25% of all drugs are metabolized by this enzyme. The *CYP2D6* gene is located on the long arm of chromosome 22 (22q13.1). Both SNP (single nucleotide polymorphism) and copy number variation (CNV) have been observed in this gene and over 80 different alleles have been described. The most important polymorphisms include *CYP2D6*2*, *CYP2D6*3*, *CYP2D6*4*, *CYP2D6*5*, *CYP2D6*6*, *CYP2D6*10*, *CYP2D6*17*, and *CYP2D6*41* [5]. Over 90% of PMs are attributable to three different defective mutations: *CYP2D6*5* (total deletion of gene), *CYP2D6*3* (adenine deletion in exon 5: rs35742686), and *CYP2D6*4* (adenine to guanine transition at the junction of intron 3 and exon 4: rs389207). *CYP2D6*17* allele found commonly in the Black population also encodes enzyme with reduced activity. The CNV in *CYP2D6* gene include deletion, duplications, and multiplications up to 13 genes in tandem. The UM metabolizers have more than one active gene on one allele (*CYP2D6*2xN* duplication).

CYP2C9 found predominately in the liver is 92% homologous with CYP2C19 but has different substrate specificity. The wild type is *CYP2C9*1* which is the normal gene with normal metabolic activity. More than 34 polymorphisms of the gene encoding CYP2C9 enzyme have been reported but the most common variants are *CYP2C*2* (5.5-fold decreased activity) and *CYP2C9*3* (27-fold decreased activity) alleles which produce enzymes with significantly reduced activity. Homozygous for *CYP2C9*3* are PMs. The *CYP2C9*3* allele occurs in approximately 6−9% of Caucasians and Asians. The *CYP2C9*2* is found in 8−20% of Caucasians but less frequently in African Americans. This allele is virtually absent in Asians [4]. Other alleles with reduced activities include *CYP2C9*4*, *CYP2C9*5*, and *CYP2C9*30*.

For CYP2C19, 2−5% Caucasian population and 20% Asian population are PMs. There are over 25 different alleles of *CYP2C19* gene but in Asian population *CYP2C19*2* and *CYP2C19*3* allele together account for 100% of defective alleles. In Caucasian 85% of PMs are homozygous for *CYP2C19*2*. In general *CYP2C19*2−*8* represent inactive version of enzyme but *CYP2C19*17* allele encodes enzyme with increased activity than the enzyme encoded by the wild type gene [5].

CYP3A isoenzymes are the predominant subfamily of CYP enzymes making it one of the most important drug metabolizing enzymes. The genes encoding CYP enzymes are expressed primarily in the liver and small intestine. The CYP3A activities are the sum of the activities of four isoenzymes; CYP3A4, CYP3A5, CYP3A7, and CYP3A43. Genes encoding CYP3A4, CYP3A5, CYP3A7, and CYP3A43 enzyme are located on a cluster on chromosome 7. At the enzyme level, CYP3A4 is the major isoform followed by CYP3A5, CYP3A43, and CYP3A7. Many polymorphisms of *CYP3A4* gene have been described but most of such polymorphisms have an uncertain impact on enzyme activities. In contrast to polymorphisms of *CYP2D6*, *CYP2C9*, and *CYP2C19* genes, which translate into wide variations in activities of enzymes encoded by these genes, only a few *CYP3A4* polymorphisms results in altered CYP3A4 enzymatic activities. Overall variation in *CYP3A4* genotype contributes only to a minor extent or only in rare cases to the interindividual variation in CYP3A4 enzymatic activity. At present *CYP3A4*22* allele appears to be the most relevant genetic variation (0.04−0.08 frequency) that encodes an enzyme with reduced activity. Currently there are two alleles (*CYP3A4*20* and *CYP3A4*26*) that lead to complete loss of function of the CYP3A4 enzyme. However, these alleles are reported only in two case reports [6]. Recently Shi et al. reported that the genetic polymorphism of CYP3A4 gene (*CYP3A4*1B*) may have an impact on the dose requirement of tacrolimus [7]. However, for other drugs no clear association between this allele and drug metabolism has been observed. More research is needed to clarify the effects (if any) of polymorphisms of CYP3A4 gene on interindividual differences in drug metabolism.

CYP3A4 and CYP3A5 enzymes share approximately 85% sequence homology and overlapping substrate specificities. Polymorphism of *CYP3A5* genes may lead to nonfunctioning enzymes with three alleles *CYP3A5*3*, *CYP3A5*6*, and *CYP3A5*7* encode nonfunctional enzymes. The most frequent is *CYP3A5*3* with a frequency ranging 0.12−0.35 in Africans and 0.88−0.97 in Caucasians [6]. Major polymorphisms of *CYP2D6*, *CYP2C9*, and *CYP2C19* genes that have most impact on various drug metabolisms are summarized in Table 7.1.

Table 7.1 **Major polymorphisms of genes encoding CYP2D6, CYP2C9, CYP2C19, and CYP2B6 enzymes**

Enzyme	Genetic allele	Enzyme activity
CYP2D6	CYP2D6*1	Wild type, normal enzymatic activity
	CYP2D6*2	Normal activity
	CYP2D6*3	Poor activity
	CYP2D6*4	Poor activity
	CYP2D6*5	No enzyme activity
	CYP2D6*10	Unstable enzyme
	CYP2D6*17	Reduced activity
CYP2C9	CYP2C9*1	Wild type, normal enzyme
	CYP2C9*2	Reduced activity
	CYP2C9*3	Reduced activity
	CYP2C9*4	Reduced activity
	CYP2C9*5	Reduced activity
	CYP2C9*30	Reduced activity
CYP2C19	CYP2C19*1	Wild type, normal enzyme
	CYP2C19*2	Poor activity
	CYP2C19*3	Poor activity
	CYP2C19*17	Increased activity
CYP2B6	CYP2B6*1	Wild type, normal enzyme
	CYP2B6*6	Poor activity
	CYP2B6*4	Increased activity

CYP2B6 enzyme is mainly expressed in the liver and has been thought to play an insignificant role in drug metabolism in the past. However, recent research indicates that polymorphisms of *CYP2B6* gene that encodes enzymes with widely different activities are clinically important because CYP2B6 enzyme approximately metabolizes 8% of clinically used drugs (over 60 drugs) including cyclophosphamide, ifosfamide, tamoxifen, ketamine, artemisinin, nevirapine, efavirenz, bupropion, sibutramine, and propofol. To date, at least 20 allelic variants and some subvariants (*1B through *29) have been described and some alleles are associated with clinically significant differences in drug metabolism and drug response [8]. *CYP2B6*4* allele encodes the enzyme with higher activity than the enzyme coded by the wild type gene (*CYP2B6*1*). Therefore, individuals with *CYP2B6*4* are UMs. In contrast *CYP2B6*6* allele encodes enzyme with poor enzymatic activity and carriers of this allele are PMs.

Pharmacogenomics of methamphetamine and related drugs

Amphetamine type stimulants include amphetamine, methamphetamine, (Ecstasy; 3,4-methylenedioxymethamphetamine (MDMA)), 3,4-methylenedioxyamphetamine (MDA), cathinone, and synthetic cathinone (bath salts). Ecstasy and methamphetamine now rank as the world's second most widely abused drugs after cannabis. Methamphetamine is metabolized by the CYP2D6 enzyme into 4-hydroxymethamphetamine which is then conjugated to form glucuronide and sulfate conjugates. Methamphetamine is also metabolized to amphetamine by CYP2D6 which is then further metabolized to 4-hydroxyamphetamine and its conjugate, norephedrine, phenyl acetone, benzoic acid, and hippuric acid. Cherner, based on a study of 52 individuals with a history of methamphetamine dependence, observed that 52 people were EM, 17 people were IMs while only 3 subjects were PMs. The authors reported that the EM group showed worse overall neurophysiological performance and were three times as likely to be cognitively impaired compared to individuals who were IM or PM. The groups did not differ in their demographics or history of methamphetamine abuse [9].

Otani et al. genotyped 202 Japanese patients with methamphetamine abuse and 337 controls and found a significant association between *CYP2D6* gene and methamphetamine dependence. The authors identified six genotypes; *CYP2D6*1/*1* (wild type, normal enzymatic activity; EM), *CYP2D6*1/*10* (EM), *CYP2D6*1/*5* (IM), *CYP2D6*5/*10* (IM), *CYP2D6*10/*10* (IM), and *CYP2D6*10/*14* (IM). No PM was observed either in the patient or control group. The patients who were dependent on methamphetamine were mostly EM with very few IM in the group. The 4-hydroxymethamphetamine may contribute to the dependence of methamphetamine. Because IM and PM metabolize methamphetamine more slowly than EM, lower CYP2D6 activity seems to confer some degree of protection against methamphetamine abuse [10]. Effects of polymorphisms of CYP2D6 on methamphetamine toxicity are listed in Table 7.2.

Sutter et al. studied the possible role of *CYP2D6* polymorphism in the development of methamphetamine related heart failure, using 56 patients, and concluded that individuals who are PMs based on *CYP2D6* genotype are less likely to develop methamphetamine induced heart failure. Although not statistically significant, a trend was observed that EMs may be at an increased risk of developing heart failure due to methamphetamine abuse [11].

MDMA is metabolized by two pathways: (1): *O*-demethylation followed by catechol-*O*-methyltransferase (COMT) catalyzed methylation and or conjugation with glucuronic acid/sulfate and (2): *N*-dealkylation, deamination, and oxidation to the corresponding benzoic acid derivatives which are finally conjugated with glycine. MDMA is metabolized to MDA by *N*-demethylation. In addition, both MDMA and MDA are further *O*-demethylated into a variety of other metabolites including 4-hydroxy-3-methoxyamphetamine, 4-hydroxy-3-methoxyamphetamine,

Table 7.2 Effects of CYP2D6 polymorphism on methamphetamine toxicity

- Extensive metabolizers based on *CYP2D6* genotype are more vulnerable to methamphetamine associated neurocognitive impairment
- Poor metabolizers based on *CYP2D6* genotype may be protected from methamphetamine abuse but EM may be at a higher risk of methamphetamine abuse
- Poor metabolizers are also less susceptible to methamphetamine induced heart failure

and other metabolites. The fact that polymorphic *CYP2D6* gene partially regulates *O*-demethylation pathways prompted a hypothesis that PMs of *CYP2D6* genotype may be at a higher risk of MDMA associated toxicity. However, because mechanism based inhibition of CYP2D6 enzyme occurs due to formation of enzyme—metabolite complex in all subjects regardless of genotype, after two consecutive dosages of MDMA all subjects become PMs of MDMA. As a result, impact of *CYP2D6* genotype in developing MDMA induced toxicity is very limited [12]. O'Donohoe also commented that there was no evidence for a major influence of genotype at *CYP2D6* on MDMA related toxicity [13]. However, drugs that are inhibitors of CYP2D6 may increase MDMA toxicity. There is a report of fatal interaction between MDMA and ritonavir, a protease inhibitor used in treating HIV infected patients, which is also an inhibitor of CYP2D6 enzyme in a male. The deceased ingested approximately 180 mg of MDMA, which should produce a plasma concentration of 0.5 mg/L. However, the concentration of MDMA in the postmortem blood was 4.56 mg/L, which was almost 10 times higher than expected. In addition, the deceased may have been a PM. Therefore, ritonavir induced inhibition of CYP2D6 enzyme may have contributed in the mechanism of death in this individual [14]. Methamphetamine is also metabolized by CYP2D6. Death in a 49-year old Caucasian man due to possible fatal interaction between protease inhibitors and methamphetamine has also been reported [15].

Wolf et al. observed a correlation between low activity of COMT enzyme (methionine substitute valine at position 158) and increased plasma cortisol levels in MDMA abusers. Moreover, low CYP2D6 enzymatic activity may also contribute to increased plasma cortisol level. The authors concluded that chronic use of MDMA may lead to hypothalamus-pituitary-adrenal-axis deregulation and that the magnitude of this may be moderated by genetic polymorphisms [16]. Atichison et al. commented that genetically determined poor metabolism of MDMA due either due to polymorphism of *CYP2D6* gene encoding absent or low activity enzyme or a low activity COMT enzyme is associated with MDMA induced hyponatremia and reduced plasma osmolality [17].

Bupropion and CYP2B6 polymorphism

Bupropion is an antidepressant approved for the treatment of major depressive disorders. This drug is also used for smoking cessation. Bupropion is a synthetic cathinone structurally related to amphetamine. Therefore, bupropion has some psychostimulant properties and as a result this drug is also abused. In the past years several case reports about recreational use of bupropion have been published. The major route of administration is via nasal insufflation but intravenous administration has also been reported. Oppek et al. reported a case of a 29-year old woman who consumed an extremely high dose of bupropion (approximately 2400 mg) intravenously together with a daily oral dose of 2400—3600 mg of pregabalin. On admission her urine drug screen was negative but her serum bupropion level was 226 μg/L (reference <166 μg/L) and hydroxy-bupropion level was 3330 μg/L (reference 480—2240 μg/L). Bupropion overdose may be associated with seizure.

Therefore, levetiracetam was administered to prevent seizure, and to support withdrawal from bupropion, quetiapine was administered [18].

Bupropion is metabolized by CYP2B6 enzyme into hydroxy-bupropion, an active metabolite. The *CYP2B6*6* allele encodes enzyme with poor activity and as a result bupropion is metabolized slowly compared to individuals carrying wild type allele. Lee at al showed that among smokers in the *CYP2B6*6* group (*CYP2B6*1/*6* or *CYP2B6*6/*6* genotype, $n = 147$) bupropion produced significantly higher abstinence rate than placebo at the end of treatment and at a 6-month follow-up compared to carriers of wild type gene (*CYP2B6*1/*1*, $n = 179$) who did not show any significant difference in smoking cessation when bupropion therapy was compared against placebo. This may be related to decreased metabolism of bupropion in *CYP2B6*6* group leading to higher plasma levels but similar levels of hydroxy-bupropion compared to carriers of wild type gene [19]. Kirchheiner et al. reported that clearance of bupropion was 1.66-fold higher in carriers of *CYP2B6*4* allele compared to carriers of wild type allele. The *CYP2B6*4* allele encodes an enzyme with higher enzymatic activity than normal enzyme encoded by the wild type allele [20]. Tomaz et al. observed that patients with *CYP2B6*4* allele had lower success with bupropion during smoking cessation. The *CYP2B6*4* variant which leads to a rapid predicted metabolic phenotype for the isoenzyme influences the pharmacological activity of bupropion [21].

Cocaine and butylcholinesterase polymorphism

Once absorbed, cocaine is rapidly metabolized into inactive metabolite ecgonine methyl ester by serum butylcholinesterase. Cocaine is also spontaneously hydrolyzed into benzoylecgonine, also an inactive metabolite. Butylcholinesterase is encoded by *BCHE* gene (located on chromosome 3) and this enzyme is synthesized in the liver. However, butylcholinesterase is distributed in plasma, intestinal mucosa, and in the white matter of the central nervous system. There are more than 65 reported mutations of *BCHE* gene although not all of them have been studied. In general polymorphism of *BCHE* gene results in enzyme with lower activities compared to enzyme encoded by the wild type of *BCHE*. In a study involving 1436 individuals (698 cocaine dependent patients and 738 controls), the authors observed a significant association between rs1803274 (AA genotype) and addiction to crack cocaine. Crack cocaine is more addictive than powdered cocaine [22]. The rs1803274 (A) allele (also known as *BCHE*539T* allele) encodes a variant of butylcholinesterase with an approximately 30% reduction in enzymatic activity compared to butylcholinesterase encoded by the wild type gene. Phase I clinical trials have shown that pure human butylcholinesterase enzyme is safe when administered in humans. A recombinant mutant of butylcholinesterase that rapidly deactivates cocaine is being developed as a treatment to recovering cocaine addicts [23].

Pharmacogenomics of opioids

Codeine, morphine, hydrocodone, hydromorphone, oxycodone, oxymorphone, and tramadol are major opioids used in pain management. Methadone is often used in drug rehabilitation programs and also for pain control. Unfortunately all of these prescription drugs are abused. Abuse of oxycodone (OxyContin) and hydrocodone (Vicodin) are also serious public health issues. Although most research has been done in the context of pain control using opioids, results of such investigations can also be translated in cases of abuse of prescription opioids.

Codeine and tramadol are metabolized by CYP2D6 enzyme. As a result, UMs of *CYP2D6* genotype are more susceptible to toxicity from codeine or tramadol. Therefore, morphine and hydromorphone, which are not metabolized by CYP2D6 enzyme, may be a better choice for pain management in patients who are UMs [24]. In contrast, PMs of *CYP2D6* genotype may receive inadequate pain control from codeine or tramadol therapy. Extensive research indicates that polymorphism of *CYP2D6* gene should be taken into consideration when codeine is prescribed for pain control, and guidelines have been published for using codeine in various groups or patients (UM, EM, IM, and PM; Table 7.3) [25]. Currently effects of *CYP2D6* gene polymorphism on codeine metabolism is best characterized among various opioids which are used for pain control as well as being abused.

Linares et al., based on population models, observed that approximately 10% of a codeine dose was converted into morphine in PMs, but approximately 40% of codeine was converted into morphine in EMs and 51% of codeine was converted into morphine in UMs. In addition, 4% of morphine generated from codeine in PMs was eventually converted into morphine-6-glucuronide. However, 39% of morphine was converted into morphine-6-glucuronide in EMs and 58% in UMs [26].

It has been estimated that 7−10% of the population are PMs based on *CYP2D6* genotype. VanderVaart et al. studied the genotypes of 45 mothers who received codeine for controlling postpartum pain. In this group 14 patients were EMs, 26 IMs, 3 were UMs (*CYP2D6*1/*2 x N*, *CYP2D6*2/*17 x N*, and *CYP2D6*2/*2 x N*) and 2 patients were PMs (*CYP2D6*4/*4* and *CYP2D6*4/*5*). The authors reported that the two patients who were PMs reported no analgesia from receiving codeine, whereas two out of three UMs reported immediate pain relief after taking codeine but discontinued codeine due to dizziness and constipation [27].

Oxycodone is approximately 50% metabolized by CYP3A4 enzyme while CYP2D6 enzyme converts oxycodone into oxymorphone. Approximately 11% of an oxycodone dose is *O*-demethylated to oxymorphone, an active metabolite which has 40-fold higher affinity for opioid receptors. Various clinical trials reported conflicting data regarding association of *CYP2D6* polymorphism and analgesic effects as well as toxicity of oxycodone [25]. However, Stamer et al. reported that metabolism of oxycodone differed between *CYP2D6* genotype. The mean oxymorphone/oxycodone ratio was 0.10 in PMs, 0.13 in IMs, 0.18 in EMs, and 0.28 in UMs. The authors concluded that the number of functional active *CYP2D6* alleles had an impact on oxycodone metabolism. The oxycodone consumption up to 12 h after surgery was highest in PMs resulting in lowest equianalgesic doses of piritramide

Table 7.3 Codeine therapy recommendation based on *CYP2D6* polymorphism

Metabolizer type	Effect on codeine metabolism	Recommendation	Commonly associated CYP2D6 allele
Poor metabolizer	Poor morphine level following codeine administration causing inadequate pain control	Codeine use may be avoided. Use of morphine or nonopioid analgesic may be more appropriate	*CYP2D6*4/*4* *CYP2D6*4/*5* *CYP2D6*4/*6* *CYP2D6*5/*5*
Intermediate metabolizer	Reduced morphine level	Codeine may be used initially but if no response, other analgesics such as morphine or nonopioid analgesic may be more appropriate	*CYP2D6*4/*10* *CYP2D6*5/*41*
Extensive metabolizers	Normal morphine level	Use of codeine is appropriate	*CYP2D6*1/*1* *CYP2D6*1/*2* *CYP2D6*1/*4* *CYP2D6*1/*10* *CYP2D6*1/*41* *CYP2D6*2/*2* *CYP2D6*2/*5*
Ultrarapid metabolizer	High risk of toxicity due to increased morphine level	Codeine use should be avoided. Morphine or nonopioid analgesics are more appropriate	*CYP2D6*1/*1 x n* *CYP2D6*1/*2 x n*

versus oxycodone for PMs. However, pain scores did not differ between genotypes [28]. Because data regarding the effect of *CYP2D6* polymorphism on analgesic efficacy as well as toxicity are conflicting, it is difficult to conclude whether *CYP2D6* phenotype affects oxycodone analgesia or risk of toxicity [25].

Hydrocodone is also metabolized into hydromorphone by CYP2D6 enzyme. Hydromorphone has 10- to 33-fold greater affinity for opiate receptors. PMs show lower peak concentration of hydromorphone after administration of hydrocodone. However, polymorphism of *CYP2D6* has not been shown to be associated with response to hydrocodone. Currently no information is available on pharmacokinetics of hydrocodone in UMs. As a result at present there is insufficient evidence to conclude that PMs may get inadequate pain control from oxycodone or UMs are at higher risk of toxicity [25].

Toxicity and fatality associated with use of codeine in ultrarapid metabolizers

Severe morphine toxicity in individuals who are UMs based on *CYP2D6* genotype is well documented in the medical literature. Madadi et al. reported fatality of a newborn infant when the mother was using codeine while breastfeeding. The boy developed difficulty in breastfeeding and lethargy at 7 days of age and was eventually taken to the emergency room on day 13 but died at the hospital. The postmortem concentration of morphine in the blood was 70 ng/mL (therapeutic 10−12 ng/mL) while acetaminophen was present at a concentration of 5.9 μg/mL. The concentration of morphine in the breast milk was 87 ng/mL. The mother was an UM of codeine due to *CYP2D6*2x2* gene duplication. However, the infant was not an UM (*CYP2D6*1/*2 genotype*). The most probable cause of death was morphine toxicity [29]. A 2-year old healthy boy who was also an UM died after receiving codeine postoperatively. His postmortem blood concentration of morphine was 32 ng/mL [30].

Kelly et al. reported three cases where two infants died after receiving codeine while one infant survived after severe toxicity. All patients received codeine after adenotonsillectomy for obstructive sleep apnea syndrome. A 4-year old boy showed postmortem morphine levels of 17.6 ng/mL, which was highly elevated based on the dosage. The boy was CYP2D6 enzyme UM (*CYP2D6*1/*2 x N*). Another 5-year old boy also died who showed blood codeine concentration of 79 ng/mL but highly elevated morphine level of 30 ng/mL in postmortem blood. It was highly likely that the child was an UM. A 3-year old girl showed severe toxicity after receiving codeine postoperatively but survived. Her blood morphine level was 17 ng/mL. She was genotyped as an EM (*CYP2D6*1/*1*) but the authors commented that EM genotype often overlaps with UM genotype [31].

CYP2D6 polymorphism and tramadol

Tramadol is metabolized by CYP2D6 to pharmacologically active *O*-desmethyltramadol (200 times more affinity than tramadol for opiate receptors). Tramadol is also metabolized by CYP2B6 and CYP3A4 enzymes into *N*-desmethyltramadol (inactive metabolite). Lassen et al. based on asystematic review of 56 studies involving tramadol and pharmacogenomics concluded that only the effects of *CYP2D6* gene polymorphisms on metabolism of tramadol and consequent effect of pain relief has been thoroughly studied and results show clinical significance [32]. Similar to codeine, PMs may not get adequate pain control from tramadol while EMs are at higher risk of tramadol toxicity, for example respiratory depression.

Clinical studies have shown that PMs often fail to exhibit analgesic effects after administration of tramadol compared to EMs. Based on a study of 300 patients who received tramadol postoperatively, Stamer et al. observed that the percentage of nonresponders was significantly higher in the PM group (46.7%) compared with the EM group (21.6%). Moreover, patients who were PMs also consumed more tramadol. The authors concluded that PMs showed a lower response rate to postoperative tramadol analgesia [33]. The *CYP2D6*10* allele is a common allele with a frequency ranging from 51.3% to 70% in the Chinese population. This allele encodes CYP2D6 enzyme with significantly reduced enzymatic activity. Wang et al. based on a study of gastric cancer patients recovering from gastrectomy observed that homozygous for *CYP2D6*10* allele (*n* = 20) required significantly more tramadol for adequate pain control in a 48 h period compared to patients who were heterozygous for *CYP2D6*10* (*n* = 26) or patients who did not carry *CYP2D6*10* allele (*n* = 17). Therefore, PMs required more tramadol for adequate pain control [34]. Susce described a case of an 85-year old woman who was a PM and had a history of problems with opioid analgesics including codeine, oxycodone, and tramadol, which are all metabolized by CYP2D6 enzyme. However, when that genetic information was transmitted to the physician in her subsequent visit to the hospital, she showed a better response to hydrocodone. The authors concluded that *CYP2D6* genotype is clinically useful in opioid pain management [35]. Based on these studies it appears that tramadol has reduced clinical efficacy in PMs.

Pharmacokinetic studies have shown higher plasma concentration of *O*-desmethyltramadol in UMs after administration of tramadol compared to EMs. As a result, UMs experience greater analgesia but also show higher incidences of side effects and toxicity from tramadol. A 5.5-year old boy underwent adenotonsillectomy under general anesthesia for obstructive sleep apnea and received in the evening eight drops of oral tramadol (20 mg). The next morning the boy was lethargic and his parents brought him to the emergency department. Although he experienced severe respiratory depression and was comatose he recovered fully the next day and was discharged. The boy was an UM with the presence of three functional alleles (*CYP2D6*2 x 2/CYP2D6*2*) and his tramadol toxicity was related to his status as an UM [36]. A 66-year old man with renal insufficiency suffered from severe respiratory depression after receiving tramadol via patient controlled analgesia. Complete recovery was achieved after administration of naloxone indicating that respiratory depression was related to opioid toxicity. Genotyping showed that the patient was an UM with gene duplication. Higher concentration of *O*-desmethyltramadol as well as slower clearance of drugs due to renal insufficiency contributed to tramadol toxicity [37].

Methadone toxicity and pharmacogenetics issues

Methadone is metabolized by both CYP3A4 and CYP2B6 isoenzymes but CYP2D6 has a minor role. Genetic polymorphism is the cause of high interindividual variability for a given dose, for example in order to achieve a methadone plasma concentration of 250 ng/mL, dosage of racemic methadone mixture may vary from 55 to 921 mg per day for a 70 kg patient without receiving any comedication [38]. Kharasch et al. showed that CYP2B6 genotypes affected methadone plasma concentrations, clearance, and metabolism. The carriers of *CYP2B6*6* allele (PMs), particularly homozygous, had higher methadone concentration, slower elimination, compared to the homozygous for wild type gene (*CYP2B6*1/*1*). However, carriers of *CYP2B6*4* allele had lower methadone concentration and faster elimination even compared with individuals carrying wild type gene. In general *CYP2B6* variants had greater influence on metabolism of (*S*)-methadone than (*R*)-methadone when administered orally compared to intravenous administration. Methadone metabolism and clearance may be significantly lower in African Americans due to larger proportion of *CYP2B6*6* carriers [39].

Levran et al. reported that carriers of *CYP2B6*6* allele metabolized methadone slower and as a result required a relatively low methadone dosage (<100 mg/day) during treatment of heroin addiction. However, no association was observed between methadone dosage and polymorphism of *CYP3A4* or *CYP2D6* genes [40]. In a study of 40 postmortem cases where methadone was involved, the authors observed that *CYP2B6*6* allele was associated with highest postmortem methadone concentration (*CYP2B6*6/*6*, homozygous, postmortem methadone concentration: 1.38 mg/L) [41]. Madadi et al. reported a case of the death of an infant (3-week old) related to methadone use by the mother (65 mg of methadone per day). The infant died after breastfeeding and postmortem investigation revealed that the infant was a homozygous for *CYP2B6*6* allele [42].

Methadone is a substrate for *P*-glycoprotein encoded by *ABCB1* gene. It has been suggested that polymorphism of *ABCB1* gene may influence methadone kinetics. However, recently Mouly et al. concluded that methadone dose was predicted by sociodemographic variables (bodyweight, fractioned dose, past cocaine dependence, and ethnicity) as well as clinical variables rather than genetic polymorphism because the authors found no correlation between polymorphism of *ABCB1* gene and methadone maintenance dose [43]. Effect of genetic polymorphism on metabolism and toxicity of hydrocodone, oxycodone, hydromorphone, tramadol, and methadone are summarized in Table 7.4.

Morphine and pharmacogenetics

Morphine is conjugated by the cation of Phase II enzyme UGT into morphine-3-glucuronide and morphine-6-glucuronide. The isoenzyme UGT2B7 is the major enzyme responsible for glucuronidation of morphine while UGT1A1 plays a minor role. There are conflicting reports regarding association between *UGT2B7* polymorphism and metabolism of morphine. Basanti et al. reported that patients who were homozygous for *UGT2B7 802 C* genotype needed significantly lower dose of morphine for pain relief [44]. However, De Gregori et al. observed no association between *UGT2B7* genotype and morphine analgesic response in acute postoperative pain. However, the authors reported association between *COMT* genetic polymorphism (*COMT* gene encodes COMT which is essential for catabolism of neurotransmitters dopamine, norepinephrine, and epinephrine) [45].

Table 7.4 Effect of genetic polymorphism on metabolism and toxicity of hydrocodone, oxycodone, hydromorphone, tramadol, and methadone

Drug	Polymorphism	Comments
Hydrocodone	CYP2D6	Currently there is insufficient information to conclude whether poor metabolizers can be expected to experience decreased analgesia or whether ultrarapid metabolizers are more susceptible to toxicity
Oxycodone	CYP2D6	Because of conflicting reports it is difficult to conclude whether CYP2D6 polymorphism is associated with analgesic effect or risk of toxicity from oxycodone use
Tramadol	CYP2B6	Tramadol is likely to have reduced clinical efficacy in poor metabolizers. Ultrarapid metabolizers show higher peak level of active metabolite O-desmethyltramadol after a dose of tramadol and as a result experience higher analgesic effects. However, ultrarapid metabolizers may expect higher incidence of side effects such as nausea and also more susceptibility to toxicity
Methadone	CYP2B6	Poor metabolizers who are carriers of CYP2B6*6 require lower dosage of methadone (<100 mg/day), but higher methadone postmortem levels have been observed in carriers of CYP2B6*6 allele. There are conflicting reports regarding effect of CYP3A4 polymorphism as well as genetic variability of ABCB1 gene on methadone metabolism and toxicity

Conclusions

Drug abuse is a polygenic disorder where several gens contribute to some extent and currently association between polymorphism of CYP2D6 and CYP2B6 with metabolism of several drugs that are also abused have been documented. There are also some associations between polymorphism of the gene encoding serum butyl-cholinesterase enzyme and cocaine toxicity as well as craving for crack cocaine. Polymorphism of genes encoding receptors, transports, as well as enzymes responsible for catabolism of neurotransmitters, may also play some role in making an individual susceptible to alcohol or drug abuse. These genetic factors are addressed in Chapter 8, Association between Polymorphisms in Genes Encoding Various Receptors, Transporters and Enzymes and Alcohol/Drug Addiction.

References

[1] Patriquin MA, Bauer IE, Soares JC, Graham DP, et al. Addiction pharmacogenetics: a systematic review of genetic variation of the dopaminergic system. Psychiatr Genet 2015;25:181−93.

[2] Nestler EJ. Epigenetic mechanism of drug addiction. Neuropharmacology 2014;76 (Pt B):259−68.

[3] Zhou SF, Liu JP, Chowbay B. Polymorphism of human cytochrome P450 enzyme and its clinical impact. Drug Metab Rev 2009;41:89−295.

[4] Johansson I, Ingelman-Sundberg M. Genetic polymorphism and toxicology-with emphasis on cytochrome P450. Toxicol Sci 2011;120:1−13.

[5] Bozina N, Bradamante V, Lovric M. Genetic polymorphism of metabolic enzymes P450 (CYP) as a susceptibility factor for drug response, toxicity and cancer risk. Arh Hig Rada Toksikol 2009;60:217−42.

[6] Werk AN, Cascorbi I. Functional gene variants of CYP3A4. Clin Pharmacol Ther 2014;96:340−8.

[7] Shi WL, Tang HL, Zhai SD. Effects of the CYP3A481b genetic polymorphism on the pharmacokinetics of tacrolimus on adult renal transplant recipients: a meta-analysis. PLoS One 2015;10:e0127995.

[8] Mo SL, Liu YH, Duan W, Wei MQ, et al. Substrate specificity, regulation, and polymorphism of human cytochrome P450 2B6. Cur Drug Metab 2009;10:730−53.

[9] Cherner M, Bousman C, Everall I, Barron D, et al. Cytochrome P450-2D6 extensive metabolizers are more vulnerable to methamphetamine associated neurocognitive impairment: preliminary findings. J Int Neuropsychol Soc 2010;16:890−901.

[10] Otani K, Ujike H, Sakai A, Okahisa Y, et al. Reduced CYP2D6 activity is a negative risk factor for methamphetamine dependance. Neurosci Lett 2008;434:88−92.

[11] Sutter ME, Gaedigk A, Albertson TE, Southard J, et al. Polymorphisms in CYP2D6 may predict methamphetamine related heart failure. Clin Toxicol (Phila) 2013;51:540−4.

[12] De la Torre R, Farre M, Roset PN, Pizarro N, et al. Human pharmacology of MDMA: pharmacokinetic, metabolism and disposition. Ther Drug Monit 2004;26:137−44.

[13] O'Donohoe A, O'Flynn K, Shields K, Hawi Z, et al. MDMA toxicity: no evidence for a major influence of metabolic genotype at CYP2D6. Addict Biol 1998;3:309−14.

[14] Henry JA, Hill IR. Fatal interaction between ritonavir and MDMA. Lancet 1998;352:1751−2.

[15] Heles G, Roth N, Smith D. Possible fatal interaction between protease inhibitors and methamphetamine. Antivir Ther 2000;5:19.

[16] Wolf K, Tsapakis EM, Pariante CM, Kerwin RW, et al. Pharmacogenetic study of change in cortisol on ecstasy (MDMA) consumption. J Psychopharamacol 2012;26:419−28.

[17] Aitchison KJ, Tsapakis EM, Huezo-Diaz P, Kerwin RW, et al. Ecstasy (MDMA)-induced hyponatremia is associated with genetic variant of CYP2D6 and COMT. J Psychopharmacol 2012;26:408−18.

[18] Oppek K, Koller G, Zwergal A, Pogarell O. Intravenous administration and abuse of bupropion: a case report and a review of literature. J Addict Med 2014;8:290−3.

[19] Lee AM, Jepson C, Hoffman E, Epstein L, et al. CYP2B6 genotype alters abstinence in a bupropion smoking cessation trail. Biol Psychiatry 2007;62:635−41.

[20] Kirchheiner J, Klein C, Meineke I, Sasse J, et al. Bupropion and 4-OH pharmacokinetics in relation to genetic polymorphism in CYP2B6. Pharmacogenomics 2003;13:619−26.

[21] Tomaz PR, Santos JR, Issa JS, Abe TO, et al. CYP2B6 rs2279343 polymorphism is associated with smoking cessation success in bupropion therapy. Eur J Clin Pharmacol 2015;71:1067−73.

[22] Negra AB, Pereira AC, Guindalini C, Santos HC, et al. Butylcholinesterase genetic variants: association with cocaine dependance and related phenotypes. PLoS One 2013;8:e80505.

[23] Lockridge O. Review of human butylcholinesterase structure, function, genetic variant, history of use in the clinic, and potential therapeutic use. Pharamcol Ther 2015;148:34−46.

[24] Haufroid V, Hantson P. CYP2D6 genetic polymorphisms and their relevance for poisoning due to amphetamines, opioid analgesics and antidepressants. Clin Toxicol (Phila) 2015;53:501−10.

[25] Crews KR, Gaedigk A, Dunnenberger HM, Leeder JS, et al. Clinical pharmacogenetic implementation consortium guidelines for cytochrome P450 2D6 genotype and codeine therapy: 2014 update. Clin Pharmacol Ther 2014;95:376−82.

[26] Linares OA, Fudin J, Schiesser WE, Daly Linares AL, et al. CYP2D6 phenotype-specific population pharmacokinetics. J Pain Palliat care Pharamcother 2015;29:4−15.

[27] VanderVaart S, Berger H, Sistonen J, Madadi P, et al. CYP2D6 polymorphisms and codeine analgesia in postpartum pain management: a pilot study. Ther Drug Monit 2011;33:425−32.

[28] Stamer UM, Zhang L, Book M, Lehmann LE, et al. CYP2D6 genotype dependent oxycodone metabolism in postoperative patients. PLoS One 2013;8:e60239.

[29] Maladi P, Koren G, Cairns J, Chitayat D, et al. Safety of codeine during breastfeeding: fatal morphine poisoning in the breastfed neonate of a mother prescribed codeine. Can Fam Physician 2007;53:33−5.

[30] Ciszkowski C, Madadi P. Codeine, ultrarapid metabolism genotype and postoperative death. N Engl J Med 2009;361:827−8.

[31] Kelly LE, Rieder M, van den Anker J, Malkin B, et al. More codeine fatalities after tonsillectomy in North American children. Pediatrics 2012;129:e1343−7.

[32] Lassen D, Damkier P, Brosen K. The pharmacogenetics of tramadol. Clin Pharmacokinet 2015;54:825−36.

[33] Stamer UM, Lehnen K, Hothker F, Bayerer B, et al. Impact of CYP2D6 genotype on postoperative tramadol analgesia. Pain 2003;105:231−8.

[34] Wang G, Zhang H, He F, Feng X. Effect of the CYP2D6*10 C188T polymorphism on postoperative tramadol analgesia in a Chinese population. Eur J Clin Pharamcol 2006;62:927−31.

[35] Susce MT, Murray-Carmichael E, De Leon J. Response to hydrocodone, codeine and oxycodone in a CYP2D6 poor metabolizer. Prog Neuropsychopharmacol Biol Psychiatry 2006;30:1356−8.

[36] Orliaguet G, Hamza J, Couloigner V, Denoyelle F, et al. A case of respiratory depression in a child with ultrarapid CYP2D6 metabolism after tramadol. Pediatrics 2015;135:e753−5.

[37] Stamer UM, Stuber F, Muders T, Musshoff F. Respiratory depression with tramadol in a patient with renal impairment and CYP2S6 gene duplication. Anesth Analg 2008;107:926−9.

[38] Li Y, Kantelip JP, Gerritsen-van-Schieveen P, Davani S. Interindividual variability of methadone response: impact of genetic polymorphism. Mol Diag Ther 2008;12:109−24.

[39] Kharasch ED, Regina KJ, Blood J, Friedel C. Methadone pharmacogenomics: CYP2B6 polymorphism determines plasma concentration, clearance and metabolism. Anesthesiology 2015;123:1142−53.

[40] Levran O, Peles E, Hamon S, Randesi M, et al. CYP2B6 SNPs are associated with methadone dose required for effective treatment of opioid addiction. Addict Biol 2013;18:709−16.

[41] Bunten H, Liang WJ, Pounder DJ, Seneviratne C, et al. ORRM1 and CYP2B6 gene variants as risk factor in methadone-related deaths. Clin Pharmacol Ther 2010;88:383−9.

[42] Madadi P, Kelly LE, Kepron C, Edwards JN, et al. Forensic investigation on methadone concentrations in deceased breastfed infants. J Forensic Sci 2016;61:576−80.

[43] Mouly S, Bloch V, Peoch K, Houze P, et al. Methadone dose in heroin-dependent patients: role of clinical factors, comedication, genetic polymorphism and enzyme activity. Br J Clin Pharmacol 2015;79:967−77.

[44] Basatami S, Gupta A, Zackrisson AL, Ahlner J, et al. Influence of UGT2B7, OPM1 and ABCB1 gene polymorphism on postoperative morphine consumption. Basic Clin Pharmacol Toxicol 2014;115:423−31.

[45] De Gregori M, Garbin G, De Gregori S, Minella CE, et al. Genetic variability at COMT but not at OPRMI and UGT2B7 loci modulates morphine analgesic response in acute postoperative pain. Eur J Clin Pharamcol 2013;69:1651−8.

Association between polymorphisms in genes encoding various receptors, transporters, and enzymes and alcohol/drug addiction

8

Introduction

Alcohol and drug addictions are psychiatric disorders associated with maladaptive behaviors where a person has persistent, compulsive, and uncontrolled use of alcohol or a drug. Moreover, alcohol abuse is often associated with poly drug abuse. Both the genetic makeup of a person and environmental factors make a person more susceptible to alcohol and/or drug abuse. The human genome contains 3.2 billion nucleotides of DNA [1]. Most of the genetic polymorphisms are single nucleotide polymorphism (SNP) and it has been estimated that more than 11 million SNPs occur in the human genome with a frequency of more than 1% (if a polymorphism occurs at a frequency less than 1% it is considered rare but when it occurs at a frequency of more than 1% it is called polymorphic). Although SNPs are the most common genetic variation, other variations including deletion, insertion, and duplication, also occur.

A genetic variation results in an altered expression and function of a protein, which may be linked to reward from alcohol and/or abused drugs and thus may be linked to alcohol and/or drug addiction. Family, twin, and linkage studies can provide information regarding a potential association between a phenotype and addiction. Genome-wide linkage studies can identify location of the genome that is associated with the particular phenotype. Moreover, through case control candidate gene association studies, contribution of a genetic polymorphism in making an individual more susceptible to alcohol or drug abuse can be identified. In addition, polymorphisms in genes that encode various enzymes responsible for alcohol and drug metabolism contribute to toxicity as well as alcohol/drug addiction. It is well known that polymorphisms of genes encoding enzymes that are responsible for metabolism of alcohol (alcohol dehydrogenase and aldehyde dehydrogenase) may protect a person from alcohol dependence or may increase the risk of alcohol dependence (depending on the particular polymorphism). Please see Chapter 6, Genetic Polymorphisms of Alcohol Metabolizing Enzymes Associated With Protection From or Increased Risk of Alcohol Abuse for more detail.

Polymorphisms of genes encoding various enzymes that metabolize drugs, including drugs of abuse, also contribute to toxicity or drug addiction. For example, certain polymorphisms in gene encoding serum butyrylcholinesterase may increase

Alcohol, Drugs, Genes and the Clinical Laboratory. DOI: http://dx.doi.org/10.1016/B978-0-12-805455-0.00008-7

susceptibility of an individual to crack cocaine addiction. Please see Chapter 7, Pharmacogenomics of Abused Drugs for detail. However, in addition to these genetic factors, polymorphisms of genes encoding various brain receptors, transporters, and enzymes linked to metabolism of neurotransmitter may also render a person more susceptible to alcohol and/or drug abuse. However, no single gene has been identified that is linked to alcohol and/or drug abuse. Therefore, alcohol and drug abuse are polygenic disorders where various genes contribute, to a very little to moderate extent, towards susceptibility of an individual to alcohol and/or drug abuse.

Heredity linked to alcohol/drug abuse

Family studies have shown that the risk of alcohol dependence is 4- to 10-fold higher in the offspring of an alcoholic parent. A meta-analysis consisting of 10,000 twin pairs have shown that heritability of alcohol use disorder is approximately 50% and other similar studies have indicated that the genetic component contributed between 40% and 60%. Alcohol dependence may also cooccur with other substance abuse such as cocaine, nicotine, and opiates. However, various nongenetic factors including condition during pregnancy (whether mother has abused alcohol and/or drugs), childhood, adolescent, and adulthood environments may play a significant role in the development of alcohol use disorder in an individual [2]. Prescott and Kendler based on studies with 3516 twins from male−male pairs, observed that the prevalence of alcoholism was substantially higher among identical pairs compared to fraternal pairs. Using liability threshold model, the authors attributed 48−58% of liability of alcoholism to inherited genetic factors. The authors concluded that genetic factors might play a more important role in the development of alcoholism in men [3].

Like alcohol addiction, drug addiction is also "familiar" indicating that such addiction tends to recur in families. However, the genetic component may vary widely depending on abused drugs. Tsuang et al., based on a study of 3372 twin pairs where both twins participated, concluded that genetic factors contributed 34% while shared environment and nonshared environmental factors contributed 34% and 38% respectively to individual's risk of developing drug use disorder [4]. Various studies indicate that the heritability range of drug addiction may vary widely depending on the particular drug, e.g., heritability may account for 39% in case of addiction for hallucinogens but heritability factor may be as high as 72% in case of cocaine addiction [5].

Overview of neurotransmitter systems with relation to alcohol and abused drugs

In general it is assumed that alcohol and drug dependence as well as addiction is an organic brain disease caused by the cumulative effects of alcohol and/or drugs on various neurotransmitters. Some drugs mimic neurotransmitters, e.g., opioids, while other abused drugs alter neurotransmission by interacting with molecular components of one or more neurotransmitter system. More than 180 neurotransmitters have been described and detailed discussion on various neurotransmitters is beyond the scope of the book. The central function of the human brain is due to the presence of 100 billion neurons, and everything humans do relies on the communication between neurons, where various neurotransmitters play important roles. A nerve cell has three basic parts; the *cell body*, containing the nucleus (also DNA), cytoplasm, and cell organelles, *dendrites* which branch off the cell body and act as contacts with neighboring neurons, and an *axon* which sends impulses and extends from the cell body to deliver impulses to another neuron. Synapses are small gaps between neurons where messages move from one neuron to another neuron mostly as a chemical signal. When a neuron is activated, a small electrical signal is generated (action potential) which travels very quickly along the axon and when the electrical signal reaches the end of the axon a chemical messenger (neurotransmitter) is released which travels through the synapse and binds to the receptor of the receiving (neighboring) neuron's dendrite. Then the entire process may be repeated again. Common neurotransmitters are acetylcholine, serotonin, dopamine, gamma-aminobutyric acid (GABA), epinephrine, norepinephrine, and glutamate. Neurotransmitters also can be divided under two broad groups: inhibitory and excitatory. Excitatory neurotransmitters stimulate neurons and the brain while inhibitory neurotransmitters have a calming effect, but some neurotransmitters may play a dual role.

Dopaminergic system

The monoaminergic neurotransmitter systems constitute the primary reward pathways in the human brain. Monoamines can be further divided into catecholamines (dopamine, epinephrine, and norepinephrine) and serotonin. Dopamine is synthesized from tyrosine which plays an important role in regulating emotional and motivational behavior through the mesolimbic dopaminergic pathway, which also includes rewards after consuming food as well as rewards related to the administration of drugs abuse. Dopamine neurons are located in the ventral tegmental area (VTA) of the brain and project into the nucleus accumbens. After receiving the appropriate signal, dopamine is released by the presynaptic neuron into the synapse where dopamine binds with a dopamine receptor. The unbound dopamine is then taken up by dopamine transporters (DATs) for future utilization or degradation.

The mesolimbic dopaminergic pathway is the major reward pathway of the brain. As a result, dysfunctions in the dopaminergic systems are involved in several pathological conditions including Parkinson's disease, Tourette's syndrome, drug addiction, and hyperactivity disorders. Dopamine binds to two families of G-protein coupled receptors. The D1 type receptors are D1 (DRD1) and D5 receptors (DRD2) while D2 type receptors are DRD2, DRD3, and DRD4. The diverse physiological functions of dopamine receptors encoded by the genes *DRD1, DRD2, DRD3, DRD4,* and *DRD5* and polymorphisms of these genes can result in change in the expression levels and may be associated with susceptibility to alcohol and/or drug abuse. The cell bodies of dopaminergic neurons are located in the hypothalamus, and the brain stem region (substantia nigra, pars compacta, and VTA). Dopamine is involved in the regulation of movement, attention, motivation, as well as reward from various activities including intake of food and abuse of alcohol and/or drugs.

DAT belongs to the family of sodium/chloride dependent transporter proteins and is responsible for the reuptake of extracellular synaptic dopamine into presynaptic neurons, thus terminating the effect of dopamine. Therefore, dopaminergic reward circuits may function differently when DAT expression level alters. The SLC6A3 gene present on chromosome 5 (5q15.3) encodes DATs responsible for sequestering dopamine back into presynaptic neurons. Dopamine-β-hydroxylase (DβH), encoded by $D\beta H$ gene, catalyzes the conversion of dopamine to norepinephrine, and several polymorphisms in the $D\beta H$ gene have been the focus of addiction research for many years. The enzyme catechol-O-methyltransferase (COMT) is involved in the metabolism of catecholamines including dopamine. Variation in COMT may influence dopamine levels in the prefrontal cortex, which may lead to alterations in the reward process as well as susceptibility to drug addiction.

Serotonergic system

Serotonin and norepinephrine are two important neurotransmitters. The serotonin, also known as 5-hydroxytryptamine (5-HT), is synthesized from tryptophan and it binds to two types of serotonin receptors; serotonin-gated ion channel (5-HT$_3$ receptors), or G-protein couples receptors (5-HT$_1$, 5-HT$_2$, and 5-HT$_{4-7}$ receptors). Serotonin is involved in the regulation of mood, sleep, appetite, and other functions. Serotonin is removed from synapses by serotonin transporters [6]. Serotonin reuptake by transporters is inhibited by SSRI antidepressants. The human serotonin transporter gene (5-hydroxytryptamine transporter gene: 5-HTT) is found on chromosome 17 (17q11.1$-$q12). Serotonin receptors are also encoded by specific genes.

Monoamine oxidase (MAO), a mitochondrial enzyme in humans, can be subclassified as monoamine oxidase A enzyme (MAOA) and monoamine oxidase B enzyme (MAOB). MAOA is responsible for metabolism of monoamine neurotransmitters including dopamine, norepinephrine, and serotonin. Human platelet MAO levels vary considerably, and platelet MAO abnormality has been linked with a number of psychiatric disorders. MAOA is encoded by an X-chromosome-linked gene ($MAOA$ gene; Xp11.23) and polymorphism of this gene affects its transcriptional activity.

Abused drugs and dopaminergic system

All abused drugs exert their initial reinforcing effects by triggering supraphysiological surges of dopamine in the nucleus accumbens either by direct or indirect mechanisms. Repeated drug administration results in neuroplastic changes in the brain [7]. While drugs of abuse increase dopamine levels in the nucleus accumbens, most drugs that are not habit-forming do not cause dopamine overflow. Psychostimulants increase dopamine levels primarily by altering dopamine clearance from extracellular space whereas opiates indirectly increase dopamine transmission by suppressing inhibitory output onto dopamine neurons [8]. In general, stimulants such as amphetamine, methamphetamine, and cocaine have their most pronounced effects on monoamine neurotransmitters such as dopamine, norepinephrine, epinephrine, and serotonin. Acute administration of amphetamine-like drugs directly stimulates release of dopamine from neurons. In addition, amphetamine-like drugs also stimulate other monogenic amines including norepinephrine, epinephrine, and serotonin. Interestingly 3,4-methylenedioxymethamphetamine (MDMA) has a potent effect on the serotonin system, which may be linked to the psychedelic effects of MDMA. However, repeated administration of these drugs results in tolerance, which is related to depletion of dopamine in the presynaptic terminals. As a result, withdrawal symptoms develop when the drug is discontinued after prolonged use.

Although amphetamines can also block dopamine reuptake, the primary mechanism of action is increased extracellular dopamine levels due to direct stimulation of dopaminergic neurons. In contrast, cocaine increases dopamine levels by blocking dopamine reuptake following normal release of dopamine by neurons. Cocaine blocks dopamine reuptake by attaching to DATs. Cocaine also increases extracellular serotonin levels. Interactions of various abused drugs and alcohol with neurotransmitter systems are summarized in Table 8.1.

Glutamate system

Glutamate which is locally synthesized from glucose is the primary excitatory neurotransmitter in the brain which binds with two types of receptors: glutamate-gated ion channel receptors (N-methyl-D-aspartate: NMDA receptor; alpha-amino-3-hydroxy-5-methyl-4-isoxazolepropionic acid-receptor and kainate receptor) and G-protein coupled glutamate receptors (three families of receptors). These receptors are also called metabotropic glutamate receptors and denoted as mGluR I–III.

Phencyclidine (PCP) is a noncompetitive NMDA-receptor antagonist, and blocks dopamine reuptake. As a result, synaptic dopamine levels are increased. PCP has a high affinity for NMDA receptors present in the cortex and limbic structures. When PCP binds with the NMDA receptor, glutamate-mediated entry of calcium in cells is inhibited. Ketamine is also an agonist of NMDA receptors.

GABA system

The chief inhibitory neurotransmitter in the central nervous system (CNS) is GABA, which is synthesized from glutamate. The neurotransmitter GABA binds to specific receptors (GABA receptors) located in the plasma membrane of neuronal cells. These receptors are heteromeric proteins complexes consisting of several homologous membrane spanning glycoprotein subunits. Two main classes of GABA receptors have been well characterized: ionotropic $GABA_A$ and $GABA_C$ receptors as well as metabotropic $GABA_B$ receptors. $GABA_A$ receptors are a family of ligand-activated chloride ion channels and a pentameric assembly out of various possible subunits: α_{1-6}, β_{1-3}, γ_{1-3}, δ, ϵ, θ, π, and ρ_{1-3}, and their splice variant. $GABA_C$

Table 8.1 Interactions of various abused drugs and alcohol with neurotransmitter systems

Neurotransmitter system	Type	Location in CNS	Functions associated with	Drugs/alcohol that interacts with the system
Dopaminergic	Both excitatory and inhibitory	Hypothalamus, cerebral cortex, mid-brain, ventral tegmental area (VTA)	Pleasure for eating food, love, interaction with friends but also euphoria from abuse of alcohol/drugs. This system also affects memory and concentration	Amphetamine, methamphetamine directly stimulates neurons to secrete dopamine but also cocaine inhibits dopamine uptake. However, all abused drugs directly or indirectly cause elevated dopamine level
Serotonin	Excitatory	Mid-brain, VTN, cerebral cortex, hypothalamus	Appetite, sleep, desire, mood	MDMA
Glutamate	Excitatory	Widely distributed	Learning, cognition, memory	Phencyclidine, ketamine, LSD
GABA	Inhibitory	Widely distributed	Anxiety, memory	Alcohol, barbiturates, benzodiazepines
Opioid receptors	Not applicable	Widely distributed in the brain and the spinal cord	Mood, sedation, rate of bodily functions	Heroin, morphine, codeine, oxycodone, oxymorphone, hydrocodone, hydromorphone, methadone, tramadol, etc.
Cannabinoid receptors	Not applicable	Cerebral cortex, hippocampus, thalamus, basal ganglia	Movement, cognition, memory	Cannabinoids and also synthetic cannabinoids (spices)
Acetylcholine	Excitatory	Hippocampus, cerebral cortex, thalamus, basal ganglia, cerebellum	Memory, attention, mood, arousal	Nicotine

Source: Impact of drugs on neurotransmission by Carl Sherman. National Institute on Drug Abuse. NIDA notes contributory writer. <http://www.drugabuse.gov/news-events/nida-notes/2007/10/impact-drugs-neurotransmission > [accessed 15.06.16].

receptors are composed of the ρ_{1-3}, subunits. The composition of most common GABA$_A$ receptor includes two α_1, two β_2, and one γ_2 subunit. When the neurotransmitter GABA binds to GABA$_A$, the conformational structure of the receptor is changed, and the membrane pore opens to allow the flow of chloride ions. GABA$_B$ receptors, which are widely distributed throughout the human brain, are G-protein coupled receptors that stimulate the opening of potassium channels. GABA$_C$ receptors, which differ in complexity of structure, abundance, distribution, and function from GABA$_A$ and GABA$_B$ receptors, can be found in retina, hippocampus, spinal cord, and pituitary tissues. GABA$_A$ receptors are encoded by 16 genes and 14 of these 16 genes are clustered on 4 chromosomes; 4p12−q13 (encoding α_2, α_4, β_1, and γ_1 subunits), 5p31−q35 (encoding α_1, α_6, β_2, and γ_2 subunits), 15q11−q13 (encoding α_5, β_3, and γ_3 subunits), and Xq28 (encoding α_3, α_4, β_4, and ϵ_1 subunits).

GABA system and pharmacological action of alcohol, barbiturates, and benzodiazepines

Unlike opioid and nicotine, which have specific receptors in the brain, there is no specific receptor for ethanol. Therefore, it has been assumed that enhanced GABA, the brain's major inhibitory neurotransmitter, glutamate (an excitatory neurotransmitter), dopamine, opioid peptides, and opioid receptors as well as serotonin neurotransmission have been associated with alcohol administration which potentially mediates some of the alcohol's reinforcing effects. The development of tolerance may be caused by GABA$_A$ receptor system. Alcohol's inhibition of the glutamatergic excitatory neurotransmitter pathway, especially at the postsynaptic NMDA receptor, may be the cause of neurotoxic effects of alcohol, particularly intoxication, blackout, and withdrawal symptoms [9].

Sedatives such as benzodiazepines and barbiturates, which are also CNS depressants, exert their effect by enhancing GABA. Barbiturates activate the GABA$_A$ receptor and as a result flow of chloride ions into neurons is increased. Barbiturates increase the time length of opening of chloride channels thus increasing inhibitory effects of GABA. Similar to barbiturates, benzodiazepines also enhance GABA activity in the brain thus having a general inhibitory effect. However, effects of barbiturates on opening of chloride channel are nonspecific but for benzodiazepines there are specific benzodiazepine receptors which are coupled with GABA$_A$ receptors. However, endogenous equivalent of benzodiazepines has not been discovered.

Opioid system

The opioid receptors and endogenous peptide ligands play an important role in neurotransmission and neuromodulation in response to alcohol, heroin, and cocaine. There are three classes of opioid receptors; μ, δ, and κ (mu, delta, and kappa), and these opioid receptors are widely expressed in the brain. There are three distinct families of opioid peptides: endorphins, encephalin, and dynorphins. Encephalin binds to delta receptor, dynorphins bind to a kappa receptor while endorphins bind to both mu and delta receptors. More recently two additional short peptides endomorphin-1 and endomorphin-2 that display high affinity for mu-receptors have been characterized. The opioid receptors are encoded by three specific genes: *OPRM1* at 6q24−q25 encodes the mu-receptor, *OPRD1* at 1p36.1−p34.3 encodes the delta receptor, and *OPRK1* at 8q11.2 encodes the kappa receptor. Endogenous cannabinoid receptors and endogenous cannabinoids also play important role in abuse of cannabinoids and synthetic cannabinoids.

Opioid drugs and opioid system

Both opioid analgesic and endogenous opiates interact with opioid receptors. Morphine, heroin, fentanyl, and codeine are strong agonists for mu-receptors but are partial agonists for delta and kappa receptors. Buprenorphine is a partial agonist of mu-receptors. Tramadol and methadone are not only agonists of mu-receptors but also inhibit uptake of norepinephrine and serotonin, thus enhancing their analgesic effect. In addition methadone is also an agonist of NMDA receptor [10]. Neurons within the VTA contain GABA. In addition, these GABA containing neurons also have mu-receptors. When opioids bind with mu-receptors, the GABA receptors release less GABA and as a result dopamine neurons are activated. The net effect is release of dopamine by these neurons and release of dopamine in the nucleus accumbens. Although dopamine release is associated with opioid-induced euphoria, there are other mechanisms by which opioids work. Inhibition of GABAergic neurons induced by binding of opioids to receptors allows descendent inhibitory serotoninergic neurons producing analgesia. At the spinal level, the analgesic effect is also produced by inhibition of release of various mediators including glutamate, substance P, and nitric oxide from nociceptive neurons [10].

Acetylcholine

Acetylcholine, a neurotransmitter found in the brain and autonomic nervous system, is the natural agonist of muscarinic and nicotinic receptors. Acetylcholine is also the first neurotransmitter discovered. Muscarinic receptors are G-protein coupled acetylcholine receptors found in the plasma membrane of neurons throughout the CNS. Nicotinic acetylcholine receptors are receptor ion channels found in the autonomic nervous system and play an important role in the mechanism of nicotine addiction.

Polymorphisms of genes in neurotransmitter systems and addiction

Although challenged by other investigators currently, dopamine hypothesis is considered as the acceptable model for explaining euphoria after drug abuse as well as development of drug tolerance (decreased effect of the drug) and addiction. Addiction is defined as a compulsive out of control drug abuse despite serious negative consequences associated with drug use, e.g., being fired from a job, violent behavior, as well as negative social stature. Addiction is also associated with a long-lasting risk of relapse which is initiated by exposure to drug related cues.

Currently it is accepted that dopaminergic system is the major site in the brain for reward and reinforcement for both natural rewards and addictive drugs. Addictive drugs, regardless of route of administration, increase the level of synaptic dopamine often by 5−10 times that of the normal level, most noticeably in nucleus accumbens, thus activating the reward circuit of the brain. Smoking or injecting an abused drug in general produces faster and higher dopamine concentration than orally ingesting the drug. Experimental evidences indicate that under physiological conditions, dopamine neurons generate a learning signal when an unexpected reward takes place with the purpose of learning so that the reward may be repeated. However, when the reward is fully predictable, dopaminergic neurons will not be activated again and the learning is ceased because behavior is now optimized. Unfortunately, the human brain is unable to distinguish between activation of the reward circuit and eventual learning cue as a result of natural physiological processes such as eating a favorite food versus activation due to drug abuse. Moreover, abused drug related activation of the reward circuit of the brain far exceeds any natural stimulus, thus generating an inappropriate learning signal that results in compulsive drug use despite negative consequences [11].

Studies have shown that in addition to the dopaminergic system other systems may also be involved in processing inappropriate learning signals general by abused drugs. Studies have indicated that a single dose of cocaine was sufficient to induce a trace of excitatory dopaminergic neurons at VTA that lasted for a week. Such a trace may also be observed after administration of one dose of morphine, nicotine, alcohol, or amphetamine. This phenomenon due to the administration of abused drug results in changes in glutamatergic transmission and such alteration in glutamatergic systems is called drug-evoked synaptic plasticity. Such plasticity may also occur at the GABAergic system and other neurotransmitter systems [12].

Repeated exposure to the abused drug alters neuroplasticity and as a result the same reward may not be achieved after taking a similar dosage of the abused drug that provided euphoria. This may be due to depletion of dopamine in neurons or depletion of dopamine receptors. This stage is called tolerance where the brain has adapted to a pattern of repeated drug abuse and a person requires much higher amounts of the drug to achieve euphoria. Finally a person is addicted to a drug when an intense craving for the drug is developed because the hippocampus and amygdala store information regarding the pleasurable feeling once obtained through drug abuse. Therefore, the individual wants to repeat that euphoria. Although both alcohol and drug addiction are psychiatric illnesses, genetic polymorphisms may result in certain alterations in neurotransmitter pathways that may increase susceptibility of a person to alcohol or drug abuse. However, genetic factors may contribute approximately 50% to the susceptibility of a person towards drug and/or alcohol abuse and environmental factors are also equally important. Because the dopaminergic pathway plays an important role in the mechanism of action of the abused drug, polymorphisms of genes that may affect dopaminergic pathways and their association with alcohol and drug abuse has been well studied.

Polymorphisms of genes that affect functions of dopaminergic pathways and addiction

As mentioned earlier, all addictive drugs stimulate dopamine release (directly or indirectly) thus increasing dopamine levels above the typical basal level, and repeated drug abuse is associated with supraphysiological levels of dopamine. Alcohol may increase dopamine levels through μ-opiate receptors present in the mesolimbic system. The D1 dopamine receptor (DRD1) is involved in the rewarding/reinforcing effects of drugs of abuse and this is also a candidate gene for possible association with alcohol dependence. D1 type family of G-protein coupled receptors such as DRD1 activate adenylyl cyclase and are involved in various brain functions including motor control, reward, and reinforcement mechanisms, as well as being involved in attention deficit hyperactive syndrome. DRD1 antagonist may reduce cocaine-seeking behavior.

Kim et al. based on genotyping of 11 polymorphisms of *DRD* gene family in 535 alcohol dependent subjects in the Korean population reported that polymorphism in the 5′-untranslated region (5′-UTR) region of *DRD1* (48 A > G: rs4532) gene located in chromosome 5 (q35.1) was associated with alcohol related problems [13]. Batel et al., based on analysis of 134 alcohol dependent patients, observed that the T allele of the rs686 polymorphism with *DRD1* gene was significantly more frequent in patients with alcohol dependence [14]. Prasad et al. also showed that rs4532 present in 5′-UTR of *DRD1* gene was associated with alcoholism in East Indian men and commented that 48 A > G SNP could be a predisposing factor for alcohol abuse [15]. Polymorphism of *DRD1* gene (rs4532, rs686, and rs265981) has been associated with substance abuse, addictive behavior and psychiatric illness. However, Zhu et al. reported that *DRD1* rs686 minor allele decreases the risk of opioid addiction in Chinese population [16].

The polymorphisms of *DRD2* gene on chromosome 11 (q22−q23) that encodes DRD2 receptor has been found to be associated with both alcohol and drug addiction. The DRD2 receptor is a G-protein coupled receptor located on postsynaptic dopaminergic neurons, which plays a role in reward pathway through the mesolimbic system. The *DRD2* gene shows primarily three kinds of polymorphism including *-141 c ins/del*, *Taq1A*, and *Taq1B* alleles. The *DRD2 Taq1A* (A1 allele causing lower DRD2 receptor density in striatum) polymorphism is located 10 kilobase-pairs downstream from the coding region of the *DRD2* gene at chromosome 11q23. In fact, the *DRD2* associated polymorphism has been more precisely located within the coding region of *ANKK1* (ankyrin repeat and kinase domain containing one) gene, which is a neighboring gene that may confer a change in amino acid sequence.

Higher frequency of the A1 allele of Taq1A near the *DRD2* gene was observed among alcoholics. Smith et al., based on metaanalysis of 42 studies with 9382 participants, observed an association between presence of one or two copies of A1 allele and alcohol dependency [17]. This polymorphism is also associated with increased risk of heroin use, cocaine dependency, psychostimulant abuse, and smoking [18].

The SNP Taq1B is closer to the regulatory and structural coding region (5′ region) of the *DRD2* gene and it may be expected that such polymorphisms may play a role in alcohol dependence. Few studies that explored association between Taq1B and alcohol dependence produced conflicting results (some studies found association while others found no association). Effect of -141 c ins/del allele on alcohol dependence is also controversial with some studies reporting no association, while other studies observed some correlation between this allele and alcohol dependence.

Several polymorphisms of DRD3 receptor genes have been reported to be associated with susceptibility to alcoholism. Although *DRD3* rs6280 (Ser9Gly; substitution of a glycine for serine residue in the extracellular receptor N-terminal domain also known as *Bal I* restriction due to a restriction site produced by the variant) polymorphism which makes the receptor more sensitive to dopamine is associated with various psychiatric disorders, association of this SNP with alcoholism is inconsistent due to conflicting results. However, *Bal I* restriction is associated with greater risk of cocaine abuse as well as nicotine abuse [18].

DRD4 receptors, G-coupled receptors encoded by the *DRD4* gene, have been linked to several psychiatric disorders (schizophrenia, bipolar disorder), neurological disorders (Parkinson's disease), and addictive behaviors (including novelty seeking). *DRD4* has a "variable number of tandem repeat" (VNTR) polymorphisms on exon 3 that may affect gene expression by binding nuclear factors. The *DRD4 VNTR* can vary from 2 to 10 with 48-bp repeats where alleles with 6 or fewer repeats are termed as "short alleles," and alleles with 7 or more repeats are termed as "long alleles." Compared with short alleles, long alleles may reduce *DRD4* gene expression. The most studied polymorphism of *DRD4* gene is a 48-bp VNTR in the third axon. In general, *DRD4 VTNR* long allele with seven or more repeats is associated with novelty seeking and drinking behavior. Ray et al. using 90 heavy drinking college students observed association between *DRD4 VNTR* long allele genotype and problem drinking as well as novelty seeking behavior [19]. A seven repeat polymorphism at exon 3 was observed more frequently in methamphetamine abusers than controls.

DAT belongs to the family of sodium/chloride dependent transporter proteins and is responsible for the reuptake of extracellular synaptic dopamine into presynaptic neurons thus terminating the effect of dopamine. Therefore, dopaminergic reward circuits may function differently when DAT expression level alters. Neuroimaging studies showed that DAT levels were significantly lower in the striatum of alcohol dependent patients compared to controls. DAT availability in the brain may be dependent on genetic variation. The *DAT* gene (*DAT1*; locus symbol SLC6A3) is present on chromosome 5q15.3. Expression of DAT is influenced by a VNTR polymorphism located in the 3'-untranslated region (3'-UTR) of the dopamine transporter (*DAT1*) gene. For VNTR, numbers ranging from 3 to 16 have been described with a 9- and 10-repeat allele being the most common. In general, many studies found no significant association between polymorphism of *DAT1* gene and alcohol dependence. However, Kohnke et al., using a group of 102 healthy subjects and 216 alcoholics, showed an association of allele A9 (9 copy repeat allele in the VNTR in the 3'-UTR of the *DAT1* gene) and alcoholism [20]. Carriers of A9 allele also showed greater response to cocaine [21]. A 30 bp functional VTNR in intron 8 of *SLC6A3* was associated with cocaine dependency in Brazilian subjects.

DβH catalyzes the conversion of dopamine to norepinephrine and several polymorphisms in the *DβH* gene have been the focus of addiction research for many years. Several studies found no association between polymorphism of *DβH* gene and alcohol dependence. However, Kohnke et al., based on a study of 102 healthy controls and 208 alcoholics, found an association between *DβH**444 G > A polymorphism, (in exon 2) with alcoholism [22]. Association of polymorphism of *DβH* gene with substance abuse is not clearly documented. Association of genetic polymorophisms in dopaminergic pathways with drug/alcohol addiction are listed in Table 8.2.

Table 8.2 Link between polymorphisms of genes encoding receptors, transporters, or enzymes involved in dopamine pathway and drug/alcohol addiction

Gene involved	Polymorphism	Association with alcohol abuse	Association with drug abuse
DRD1	5'-UTR: *DRD1* (48 A > G: rs4532*G)	Associated with alcohol abuse	May be associated with poly drug abuse but conflicting results
DRD2	*Taq1A/ANKK1*	Associated with alcoholism	Associated with stimulant, cocaine, and heroin abuse. May increase smoking risk
DRD3	*DRD3* rs6280 (Ser9Gly; Bal/I restriction)	Conflicting results	Greater risk of cocaine abuse
DRD4	*DRD4* VNTR Long allele with seven or more repeats of 48 bp	Associated with problem drinking/ alcoholism and novelty seeking behavior	Seven repeat polymorphism in exon 3 observed more often in methamphetamine abusers
DAT1	*DAT1* gene Allele A9	May be associated with alcoholism in certain population	Carriers of A9 allele also showed greater response to cocaine
DβH	*DβH**444 G > A	Conflicting result	No clear association with drug abuse
MAOA	3-Reapeat allele of *MAOA-μVNTR*	May be associated with alcoholism	Associated with substance abuse as well as impulsive and antisocial behavior
COMT	*COMT Val158Met* polymorphism	Conflicting results	Allele causing higher enzymatic activity is associated with polysubstance abuse including heroin, methamphetamine, and marijuana

MAOA is encoded by an X-chromosome-linked gene (*MAOA* gene; Xp11.23) and polymorphism of this gene affects its transcriptional activity. The locus termed as *MAOA*-linked polymorphic region is a VNTR which is located approximately 1.2 kb upstream from *MAOA* start codon and within the gene's transcriptional control region. Alleles of this *VTNR (MAOA-µVTNR)* have different numbers of copies of 30 bp repeated sequence present in 3, 3.5, 4, or 5 copies. The three-repeat allele is associated with lower MAOA activity and low MAO activity has been related to traits associated with a high-risk of alcoholism, drug abuse, and impulsive behavior, but there are conflicting results regarding association of this polymorphism either with alcohol or drug abuse.

COMT is an enzyme that metabolizes epinephrine, norepinephrine, and dopamine. COMT enzyme is encoded by *COMT* gene located on chromosome 22 (22q11.21) and produces two versions of this enzyme. The longer form called membrane bound COMT is mainly produced by the nerve cells in the brain. A shorter form of this enzyme called soluble COMT is found in liver, kidneys, and blood. Polymorphism of *COMT* gene may cause mental illness such as schizophrenia. As a result of polymorphism of *COMT* gene (nucleotide change adenine to guanine), in the longer form of the enzyme the amino acid variation occurs at position 158 (Val158Met; indicating amino acid at position 158 could be either valine or methionine). In the shorter form of this enzyme the variation occurs at position 108 (Val108Met). The enzyme containing valine is three to four times more active than the enzyme containing methionine. The effect of Val158Met polymorphism on alcohol addiction is contradictory, with some studies reporting association with this polymorphism with alcohol abuse but other studies observed no association. However, there are associations between increased COMT activity (valine at 158) and polysubstance abuse including addiction to heroin and methamphetamine. The allele (valine at 158) producing high activity enzyme was also directly associated with susceptibility to cannabis dependence [23].

Polymorphism of genes associated with serotonergic system and addiction

It has been postulated that polymorphism of the gene encoding serotonin transporter protein may be associated with alcohol and drug addiction. The human serotonin transporter gene (5-hydroxytryptamine transporter gene: *5-HTT: SLC6A4*) found on chromosome 17 (17q11.1−q12) has a biallelic functional polymorphism in its *5-HTT*-linked promoter region (*5-HTTLPR*) which is composed of a 44 bp insertion (long allele: L-allele) or deletion (short allele: S-allele) that regulates the transcription of serotonin transporter. The S-allele is associated with reduced serotonin transporter protein expression but L-allele is associated with increased expression of presynaptic serotonin transporter protein, resulting in more efficient serotonin reuptake and reduction of synaptic serotonin level compared to individuals with S-allele.

The S-allele has been associated with alcohol dependence, affective disorders, as well as several personality traits including anxiety, depression, impulsiveness, and risk of suicide. Feinn et al. conducted metaanalysis of data from 17 published studies (including 3489 alcoholics and 2325 controls) and concluded that the frequency of the S-allele at *5-HTTLPR* was significantly associated with alcohol dependence (odd ratio (OR): 1.18) [24]. Kweon et al. observed higher frequency of L-allele at *5-HTTLPR* in alcohol dependent male Korean patients than normal controls [25]. Gerra et al. reported that homozygous S-allele frequency was higher among heroin dependent individuals than normal controls and concluded that such polymorphism may be associated with increased risk of drug abuse [26] (Table 8.3).

In addition to serotonin transporter gene polymorphism, serotonin receptor gene polymorphism has also been studied in order to find potential association with alcohol use disorder. Although some investigators reported no association between serotonin receptor gene polymorphism and alcoholism, Cao et al., using meta-analysis, observed an association between polymorphism of *HTR2A* (rs6313; 102T/C at exon 1) gene and susceptibility to alcohol dependence [27]. In another study, the authors using metaanalysis observed association between *HTR1B* gene polymorphisms (rs130058) with alcohol cocaine and heroin dependence in the combined European, Asian, Hispanic, and African populations [28]. Yang and Li reported that one haplotype formed by SNPs rs3891484 and rs3758987 in *HTR3B* was associated with alcohol dependence in African American subjects [29]. Levran et al. reported an association between *HTR3B* gene polymorphism (rs11606194) and heroin addiction in a European ancestry subgroup [30].

Polymorphism of genes associated with GABA system and addiction

The chief inhibitory neurotransmitter in the CNS is GABA. The neurotransmitter GABA binds to specific receptors (GABA receptors) located in the plasma membrane of neuronal cells. Neurotransmitter GABA as well as GABA receptors has long been implicated in mediating at least some pharmacological actions of alcohol. GABA receptors are also molecular target for benzodiazepines and barbiturates both of which show some cross-dependence with alcohol. Fehr et al. based on a study of 257 German alcohol dependent patients and 88 healthy controls observed that *GABRA2* gene is a susceptible gene for alcohol dependence in European population [31]. Zintzaras performed metaanalysis of 14 variants of GABRA2 gene reported in 8 studies and concluded that variants in the *GABRA2* gene are associated with alcoholism [32]. Enoch et al. based on a study of 547 Finnish Caucasian men (266 alcoholics) and 311 community-derived Plains Indians men and women (181 alcoholics) concluded that *GABRA2* and *GABRG1* haplotypes appear to be independent predictors of alcoholism in Finnish and Plains Indian population [33]. Loh et al. observed association between *GABRG2* gene and alcohol dependence comorbid with antisocial personality disorder in a study based on Japanese population [34]. Nishiyama reported an association between *GABRG2* gene haplotype and increased risk of methamphetamine abuse [35].

Glutamic acid decarboxylase (GAD) is the rate limiting enzyme in the conversion of glutamate to GABA. Two isoforms of GAD have been identified; GAD1 and

Table 8.3 Link between polymorphisms of genes encoding receptors, transporters, or enzymes involved in serotonin pathway and addiction

Gene involved	Polymorphism	Association with alcohol abuse	Association with drug abuse
5-*HTT* (serotonin transporter gene)	5-*HTTLPR*, short (S)-allele, and long (L)-allele	S-allele is associated with alcohol dependence while L-allele is also associated with alcohol dependence among Korean male population	S-allele increases risk of drug abuse especially heroin abuse
5-*HTR2A* (serotonin receptor gene)	SNP (rs6313: 102T/C)	Associated with schizophrenia but also with alcohol dependence	Susceptibility to drug abuse
HTR1B (serotonin receptor gene)	SNPs (rs130058)	Associated with alcohol dependence	Associated with drug dependence
HTR3B (serotonin receptor gene)	Haplotype formed by SNPs (rs3891484 and rs3758987)	Associated with alcohol dependence in African Americans	
HTR3B (serotonin receptor gene)	Rs11606194		Associated with heroin addiction in European ancestry

GAD2. GAD1 is associated with cytosolic GABA production and is responsible for maintaining basal GABA level while GAD2 is mostly involved in synaptosomal GABA release and can be rapidly activated on demand for GABA. However, GAD1 is the primary rate limiting enzyme regulating GABA level under normal circumstances. Based on a study of 370 heroin dependent subjects and 389 healthy controls, Wu et al. showed that polymorphisms of the glutamate decarboxylate 1 gene (*GAD1* gene) were associated with heroin dependence in Han Chinese subjects [36].

Polymorphism of genes encoding opioid receptors and addiction

The opioid receptors and endogenous peptide ligands play an important role in neurotransmission and neuromodulation in response to alcohol, heroin, and cocaine. Human and animal experiments have indicated that there is a correlation between endogenous opioids, especially beta-endorphin and alcohol abuse. Consumption of alcohol stimulates beta-endorphin levels in specific regions of the brain functionally connected with the mesolimbic reward system. However, chronic alcohol consumption results in desensitization of the system in the beta-endorphin neuronal cell population. Plasma levels of beta-endorphin are decreased in chronic alcohol abusers. Studies have shown that individuals belonging to a high-risk group for alcohol abuse had lower basal levels of beta-endorphin compared to individuals with low risk of alcohol abuse [37].

Because mu-opioid receptor is the primary target of opioids, genetic polymorphism of gene (*OPRM1*) encoding this receptor may be associated with addiction. A coding variation in *OPRM1* (118 A > G; rs1799971) has been extensively studied because it alters amino acid position 40 in the mu-receptor protein from asparagine to aspartate (Asp40). This is also the most common polymorphism in the OPRMI gene (frequency varies widely between 2% and 49% among different ethnic groups). When this substitution occurs (118G allele), the mu-receptor has a higher affinity for beta-endorphin, although this finding has been challenged. This allele has been observed among alcohol dependent subjects. Another polymorphism *OPRM1* gene (17C > T), which occurs in range of 0.5–21% across different populations, results in change of an alanine residue at position 6 of the receptor protein to valine residue has also been associated with alcohol dependence. Alcohol dependent patients with one or two copies of 118G allele (Asp40) who are treated with opioid antagonist naltrexone have a significantly lower rate of relapse, making naltrexone pharmacotherapy more effective [38].

The 118G allele has been shown to be associated with greater risk of opiate addiction in Swedish and also in Han Chinese populations. This allele is also is a risk factor for heroin addiction in Swedish population. The second most common polymorphism of *OPRM1* gene (17C > T) is also associated with greater risk of opiate dependency. Manini et al. reported that patients with 118G allele had worst clinical severity after acute drug overdose [39]. The kappa-opioid receptor is encoded by

OPRK1 gene and this receptor is also been implicated in response to opiates. Gerra et al. observed that polymorphism of *OPRK1* gene (36G > T) occurred in significantly higher frequency in heroin addicts ($n = 106$) compared to healthy control subjects ($n = 70$) [40]. In another study, based on 1063 European Americans, the authors observed that polymorphisms of gene (*OPRD1*) encoding delta-opioid receptors were associated with opioid dependence. The 921 T > C allele was associated with greater risk of opioid addiction. The 80G > T polymorphism was also associated with higher risk of opioid abuse. However, the haplotype containing both the 80G > T and 921C > T polymorphisms increases the risk of alcohol dependence, opioid dependence, and cocaine dependence [41].

The polymorphism of proenkephalin gene (*PENK*) encodes the endogenous opioid has been associated with heroin addiction. Nikoshkov et al. reported that heroin abuse was significantly associated with polymorphic 3'-UTR dinucleotide (CA) repeat, where 79% of subjects homozygous for 79-bp allele were heroin abusers [42].

Polymorphism of genes encoding cannabinoid receptors and addiction

The endocannabinoid system consists of cannabinoid receptors, endogenous cannabinoids, and enzymes for the synthesis as well as degradation of endocannabinoid. There are two well-characterized G-protein coupled cannabinoid receptors CB1 and CB2. CB1 receptors are mostly expressed in the CNS whereas CB2 receptors are found in immune cells and peripheral tissues. Therefore, CB2 is also referred to as a peripheral cannabinoid receptor. Two fatty acid derivatives, namely arachidonylethanolamide and 2-arichidonylglycerol, have been isolated from nerve and peripheral tissue, which are endocannabinoid. Rodent experiments have shown that CB1 is involved in the neural circuitry regarding alcohol intake and motivation to consume alcohol. Chronic consumption of alcohol results in downregulation of CB1 receptor binding and its signal transduction capacity, which may be due to increased synthesis of CB1 receptor agonist arachidonylethanolamide and 2-arichidonylglycerol due to chronic alcohol consumption. Therefore, CB1 receptor gene polymorphism may play a role in development of alcoholism.

CB1 receptor is encoded by cannabinoid receptor gene 1 (*CNR1*) located on the chromosome 6 (6q14–q15). *CNR1* seems to be a promising candidate gene for association with alcohol and substance abuse. Zuo et al. studied 451 healthy control subjects and 550 substance abuse (alcohol or drug dependent) patients and observed that two SNPs in *CNR1* gene (SNP3: rs6454674 and SNP8; rs806368) were associated with alcohol and drug dependence [43]. Marcos et al. reported an interaction between G-allele of rs6454674 SNP and C-allele of rs806368 SNP in alcohol dependence [44]. A polymorphism of *CNR1* gene (rs2023239) has been associated with liability to cannabis dependence. Moreover, *CNR1* rs2023239 polymorphism may predispose smaller hippocampal volume after heavy cannabis use [45]. Ishiguro et al. observed association between cannabinoid receptor 2 gene polymorphism and alcoholism in the Japanese population [46].

Conclusion

As mentioned earlier, there is no single gene that is associated with alcohol and/or drug abuse. There are various genes that may contribute to some extent to increased susceptibility of an individual towards alcohol and/or drug abuse. Sometimes, the same genetic polymorphisms may contribute to increased risk of both alcohol and drug abuse. In addition, multiple genetic polymorphisms may act in synergy to increase such risks. In this chapter a brief overview of this topic is presented because detailed discussion on this topic is beyond the scope of this book. Moreover, there are also conflicting results regarding various polymorphisms and their association with alcohol and drug abuse, and sometimes such conflicts are due to small sample sizes or ethnic differences in the subjects studied.

References

[1] Venter JC, Adams MD, Myers EW, Li PW, et al. The sequence of human genome. Science 2001;291:1304−51.
[2] Diaz-Anzaldua A, Diaz-Martinez A, Diaz-Martinez LR. The complex interplay of epigenetics, and environment in the predisposition to alcohol dependence. Salud Mental 2011;34:157−66.
[3] Prescott CA, Kendler KS. Genetic and environmental contributions to alcohol abuse and dependence in a population based sample of male twins. Am J Psychiatry 1999;156:34−40.
[4] Tsuang MT, Lyons MJ, Eisen SA, Goldberg J, et al. Genetic influence on DSM-III-R drug abuse dependence: a study of 3,372 twin pairs. Am J Med Genet 1996;67:473−7.
[5] Goldman D, Oroszi G, Ducci F. The genetics of addictions: uncovering the genes. Nat Rev Genet 2005;6:521−32.
[6] Valenzuela CF, Puglia MP, Zucca S. Focus on: neurotransmitter systems. Alcohol Res Health 2011;34:106−20.
[7] Volkow ND, Morales M. The brain on drugs: from reward to addiction. Cell 2015;162:712−25.
[8] Oliva I, Wanat MJ. Ventral tegmental area afferents and drug dependent behavior. Front Psychiatry 2016;7:00030.
[9] Enoch MA, Goldman D. The genetics of alcoholism and alcohol abuse. Curr Psychiatry Rep 2001;3:144−51.
[10] Ghelardini C, Di Cesare Mannelli L, Bianchi E. The pharmacological basis of opioids. Clin Cases Miner Bone Metab 2015;12:219−21.
[11] Hyman SE, Malenka RC. Addiction and the brain: the neurobiology of compulsion and its persistence. Nat Rev Neurosci 2001;2:695−703.
[12] Luscher C. The emergence of a circuit model for addiction. Annu Rev Neurosci 2016;39:257−76.
[13] Kim DJ, Park BL, Yoon S, Lee HK, Joe KH, Cheon YH, et al. 5′-UTR polymorphism of dopamine receptor D1 (DRD1) associated with severity and temperament of alcoholism. Biochem Biophys Res Commun 2007;357:1135−41.
[14] Batel P, Houch H, Daoust M, Ramoz N, Naassila M, Gorwood P. A haplotype of the DRD1 gene is associated with alcohol dependence. Alcohol Clin Exp Res 2008; 32:567−72.

[15] Prasad P, Ambekar A, Vaswani M. Case-control association of dopamine receptor polymorphisms in alcohol dependence: a pilot study with Indian males. BMC Res Notes 2013;17:418.

[16] Zhu F, Yan C, Wen YC, Wang J, et al. Dopamine D1 receptor gene variation modulates opioid dependence risk by affecting transition to addiction. PLos One 2013; 8:e70805.

[17] Smith L, Watson M, Gates S, Ball D, et al. Meta-analysis of the association of the Taq 1A polymorphism with the risk of alcohol dependency: a huGE gene-disease association review. Am J Epidemiol 2008;167:125−38.

[18] Khokhar JY, Ferguson CS, Zhu A, Tyndale RF. Pharmacogenetics of drug dependence: role of variation in susceptibility treatment. Annu Rev Pharmacol Toxicol 2010;50: 39−61.

[19] Ray LA, Bryan A, Mackillop J, McGeary J, Hesterberg K, Hutchison KE. The dopamine D receptor (DRD4) gene exon III polymorphism, problematic alcohol use and novelty seeking: direct and mediated genetic effect. Addict Biol 2009;14:238−44.

[20] Kohnke MD, Batra A, Kolb W, Kohnke AM, Lutz U, Schick S, et al. Association of the dopamine transporter gene with alcoholism. Alcohol Alcohol 2005;40:339−42.

[21] Brewer III AJ, Nielsen DA, Spellicy CJ, Hammon SC, et al. Genetic variation of the dopamine transporter (DAT1) influences the acute subjective responses to cocaine in volunteers with cocaine use disorder. Pharmacogenet Genomics 2015;25:296−304.

[22] Kohnke MD, Kolb W, Kohnke AM, Schick S, Bartra A. DBH*444G/A polymorphism of the dopamine beta-hydroxylase gene is associated with alcoholism but not with sever alcohol withdrawal symptoms. J Neural Transm (Vienna) 2006;113:869−76.

[23] Baransel Isir AB, Oquzkan S, Nacak M, Gorucy S, et al. The catechol O-methyl transferase Val 158Met polymorphism and susceptibility to cannabis dependence. Am J Forensic Med Pathol 2008;29:320−2.

[24] Feinn R, Nellissery M, Kranzler HR. Meta-analysis of the association of a functional serotonin transporter promotor polymorphism with alcohol dependence. Am J Med Genet B Neuropsychiatr Genet 2005;133:79−84.

[25] Kweon YS, Lee HK, Lee CT, Pae CU. Association of the serotonin transporter gene polymorphism with Korean male alcoholics. J Psychiatr Res 2005;39:371−6.

[26] Gerra G, Garofano L, Santo G, Bosari S, et al. Association between low activity serotonin transporter genotype and heroin addiction: behavioral and personality correlates. Am J Med Genet B Neuropsychiatr Genet 2004;126B:37−42.

[27] Cao J, Liu X, Han S, Zhang CK, Liu Z, Li D. Association of the HTR2A gene with alcohol and heroin dependence. Hum Genet 2014;133:357−65.

[28] Cao J, LaRocque R, Li D. Associations of the 5-hydroxytryptamine (serotonin) receptor 1B gene (HTR1B) with alcohol, cocaine and heroin abuse. Am J Med Genet B Neuropsychiatr Genet 2013;162B:169−76.

[29] Yang J, Li MD. Association and interaction analyses of 5-HT3 receptor and serotonin transporter genes with alcohol, cocaine and nicotine dependence using SAGE data. Hum Genet 2014;133:905−18.

[30] Levran O, Peles E, Randesi M, Correa de Rosa J, et al. Susceptibility loci for heroin and cocaine addiction in the serotonergic and adrenergic pathway in populations of different ancestry. Pharmacogenomics 2015;16:1329−42.

[31] Fehr C, Sander T, Tadic A, Lenzen KP, Anghelescu I, Klawe C, et al. Confirmation of association of the GABRA2 gene with alcohol dependence by subtype-specific analysis. Psychiatr Genet 2006;16:9−17.

[32] Zintzaras E. Gamma-aminobutyric acid α receptor, a-2 (GABRA2) variants as individual marker for alcoholism: a meta-analysis. Psychiatr Genet 2012;22:189−96.
[33] Enoch MA, Hodgkinson CA, Yuan Q, Albaugh B, Virkkunen M, Goldman D. GABRG1 and GABRA2 as independent predictors for alcoholism in two populations. Neuropsychopharmacology 2009;34:1245−54.
[34] Loh EW, Higuchi S, Matsushita S, Murray R, Chen CK, Ball D. Association analysis of the GABA(A) receptor subunit genes cluster on 5q33-34 and alcohol dependence in a Japanese population. Mol Psychiatry 2000;5:301−7.
[35] Nishiyama T, Ikeda M, Iwata N, Suzuki T, et al. Haplotype association between GABAA receptor gamma2 subunit (GABRG2) and methamphetamine use disorder. Pharmacogenomics J 2005;5:89−95.
[36] Wu W, Zhu YS, Li SB. Polymorphisms in the glutamate decarboxylase 1 gene associated with heroin dependence. Biochem Biophys Res Commun 2012;422:91−6.
[37] Zalewska-Kaszubska J, Czarnecka E. Deficit in beta-endorphin peptide and tendency to alcohol abuse. Peptides 2005;26:701−5.
[38] Setiawan E, Pihl RO, Benkelfat C, Leyton M. Influence of OPRM1 A118G polymorphism on alcohol induced euphoria, risk of alcoholism and the clinical efficacy of naltrexone. Pharmacogenomics 2012;13:1161−72.
[39] Manini AF, Jacobs MM, Viahov D, Hurd YL. Opioid receptor polymorphism A118G associated with clinical severity in a drug overdose population. J Med Toxicol 2013; 9:148−54.
[40] Cerra G, Leonardi C, Cortese E, D'Amore A, et al. Human kappa opioid receptor gene (OPRK1) polymorphism is associated with opiate addiction. Am J Med Genet B Neuropsychiatr Genet 2007;144B:771−5.
[41] Zhang H, Kranzler HR, Yang BZ, Luo X, et al. The OPRD1 and OPRK1 loci in alcohol or drug dependence: OPRD1 variation modulates substance dependence risk. Mol Psychiatry 2008;3:531−43.
[42] Nikoshkov A, Drakenberg K, wang X, Horvath MC, et al. Opioid neuropeptide genotypes in relation to heroin abuse: dopamine tone contributes to reversed mesolimbic proenkephalin expression. Proc Natl Acad Sci USA 2008;105:786−91.
[43] Zuo L, Kranzler HR, Luo X, Covault J, Gelernter J. CNR1 variation modulates risk for drug and alcohol dependence. Bol Psychiatry 2007;62:616−26.
[44] Marcos M, Pastor I, de la Calle C, Barrio-Real L, Laso FJ, Gonzalez-Sarmiento R. Cannabinoid receptor 1 gene is associated with alcohol dependence. Alcohol Clin Exp Res 2012;36:267−71.
[45] Schacht JP, Hutchison KE, Filbey FM. Associations between cannabinoid receptor -1 (CNRI) variation and hippocampus and amygdala volumes in heavy cannabis users. Neuropsychopharmacology 2012;37:2368−76.
[46] Ishiguro H, Iwasaki S, Teasenfitz L, Higuchi S, Horiuchi Y, Satio T, et al. Involvement of cannabinoid CB2 receptor in alcohol preference in mice and alcoholism in humans. Pharmacogenomics 2007;7:380−5.

Methods of alcohol measurement

Introduction

Alcohol levels are measured in various bodily fluids including blood, breath, urine, and saliva. In addition, transdermal alcohol sensors are used in the criminal justice system. Alcohol measurements in various biological matrixes are summarized in Table 9.1. Blood alcohol is measured in both medical and legal situations while breath alcohol is measured only to identify a driver potentially driving with impairment. Although driving while intoxicated and driving under the influence (DUI) are very similar in nature, in some states DUI may indicate a lesser degree of impairment. Currently, in all states in the United States, the legal limit of driving is 0.08% alcohol in whole blood (serum alcohol level is higher than whole blood).

In general, alcohol is eliminated from blood following zero order kinetics and the average rate of elimination is 15 mg/dL/h, and ethanol in blood can be detected for 4–8 h after consumption depending amount of alcohol consumed. Interestingly, disappearance of alcohol from breath is similar to blood alcohol. Jones et al. reported that average disappearance rate of alcohol from venous blood was 15.2 mg/dL/h while average rate of disappearance of alcohol from breath was equivalent to 16.3 mg/dL/h of blood alcohol [1]. However, alcohol can be detected in urine longer than blood but only a small fraction of alcohol is excreted unchanged in urine. Alcohol testing in various specimens are listed in Table 9.1.

Alcohol measurement in blood

In general, whole blood alcohol level is determined using gas chromatography (GC) in a forensic laboratory while serum or plasma blood alcohol is determined in a hospital laboratory either by an enzymatic method or by using a GC. Because the legal limit for driving is 0.08% (80 mg/dL) of whole blood, if serum alcohol is used as evidence, it must be converted into whole blood alcohol. Rainey reported that the ratio between serum and whole blood alcohol ranged from 0.88 to 1.59 but the median value was 1.15. Therefore, dividing serum alcohol value by 1.15 provides whole blood alcohol concentration, or multiplying serum alcohol by 0.87 should also provide whole blood alcohol concentration [2]. In the United States alcohol concentration is reported as mg/dL but in many other countries alcohol concentration is expressed as mmol/L. The molecular weight of ethanol is 46. Therefore if ethanol concentration is expressed as mmol/L, it should be multiplied by 4.6 in order to get alcohol concentration in mg/dL.

Alcohol, Drugs, Genes and the Clinical Laboratory. DOI: http://dx.doi.org/10.1016/B978-0-12-805455-0.00009-9

Table 9.1 **Alcohol testing in various specimens**

Biological matrix for alcohol measurement	Comments
Whole blood or serum	Most common specimen for alcohol measurement. Alcohol is measured for medical purposes using serum (enzymatic method or gas chromatography) but legal alcohol is usually measured in whole blood using headspace gas chromatography
Urine	Not a common specimen for alcohol measurement but this matrix is usually used for legal alcohol determination and rarely for medical purposes
Breath	Exclusively used for legal purposes to identify drivers who are driving under the influence of alcohol with blood levels exceeding the legal limit (0.08%). Breathalyzers may utilize colorimetry, infrared spectroscopy, fuel cell technology, or mixed technology (infrared and fuel cell). Ignition lock devices also measure alcohol in exhaled breath and use similar techniques
Saliva	Saliva is an uncommon matrix for alcohol measurement
Swat	Transdermal alcohol sensor such as SCRAM is based on electrochemical determination of alcohol (fuel cell technology), which is excreted transdermally (approximately 1% of total alcohol consumed). Transdermal sweat alcohol is exclusively utilized in the criminal justice system

Gas chromatography: the gold standard

The gold standard for determination of blood alcohol is GC or gas chromatography/ mass spectrometry (GC/MS). Usually headspace GC is used for determination of alcohol in whole blood. However, direct injection of sample has also been described. Jain et al. described a gas chromatographic method where blood can be injected directly to a column after addition of isobutanol as the internal standard [3]. Smith et al. described determination of ethanol along with methanol, isopropanol, and acetone using capillary GC and direct sample injection. The author used 1-propanol (*n*-propanol) as the internal standard. Baseline separation was obtained between ethanol, other analytes, and the internal standard [4].

Several authors also used GC/MS for analysis of ethanol and related volatiles in biological specimens. Wasfi et al. developed static headspace capillary column gas chromatography combined with mass spectrometry (GC/MS) for analysis of ethanol along with acetone, methanol, acetaldehyde, and acetic acid in blood, using *n*-propanol as the internal standard [5]. Cordell et al. described a static headspace GC coupled with MS for quantitative analysis of acetaldehyde, methanol, ethanol, and acetic acid in headspace microvolume of blood using *n*-propanol as the internal standard [6]. Xiao et al. described a GC/MS method for analysis of whole blood ethanol using *n*-propanol as the internal standard. The mass spectrometer was operated in selected ion monitoring mode (ionization source: electron ionization), monitoring m/z 31 and 45 for ethanol and 31 and 59 for the internal standard. The method was linear for whole blood ethanol concentration between 4 and 126.3 mg/dL [7].

Methods based on alcohol dehydrogenase

In hospital laboratories, ethyl alcohol is also analyzed using enzymatic methods and automated analyzers. Enzyme-based automated methods are generally not applicable for analysis of whole blood. Enzymatic alcohol assay is based on the principle of conversion of alcohol to acetaldehyde by alcohol dehydrogenase and in this process nicotinamide adenine dinucleotide (NAD) is converted into NADH.

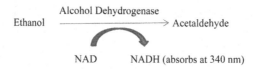

While NAD has no absorption at ultraviolet light at 340 nm wavelength, NADH absorbs at 340 nm. Therefore, an absorption peak is observed when alcohol is converted into acetaldehyde due to simultaneous conversion of NAD into NADH. The intensity of the peak is proportional to the amount of alcohol present in the specimen. If no alcohol is present, no peak is observed. However, other detection methods instead of direct UV detection at 340 nm have also been utilized in commercially available kits for serum or plasma alcohol analysis. Usually methanol, isopropyl alcohol, ethylene glycol, and acetone have a negligible effect on alcohol determination using enzymatic methods, but propanol if present may elevate true alcohol value by 15−20%. Although isopropyl alcohol, which is used as rubbing alcohol, is common in households, propanol is used in much lower frequency in household products.

The major interference in the enzymatic alcohol method is the interference of lactate dehydrogenase (LDH) and lactate, which may cause false positive alcohol levels in a patient suffering from lactic acidosis. In addition, enzymatic alcohol assay is unsuitable for determination of alcohol in postmortem serum due to high concentrations of LDH and lactate. Therefore, only GC can be used for measuring alcohol in a postmortem specimen. Badcock and O'Reilly reported false positive ethanol levels in the postmortem plasma of infants who died from sudden infant death syndrome using enzyme multiplied immunoassay technique (EMIT) alcohol assay, which utilizes alcohol dehydrogenase. The authors suspected elevated LDH and lactate as interfering substances causing such interferences and established that LDH concentration of 2800 U/L or higher and lactate concentration of 20 mmol/L or higher was needed for a false positive alcohol result. The mean plasma LDH value in sera of infants with falsely elevated alcohol by the EMIT assay was 6430 U/L, while mean plasma lactate level was 91 mmol/L, explaining the observed interference [8]. Lactate concentrations also tend to increase in trauma patients. Dunne et al. reported that 27% (3536) of 13,102 patients they studied had a positive alcohol screen (mean alcohol: 141 mg/dL; range: 10−508 mg/dL) [9]. In contrast, Winek et al. compared alcohol concentration obtained by an enzyme assay (Dimension Analyzer, Siemens Diagnostics) and GC in trauma patients and observed no false positive result using the enzyme assay [10]. Contrasting results may be related to differences in lactate concentrations in patients in two different studies.

Although elevated lactate and LDH are the major cause of interference in enzymatic alcohol method, other interferences have also been reported. Gharapetian et al. observed false positive ethanol levels in three patients with acetaminophen induced hepatocellular necrosis using EMIT alcohol assay and ADVIA 1650 analyzer (Siemens Diagnostics). However, when ethanol was measured by GC or Dade Behring Dimension Flex alcohol cartridge, no ethanol was detected in these specimens. The authors speculated that endogenous dehydrogenases and substrates other than LDH and lactate may be implicated in the NADH production causing false positive test results in these three patients using ADVIA 1650 analyzer [11]. Nonspecific interference in enzymatic alcohol assay has also been reported.

Breath alcohol measurement

Breath alcohol is measured using breathalyzers, which have been used as a reliable estimate of blood alcohol concentration since the 1970s. Evidentiary breathalyzers, which are approved by National Highway Traffic Safety Administration, are reliable for breath alcohol measurement and values are admissible to court as evidence. Although interlock devices in the car also work on the principle of breathalyzers, such devices are not designed for legal alcohol testing. The principle of breath alcohol measurement is partition of alcohol between blood and alveolar air. The estimated ratio between breath alcohol and blood alcohol is 1:2100 and this ratio is utilized in various breathalyzers to calculate blood alcohol level based on the concentration of ethanol in exhaled air by multiplying breath alcohol concentration expressed in mg/L with 2100 to produce blood alcohol concentration in mg/L (or multiply by 210 to obtain blood alcohol concentration in mg/dL). Some breathalyzer software may automatically calculate blood alcohol value from observed breath alcohol level.

How breathalyzers work?

Breathalyzers are based on various technologies. While most breathalyzers are based on a single technology, some analyzers may involve two different technologies in order to achieve higher precision and accuracy. These technologies are summarized

Table 9.2 Examples of breathalyzers based on different technologies

Technology	Examples of breathalyzers
Analyzers based on colorimetric detection due chemical reaction of reagents with alcohol	Breathalyzer 900, breathalyzer 1100
Infrared based technology	Intoxilyzer 5000, Intoxilyzer 8000, Data Master cdm
Fuel cell based technology	Alcotest models 6510, 6810, 7410, etc.
	Alco-Sensor III and IV
Mixed technology (infrared and fuel cell)	Intox EC/IR

in Table 9.2. The earliest developed breathalyzer was based on reaction of alcohol if present in the exhaled air with a cocktail of chemicals containing sulfuric acid, potassium dichromate, silver nitrate, and water. Silver nitrate catalyzes the reaction between alcohol and potassium dichromate in acidic medium. As a result the yellow color of the cocktail due to presence of potassium dichromate turns into green and the amount of alcohol in the exhaled air is estimated from the intensity of green color. This colormetric principle was adopted in the Breathalyzer first developed and marketed by Smith and Wesson and later sold to a German Company called Draeger. The old Breathalyzer 900 model was replaced by newer versions such as model 1100. However, this technology is subjected to interferences from a variety of substances.

There are many evidentiary breathalyzers that are based on the principle of infrared spectroscopy (IR spectroscopy) for quantitative determination of alcohol in exhaled air. The Intoxilyzer was originally developed by Omicron in Palo Alto, CA, and later sold to CMI, Inc., in Owensboro, KY. The earlier models were 4011 A, 4011 S, and then Intoxilyzer 5000 which is used as an evidentiary breath alcohol analyzer and more recently a Intoxilyzer 8000 model is commercially available. In addition to Intoxilyzer, Data Master cdm (National Patent Analytical System, Mansfield, OH), which can also be used as the evidentiary breathalyzer, is based on IR spectroscopy technology where alcohol is detected using two different wavelengths (3.37 and 3.44 μm).

There are several different brands of evidentiary breathalyzers which are based on the principle of fuel cell technology, e.g., Alcotest Models 6510, 6810, and 7410 (National Drager, Durango, Colorado), and Alco-Sensor III and IV (Intoximeters, Inc., St. Louis, MO). The fuel cell is a porous disk coated with platinum oxide (also called platinum black) on both sides. The porous layer is impregnated with an acidic solution containing various electrolytes so that charged particles such as hydrogen ions can travel through that medium. In addition, both sides of the disk containing platinum oxide are connected through a platinum wire. The manufacturer mounts this fuel cell in a case along with the entire assembly so that when a person blows to the disposable mouthpiece the air can travel through the fuel cell. If any alcohol is present in the exhaled air, then the alcohol is converted into acetic acid, hydrogen ion, and electrons on the top surface by the platinum oxide. Then hydrogen ions travel to the bottom surface and are converted into water by combining with oxygen present in the air. In this process, an electric current is generated and the microprocessor of the instrument then converts that current to equivalent breath alcohol as well as calculated blood alcohol.

Some evidentiary breathalyzers are based on both fuel cell and IR spectroscopy technology, giving them good sensitivity and specificity. Various models of Intox EC/IR I desktop evidentiary alcohol breath analyzers, also manufactured by Intoximeters, Inc., combine reliable fuel cell analysis with infrared technology. Semiconductor alcohol sensors are utilized in inexpensive breathalyzers marketed to the general public. However, sensor response is nonspecific to alcohol and response may be nonlinear. For example, semiconductor sensors will respond to particles and gases present in cigarette smoke [12].

Breath alcohol test is a single exhalation maneuver where a subject is asked to inhale air (preferably a full inhalation to total lung capacity) and then exhale (preferably a full exhalation to residual volume) into the breathalyzer instrument. The assumption is that alcohol concentration in exhaled breath is equal to that in alveolar air. In general ethanol levels in end-exhaled air is always lower than alveolar air. When performing a breath alcohol test, the subject is asked to inhale ambient air and exhale into the breathalyzer (usually 1.1−1.5 L of exhaled air is needed for the test). Therefore, a smaller subject with smaller lung capacity must exhale a greater fraction of air in their lungs to fulfill minimum volume requirement of the analyzer and as a result, the alcohol breath test may overestimate the blood alcohol level in the smaller subject compared to a larger subject with larger lung capacity [13].

Issues with breathalyzers

There are several issues that may produce a misleading breathalyzer reading. Sometimes a driver stopped by the police may use mouthwash to hide any alcoholic breath. Because some mouthwashes contain alcohol, use of a mouthwash prior to taking a breath alcohol analysis may cause falsely elevated breath alcohol result. However, residual alcohol evaporates from the mouth rapidly and a mandatory 15 min waiting time in the police station when no food or drink is allowed eliminates possibility of an elevated test result. Fessler et al. studied the effect of alcohol based substances such as mouthwash, cough mixture, and breath spray just prior to breath alcohol measurement using Drager Evidentiary portable breathalyzer and 25 volunteers. The authors concluded that a 15 min waiting period was necessary to ensure an accurate result [14]. Logan et al. evaluated the effect of asthma inhalers and nasal decongestant sprays on breath alcohol test and observed that the only product that had any effect on the breath alcohol test was Primatene Mist containing 34% ethyl alcohol, but alcohol was eliminated from the breath within 5 min. The authors concluded that a 15 min waiting period eliminated the possibility of a falsely elevated result [15]. Some energy drinks contain low amounts

Table 9.3 Interferences in breath alcohol test

- Propyl alcohol
- Isopropyl alcohol
- Methanol
- Toluene
- Xylene
- Ketogenic diet
- Glue sniffing

of alcohol but again, 15 min waiting time is sufficient to eliminate the possibility of a false positive test result using breathalyzer [16].

Laakso et al. studied the effect of various volatile solvents for potential interference with breath alcohol analysis using Drager 7110 evidentiary breathalyzer and concluded that acetone, methyl ethyl ketone, methyl isobutyl ketone, ethyl acetate, and diethyl ether did not interfere with breath alcohol measurement significantly but propyl alcohol and isopropyl alcohol had significant effects on breath alcohol measurement [17]. In addition, consuming the ketogenic diet may cause false positive test results [18]. Glue sniffing may also cause false positive breath alcohol test result because glue contains aliphatic hydrocarbons, ethyl acetate, and toluene [19]. Methanol poisoning is dangerous because it may cause death or blindness. Methanol poisoning may cause false positive test results with breathalyzer. In one report the authors observed that toluene, xylene, methanol, and isopropyl alcohol in exhaled air can be mistakenly identified as breath alcohol by the Intoxilyzer 5000 evidentiary breathalyzer [20]. Common interferences in breathalyzers are summarized in Table 9.3.

Urine alcohol determination

Urine ethanol determination is less common than breath alcohol tests or blood alcohol tests. In some workplaces drug testing urine alcohol tests may be conducted to monitor abstinence of a person through alcohol. Urine alcohol test may also be used by social service agencies, the criminal justice system, or in alcohol rehabilitation programs. Fraser et al. reported that only 1.6% specimens collected by social service agency in Nova Scotia, Canada, from parents with a history of drug abuse showed positive alcohol result [21].

In general, after consuming a moderate amount of alcohol, approximately 2% of the dose could be recovered in the urine after 7 h. Uncontrolled diabetes mellitus may cause glycosuria and if yeast infection is present, in vitro production of alcohol may result after collection because *Candida albicans* can produce alcohol from glucose. Therefore, storing urine at 4°C and using 1% sodium fluoride or potassium fluoride as a preservative is essential to avoid such in vitro generation of alcohol after collecting urine specimens. Most urine alcohol tests are performed for legal purposes. Therefore, headspace GC is the preferred analytical method for urine alcohol testing. However, serum enzymatic alcohol assay can be modified to measure urine alcohol using automated analyzers.

Saliva alcohol determination

Urine, sweat, and saliva are all body fluids derived from serum and contain alcohol. Saliva can be collected noninvasively and can be used for determination of alcohol concentration although the breath alcohol test is more commonly used compared to saliva alcohol testing. Nevertheless, saliva alcohol may be used to monitor abstinence although monitoring ethyl glucuronide, an alcohol biomarker, is superior to direct alcohol measurement in showing abstinence due to a longer window of detection of ethyl glucuronide compared to saliva alcohol. In general, ethanol levels in saliva correlate with blood alcohol levels [22].

Onsite alcohol testing devices such as quantitative ethanol detector saliva alcohol tests can be used to measure saliva ethanol level. The test is based on enzymatic oxidation of alcohol by alcohol dehydrogenase. Saliva is collected using a cotton swab, which can be inserted into the analyzer. Each test could be read by a color bar and the test has a built-in quality control check that indicates if the test is performed properly. The test can measure saliva ethanol levels up to 150 mg/dL. Jones commented that alcohol levels determined by the QED device correlated well with blood and breath alcohol levels, indicating that this device could be used for quick analysis of ethanol in saliva [23]. However, Bendtsen et al. did not observe a good correlation between QED saliva ethanol and breath or blood alcohol levels [24].

Alco-Screen saliva dipstick is an inexpensive and easy to use colorimetric test that provides a semiquantitative estimation of alcohol. Schwartz et al. compared salivary alcohol levels with blood alcohol levels in 53 patients suspected of ingesting alcohol. The authors concluded that although correlation was good with blood alcohol levels of around 100 mg/dL, for lower alcohol levels between 20 and 50 mg/dL, performance of Alco-Screen test was unsatisfactory [25]. Recently Cirado-Garcia et al. reported GC-differential mobility spectrometry for detection of alcohol, ethylene glycol, and gamma-hydroxybutyric acid in human plasma [26]. Jung et al. described a simple colorimetric device attached to a smartphone for analysis of salivary alcohol [27].

Transdermal alcohol sensors

Some alcoholic individuals are viewed as posing a risk to the general public, and as a result court may order them to completely abstain from alcohol. Approximately 1% of ingested alcohol is excreted through the skin, mostly through "insensible perspiration," which is vapor that escapes through the skin when a person sweats, but it cannot be detected by the olfactory system. There is a good correlation between alcohol concentrations in vapor above the skin and blood alcohol. Therefore, transdermal alcohol could be measured by putting a portable electrochemical sensor directly above the skin and the alcohol levels in insensible perspiration can be used to estimate blood alcohol level. Secure Continuous Remote Alcohol Monitor (SCRAM) is the first ankle worn transdermal alcohol monitoring device (Alcohol Monitoring System, Littleton, CO). Wrist transdermal alcohol sensor (WrisTAS was developed initially by Giner, Inc. (Newton, MA) [28]. Another transdermal alcohol detection device which is also an ankle worn device is commercially available for transdermal alcohol monitoring from BI Incorporated (Boulder, CO). However, there is a lag time of between 33 and 60 min between observation of peak blood alcohol and peak transdermal alcohol depending on amount of alcohol consumed [29].

SCRAM device uses fuel cell technology which is a similar technique widely used in breathalyzer. The device measures alcohol concentration every 60 min unless a measurable alcohol level is detected and then taking samples every 30 min until the reading drops below 0.02% (20 mg/dL). The device also records the temperature and skin reflectance using infrared light to provide data that detects attempts to remove the device, or tampering. The device automatically transmits information stored in the ankle bracelet via a modem to a secure web server through a telephone line. Barnett et al. studied performance of SCRAM device using 66 heavily drinking adults who wore the device between 1 and 28 days and reported their alcohol consumption daily by web-based survey. On days when bracelets were functional, 502 out of 690 drinking episodes (72.8%) were detected by remote sensing data and no gender difference was observed. However, for consumption of fewer than five drinks, women's drinking episodes were more likely to be detected than men's drinking episodes due to higher transdermal alcohol levels in women, but for five or more drinks, no gender difference was observed [30]. Currently, transdermal devices do have some limitations and more research is needed for further improvement of such devices [31].

Can alcohol be produced endogenously?

Endogenous production of alcohol (auto-brewery syndrome) is a common defense strategy adopted by some individuals charged with DUI of alcohol. A small amount of alcohol is produced endogenously but it should not alter blood alcohol levels. Jones et al. reported that endogenous alcohol levels varied from none detected to 1.6 μg/mL (0.16 mg/dL), which is negligible [32]. Madrid et al. studied eight patients with liver cirrhosis and observed that during fasting no patient showed any endogenous ethanol level but after meals two patients showed serum alcohol levels of 11.3 and 8.2 mg/dL while another four patients showed negligible values [33]. In general, healthy individuals as well as patients with metabolic disease such as diabetes, hepatitis, or cirrhosis showed blood alcohol levels ranging from 0 to 0.08 mg/dL due to endogenous production of alcohol, which is negligible.

The dermal absorption of alcohol is usually negligible. However, keratinized stratum, which gives adult skin a barrier, begins to develop in the seventh month of fetal life and poorly keratinized skin of a preterm baby may be a poor barrier for alcohol. Haprin and Rutter described a case of a premature infant with 27 weeks of gestation who developed severe hemorrhagic skin necrosis on the back and buttocks after umbilical arterial catheterization. The infant showed a blood ethanol level of 259 mg/dL and a blood methanol level of 26 mg/dL. Before catheterization baby's skin was cleaned with methylated spirit, which caused elevated blood ethanol and methanol due to percutaneous absorption [34].

Conclusions

Alcohol testing may be for medical or legal purposes. In general, blood alcohol measured by headspace GC is the gold standard and is the preferred method for legal alcohol determination. The legal limit of driving in all states is 0.08% whole blood. Sometimes medical alcohol determined by an enzymatic method may be admissible to court as evidence, but medical alcohol determined in serum is higher than whole blood alcohol and serum blood alcohol must be converted into whole blood alcohol in order to determine if the defendant exceeds the legal limit for driving. Breath alcohol determination using an evidentiary breathalyzer is also admissible to a court as evidence. More recently transdermal alcohol sensors are used in the criminal justice system, to monitor sobriety of an individual. However, these devices have certain limitations.

References

[1] Jones AW, Norberg A, Hahn RG. Concentration-time profiles of ethanol in arterial and venous blood and end-expired breath during and after intravenous infusion. J Forensic Sci 1997;42:1088−94.
[2] Rainey P. Relation between serum and whole blood ethanol concentrations. Clin Chem 1999;39:2288−92.
[3] Jain NC. Direct blood injection method for gas chromatographic determination of alcohols and other volatile compounds. Clin Chem 1971;17:82−5.
[4] Smith NB. Determination of volatile alcohols and acetone in serum by non-polar capillary gas chromatograph after direct sample injection. Clin Chem 1984;30:1672−4.
[5] Wasfi A, Al-Awadhi AH, Al-Hatali ZN, Al-Rayami FJ, Al-Katheeri NA. Rapid and sensitive static headspace gas chromatography-mass spectrometry method for the analysis of ethanol and abused inhalants in blood. J Chromatogr B Analyt Technol Biomed Life Sci 2004;799:331−6.
[6] Cordell RL, Pandya H, Hubbard M, Turner MA, Monks PS. GC-MS analysis of ethanol and other volatile compounds in micro-volume blood samples-quantifying neonatal exposures. Ann Bioanal Chem 2013;405:4139−47.

[7] Xiao HT, He L, Tong RS, Yu JY, Chen L, Zpou J, et al. Rapid and sensitive headspace gas chromatography-mass spectrometry method for the analysis of ethanol in the whole blood. J Clin Lab Anal 2014;28:386–90.

[8] Badcock NR, O'Reilly DA. False positive EMIT-st ethanol screen with post-mortem infant plasma. Clin Chem 1992;38:434.

[9] Dunne JR, Tracy JK, Scalea TM, Napolitano L. Lactate and base deficit in trauma: does alcohol or drug use impair predictive accuracy? J Trauma 2005;58:959–66.

[10] Winek CL, Wahba WW, Windisch R, Winek CL. Serum alcohol concentrations in trauma patients determined by immunoassays versus gas chromatography. Forensic Sci Int 2004;139:1–3.

[11] Gharapetain A, Holmes DT, Urquhart N, Rosenberg F. Dehydrogenases interference with enzymatic ethanol assays: forgotten but not gone. Clin Chem 2008;54:1251–2.

[12] Swift R. Direct measurement of alcohol and its metabolites. Addiction 2003;98 (Suppl. 2):73–80.

[13] Hlastala MP, Anderson JC. The impact of breathing pattern and lung size on the alcohol breath test. Ann Biomed Eng 2007;35:264–72.

[14] Fessler CC, Tulleners FA, Howitt DG, Richrads JR. Determination of mouth alcohol using the Drager Evidential Portable Alcohol System. Sci Justice 2008;48:16–23.

[15] Logan BK, Distefano S, Case GA. Evaluation of the effect of asthma inhalers and nasal decongestant sprays on a breath alcohol test. J Forensic Sci 1998;43:197–9.

[16] Lutmer B, Zurfluh C, Long C. Potential effect of alcohol content in energy drinks on breath alcohol testing. J Anal Toxicol 2009;33:167–9.

[17] Laakso O, Pennanen T, Himbwerg K, Kuitunen T, Himberg JJ. Effect of eight solvents on ethanol analysis by Drager 7110 evidentiary breathalyzer. J Forensic Sci 2004;49:1113–16.

[18] Jones AW, Rossner S. False positive breath alcohol test after a ketogenic diet. Int J Obesity (London) 2007;31:559–61.

[19] Aderjan R, Schmitt G, Wu M. Glue solvent as the cause of breath alcohol value of 1.96 permille. Blutalkohol 1992;29:360–4. [article in German].

[20] Caldwell JP, Kim ND. The response of the Intoxilyzer 5000 to five potential interfering substances. J Forensic Sci 1997;42:1080–7.

[21] Fraser AD. Urine drug testing for social service agencies in Nova Scotia, Canada. J Forensic Sci 1998;43:194–6.

[22] Gubala W, Zuba D. Gender differences in the pharmacokinetics of ethanol in saliva and blood after oral ingestion. Pol J Pharamcol 2003;55:639–44.

[23] Jones AW. Measuring ethanol in saliva with QED enzymatic test device: comparison of results with blood and breath alcohol concentrations. J Anal Toxicol 1995;19:169–74.

[24] Bendtsen P, Hultberg J, Carlsson M, Jones AW. Monitoring ethanol exposure in a clinical setting by analysis of blood, breath, saliva and urine. Alcohol Clin Exp Res 1999;23:1446–51.

[25] Schwartz RH, O'Donnell RM, Thorne MM, Getson PR, Hicks JM. Evaluation of colorimetric dipstick to detect alcohol in saliva: a pilot study. Ann Emerg Med 1989;18:1001–3.

[26] Cirado-Garcia L, Ruszkiewicz DM, Eiceman GA, Thomas CL. A rapid and non-invasive method to determine toxic levels of alcohols and g-hydroxybutyric acid in saliva samples by gas chromatography-differential mobility spectrometry. J Breath Res 2016;10:017101.

[27] Jung Y, Kim J, Awofeso O, Kim H, et al. Smartphone based colorimetric analysis for detection of saliva alcohol concentration. Appl Opt 2015;54:9183–9.

[28] Hawthrone JS, Wojcik MH. Transdermal alcohol measurement: a review of literature. Can Soc Forensic Sci J 2006;39:65–71.
[29] Webster GD, Gabler HC. Feasibility of transdermal ethanol sensing for the detection of intoxicated drivers. Annu Proc Assoc Adv Automot Med 2007;51:449–64.
[30] Barnett NP, Meade EB, Glynn TR. Predictors of detection of alcohol use episodes using a transdermal alcohol sensor. Exp Clin Psychopharmacol 2014;22:86–96.
[31] Leffingwell TR, Cooney NJ, Murphy JG, Luczak S, Rosen G, Dougherty DM, et al. Continuous objective monitoring of alcohol use: twenty-first century measurement using transdermal sensors. Alcohol Clin Exp Res 2013;37:16–22.
[32] Jones AW, Mardg G, Anggard E. Determination of endogenous ethanol in blood and breath by gas chromatography-mass spectrometry. Pharamcol Biochem Behav 1983;18(Suppl. 1):267–72.
[33] Madrid AM, Hurtado C, Gatica S, Chacon I, Toyos A, Defilippi C. Endogenous ethanol production in patients with liver cirrhosis, motor alteration and bacterial overgrowth. Rev Med Chil 2002;130:1329–34.
[34] Harpin V, Rutter N. Percutaneous alcohol absorption and skin necrosis in a preterm infant. Arch Dis Child 1982;57:477–9.

Laboratory methods for measuring drugs of abuse in urine

Introduction

There are two types of drugs of abuse testing: medical drug testing and legal drug testing. Medical drug testing is often conducted in a hospital clinical laboratory to screen for presence of any drug in the urine specimen of a person admitted to the emergency department with a suspicion of drug overdose. Moreover, a physician may conduct a urine drug test to ensure compliance of a patient with opioid pain medication or therapy with benzodiazepine. Medical drug testing may be conducted in a hospital laboratory setting using an automated analyzer and U.S Food and Drug Administration (FDA) approved immunoassays, or using a suitable FDA approved point of care device in a physician's office setting. Results obtained during medical drug testing cannot be used in any legal context and such results are also protected by patient's privacy act such as Health Insurance Portability and Accountability Act regulations. Legal drug testing has more stringent regulations than medical drug testing. Workplace drug testing is considered as legal drug testing because results can be used to deny employment to a new hire, or a current employee can be terminated based on positive drug testing results.

Medical versus legal drug testing

Legal drug testing was initiated by President Reagan, who issued executive order number 12,564 on September 15, 1986. This executive order directed drug testing for all federal employees who are involved in law enforcement, national security, protection of life and property, public health, and other services requiring a high degree of public trust. Following this executive order, the National Institute of Drug of Abuse was given the responsibility of developing guidelines for federal drug testing. Currently Substance Abuse and Mental Health Services Administration (SAMHSA), affiliated with Department of Health and Human Services of the Federal Government, is responsible for providing mandatory guidelines for federal work place drug testing. Bush summarized guidelines for legal drug testing [1].

Although Reagan's executive order was not intended for private employers, currently a majority of fortune 500 companies have policies for workplace drug testing. Drug abuse costs American industry and public an estimated $100 billion a

Alcohol, Drugs, Genes and the Clinical Laboratory. DOI: http://dx.doi.org/10.1016/B978-0-12-805455-0.00010-5

year, but workplace drug testing can provide a better work environment, improves
the morale of employees, and is very effective in preventing work related accidents.
Therefore, developing a cost effective corporate work place drug testing program
which meets federal guidelines, is capable of standing legal challenge and is also
accepted by employees, is the objective of any workplace drug testing program [2].
Several publications have established large negative correlations between workplace
drug testing and employee substance abuse [3].

In medical drug testing, informed consent may not be taken from a patient. An
overdosed patient admitted to the emergency department may not be able to grant
an informed consent anyway. In contrast, in workplace or any other legal drug
testing program, obtaining an informed consent prior to testing is mandatory.
Another major difference between medical and legal drug testing is that in medical testing an initial positive screening result obtained by using immunoassays
may not be confirmed by using gas chromatography combined with mass spectrometry (GC/MS), but in legal drug testing GC/MS confirmation is mandatory.
In addition, a chain of custody must be maintained in legal drug testing indicating
all personnel that have possession of the specimen from the time of collection to
the time of reporting results. Chain of custody is not usually initiated in medical
drug testing. Therefore, a medical drug testing result may not be able to stand a
legal challenge.

Commonly tested drugs

Traditionally, five SAMHSA mandated drugs for federal workplace drug testing
include amphetamine, cocaine (tested as benzoylecgonine, the inactive metabolite),
opiates, phencyclidine (PCP), and marijuana tested as 11-nor-9-carboxy-Δ^9-tetrahy-
drocannabinol (THC-COOH) the inactive metabolite of marijuana. In a 2015 revision to proposed guidelines, SAMHSA recommended additional testing for
oxycodone, oxymorphone, hydrocodone, and hydromorphone [4]. Although these
drugs are more frequently tested, currently there is no industry standard and different laboratories may have different panels for drug testing [5]. Some private
employers may test for additional drugs in their workplace drug testing protocols
and such comprehensive drug panels may include barbiturates, benzodiazepines,
methadone, methaqualone, and propoxyphene.

Cut-off concentrations and detection window
of drugs in urine

For drug testing in urine, depending on the particular drug, either the parent drug or
its metabolite is targeted. For SAMHSA mandated drugs, recommended cut-off
concentrations for both immunoassay and GC/MS of various drugs are available.

Table 10.1 Screening and confirmation cut-off concentrations of various drugs

Drug class/drug	Target analyte in urine	Screening cut-off (ng/mL)	Confirmation cut-off
Amphetamine/ methamphetamine[a]	Amphetamine/ methamphetamine	500	250 ng/mL
MDMA/MDA/ MDEA[a]	MDMA	500	250 ng/mL for MDMA/ MDA/MDEA
Cocaine[a]	Benzoylecgonine	150[b]	100 ng/mL
Opiates[a]	Morphine	2000[b]	2000 ng/mL for either drug
Heroin[a]	6-Monoacetyl-morphine	10	10 ng/mL
Marijuana[a]	THC-COOH[c]	50	15 ng/mL
Phencyclidine[a]	Phencyclidine	25	25 ng/mL
Barbiturates[d]	Secobarbital	200/300	200 ng/mL
Benzodiazepines[d]	Oxazepam/nor-diazepam and others	200/300	200 ng/mL
Hydrocodone/ hydromorphone[e]	Hydrocodone	300	100 ng/mL for either drug
Oxycodone/ oxymorphone[e]	Oxycodone	100	50 ng/mL for either drug
Propoxyphene[d]	Propoxyphene	300	300 ng/mL
Methadone[d]	Methadone or EDDP	300	100 ng/mL

MDMA, 3,4-methylenedioxymethamphetamine; MDA, 3,4-methylenedioxyamphetamine; MDEA, 3,4-methylenedioxyethylamphetamine.
[a]Included in original SAMHSA guidelines. For amphetamine analysis, methamphetamine is the target drug but for reporting positive methamphetamine, its metabolite amphetamine must be present at a concentration of 100 ng/mL or higher.
[b]Private employer may use 300 ng/mL cut-off for screening and confirmation.
[c]THC-COOH, 11-nor-Δ^9-tetrahydrocannabinol-9-carboxylic acid.
[d]Non-SAMHSA drugs.
[e]From new SAMHSA proposed guidelines (2015).

In general, such guidelines are also followed in medical drug testing. Screening and confirmation cut-off of common drugs that are tested in both medical legal drug testing are given in Table 10.1. Usually a drug or its metabolites can only be detected in urine for a limited time after last abuse. However, detection time also varies according to the dosage administered, as well as characteristics of screening and confirmation assay. For example, marijuana (Δ^9-tetrahydrocannabinol, THC) tested as marijuana metabolite (THC-COOH) is detectable in urine for 2−4 days (using 50 ng/mL cut-off) but for more frequent use, it may be detected for up to 1 month. Widows of detection of various drugs in urine are summarized in Table 10.2.

Table 10.2 Window of detection of SAMHSA mandated drugs in urine

Drug	Detection window
Amphetamine/ methamphetamine	2 days
MDMA	2 days
Cocaine as benzoylecgonine	2–4 days
Opiates	Morphine/codeine: 3 days
Heroin as 6-monoacetyl morphine	12 hours to 1 day
Heroin as morphine	2 days
Hydrocodone/hydromorphone	3 days
Methadone	3 days
Oxycodone/oxymorphone	3 days
Marijuana as THC-COOH	2–3 days after single use, 30 days for chronic use
Propoxyphene	3 days
Phencyclidine	8 days
Barbiturates	Short acting (pentobarbital, secobarbital, etc.): 3 days Long acting (phenobarbital): 15 days
Benzodiazepine	Short acting (e.g., triazolam): 2 days Intermediate acting (e.g., lorazepam, temazepam): 5 days Long acting (e.g., diazepam): 10 days

Methodologies for drug testing

Immunoassays are widely used as the first step of drug screening in both medical and workplace drug testing programs. Immunoassays can be easily automated and several drugs can be analyzed using one urine specimen and results can be directly downloaded in laboratory information system. In general, competitive immunoassays are used for drugs of abuse testing. Various commercially available immunoassays are available for drug testings including fluorescence polarization immunoassays (FPIAs), enzyme multiplied immunoassay technique (EMIT), cloned enzyme donor immunoassay (CEDIA), turbidimetric immunoassay, kinetic interaction of microparticle in solution (KIMS). The ONLINE Drugs of Abuse Testings immunoassays marketed by Roche Diagnostics (Indianapolis, IN) are based on KIMS format. All of these immunoassays are homogenous immunoassays where separation between bound and free label is not necessary before measuring the signal.

In the heterogeneous immunoassays format the bound label is physically separated from the unbound labels before signal is measured. The separation is often done magnetically, where the reagent analyte (or its analog) is provided as coupled to paramagnetic particles (PMPs), and the antibody is labeled. Conversely, the antibody may be also provided as conjugated to the PMP, and the reagent analyte may carry the label. After separation and wash, the bound label is reacted with other reagents to generate the signal. This is the mechanism in many chemiluminescent immunoassays, where the label may be a small molecule which generates the chemiluminescent signal. The label also may be an enzyme (enzyme immunoassay, EIA, or enzyme-linked immunosorbent assay, ELISA) which generates chemiluminescent, fluorometric, or colorimetric signal.

Usually multiple calibrators (four to six levels) are recommended for accurate measurements of the analyte across the entire assay range in an immunoassay although two point calibrations are also used. Most automated assay systems can store a calibration curve depending on the assay stability on that system. Therefore, when a sample is analyzed during the period denoted by calibration stability, the assay signal is automatically converted into analyte concentration via the stored calibration curve. Drugs of abuse assays are often used to report "qualitative" results, i.e., positive or negative with respect to a certain analyte concentration (the "cutoff" level). Thus, many of the assays come in qualitative or quantitative formats and in most cases such formats are defined by assay protocol and calibration. In qualitative formats, the calibration can be simplified to two calibrators, centering on the cut-off point, thus providing the most accuracy around that point. The algorithm compares the signal observed with a sample with that of the cutoff calibrator and reports the result as positive or negative. Semiquantitative results can be reported with a calibration curve containing a minimum of three calibrator samples; often the combination of the zero-calibrator, together with two or more calibrators at or near cutoff level, is used to generate a calibration curve. Obviously, such assay formats will have increased inaccuracy at analyte concentrations much higher than the cut-off concentration.

In general, immunoassays used for drug of abuse testing target a specific drug or a metabolite. The major limitation of immunoassays is that an antibody may cross-react with a structurally similar drug causing false positive test results. Therefore, initial drug screening should be confirmed by GC/MS or liquid chromatography combined with mass spectrometry (LC−MS) or tandem mass spectrometry (LC−MS/MS). Eichhorst proposed use of LC−MS for rapid screening and confirmation of the presence of abused drugs in urine specimen as an alternative to immunoassay screening [6].

Analysis of amphetamine class

In general, immunoassays for amphetamines can detect not only amphetamine and methamphetamine but also 3,4-methylenedioxymethamphetamine (MDMA). However, certain amphetamine immunoassays may have lower capability of detecting MDMA and 3,4-methylenedioxyamphetamine (MDA) due to lower cross-reactivity of the antibody used for MDMA and MDA. Poklis et al. reported that the EMIT d.a.u monoclonal amphetamine/methamphetamine immunoassay has a cutoff concentration of 3000 ng/mL for racemic MDMA but only 800 ng/mL for MDA. The assay had higher sensitivity for detecting the S(+) isomer of both

MDMA and MDA [7]. The Roche Abuscreen ONLINE amphetamine immunoassay also has low cross-reactivity toward MDMA but higher cross-reactivity of MDA [8]. However, MDMA is metabolized to MDA and this assay may be able to identify individuals abusing MDMA.

Amphetamine immunoassays may not be sensitive enough to detect amphetamine-like designer drugs other than MDMA and MDA. Kerrigan et al. evaluated cross-reactivities of 11 designer drugs with 9 various commercially available immunoassays. These 11 designer drugs included in the study were 2,5-dimethoxy-4-bromophenylethylamine (2C-B), 2,5-dimethoxyphenethylamine (2C-H), 2,5-dimethoxy-4-iodophenethylamine (2C-I), 2,5-dimethoxy-4-ethylthio-phenethylamine (2C-T-2), 2,5-dimethoxy-4-isopropylthiophenethylamine, 2,5-dimethoxy-4-propylthiophenethylamine (2C-T-7), 2,5-dimethoxy-4-bromo-amphetamine (DOB), 2,5-dimethoxy-4-ethylamphetamine (DOET), 2,5-dimethoxy-4-iodoamphetamine (DOI), 2,5-dimethoxy-4-methylamphetamine (DOM), and 4-methylthioamphetamine (4-MTA). Cross-reactivities of these designer drugs with immunoassays studied were <0.4% and even at a concentration of 50,000 ng/mL. Therefore, these designer drugs cannot be detected by amphetamine immunoassays. However, 4-MTA was the only drug that demonstrated 5% cross-reactivity with the Neogen amphetamine ELISA assay (Lexington, KY) but a significant 200% cross-reactivity with the Immunalysis amphetamine ELISA assay (Pomona, CA) [9].

Apollonio et al. reported that 4-MTA had 280% cross-reactivity with the Bio-Quant Direct ELISA assay for amphetamine [10]. Petrie et al. concluded that some amphetamine like designer drugs at concentrations 20,000 ng/mL may produce positive result with various amphetamine immunoassays but existing immunoassays unevenly detect amphetamine-like designer drugs, particularly the 2C series, piperazine, and beta-keto class (synthetic cathinone; bath salts) [11]. However, a specific immunoassay is available for screening of bath salts if present in urine (see chapter: Designer Drugs Including Bath Salts and Spices). In addition, LC−MS or the GC/MS methods are capable of detecting the presence of these drugs or their metabolites in urine specimens. Kerrigan et al. described a GC/MS protocol for analysis of 2C-B, 2C-H, 2C-I, 2C-T-2, 2C-T-7, 4-MTA, DOB, DOET, DOI, and DOM in urine specimens [12]. The presence of synthetic cathinone in urine can also be confirmed by GC/MS or LC−MS/MS.

Amphetamine and methamphetamine have optical isomers designated d (or $+$) for dextrorotatory and l (or $-$) for levorotatory and the d isomers, the more physiologically active compounds, are the intended targets of immunoassays because d isomers is abused. Ingestion of medications containing the l isomer can cause false−positive results. For example Vicks inhaler contains the active ingredient l-methamphetamine and extensive use of this product may cause false−positive results for immunoassay screening. Specific isomer resolution procedures must be performed to differentiate the d and l isomers because routine confirmation by GC/MS does not identify isomer composition unless chiral derivatization of amphetamine and methamphetamine is performed prior to GC/MS confirmation. Poklis et al. reported relatively high concentrations of l-methamphetamine observed in two subjects (1390 and 740 ng/mL respectively) after extensively inhaling Vicks inhaler every hour for several hours. Nonetheless, urine specimens tested negative by the EMIT II amphetamine/methamphetamine assay even after such extensive use of Vicks inhaler [13].

However, many over the counter cold medications containing ephedrine or pseudoephedrine may cause false positive amphetamine test result due to cross-reactivity with assay antibodies. Ranitidine is a H_2 receptor blocking agent (antihistamine) which reduces acid production by the stomach and is available over the counter without any prescription. Dietzen et al. reported that ranitidine, if present in urine at a concentration over 43 μg/mL, may cause a false positive amphetamine screen test result using Beckman SYNCHRON immunoassay reagents (Beckman Diagnostics, Brea, CA). This concentration of ranitidine is expected in patients taking ranitidine at the recommended therapeutic dosage [14]. Casey et al. reported that bupropion, a monocyclic antidepressant and an aid for smoking cessation, may cause false positive screen results using the EMIT II amphetamine immunoassay [15]. Trazodone, an antidepressant, interferes with both amphetamine and MDMA assays. Baron et al. demonstrated that the trazodone metabolite metachlorophenylpiperazine is responsible for the interference [16].

Labetalol, a beta-blocker commonly used for control of hypertension in pregnancy, can cause false positive amphetamine screen results using an immunoassay. A labetalol metabolite, which is structurally similar to amphetamine and methamphetamine, is responsible for the interference [17]. The antidepressant desipramine and the antiviral agent amantadine also interfere with amphetamine immunoassays [18]. Vorce et al. showed that dimethylamylamine (DMAA), aliphatic amine naturally found in geranium flowers but also used in body building natural supplements such as Jack3d and OxyELITE Pro may cause false positive test results with a KIMS amphetamine assay (Roche Diagnostics) and the EMIT II Plus amphetamine assay if present at a concentration of 6900 ng/mL, due to structural similarity of DMAA with amphetamine. DMMA has been promoted as a safe alternative to ephedrine. The authors further analyzed 134 urine specimens which were tested false positive for amphetamine but confirmed negative by GC/MS and did not contain any known drugs that may cause false positive amphetamine test results and observed the presence of DMAA in 92.3% of specimens, with concentrations varying from 2500 to 67,000 ng/mL [19]. Common drugs that may cause false positives with amphetamine immunoassays are listed in Table 10.3.

Confirmation of amphetamine class

In general amphetamine immunoassay positive specimens are confirmed by using GC/MS. Amphetamine and methamphetamine can be extracted from urine using solid phase extraction or liquid—liquid extraction. However, derivatization is needed prior to GC/MS analysis. For nonchiral derivatization, commonly used agents include pentafluoropropionic anhydride, heptafluorobutyric anhydride, trifluoroacetic anhydride, 4-carboethoxyhexafluorobutyryl chloride, N-methyl-N-tert-butyldimethylsilyl trifluoroacetamide, N-trifluoroacetyl-1-propyl chloride, 2,2,2-trichloroethyl chloroformate, etc. However, pentafluoropropionic anhydride

Table 10.3 Common drugs that may cause false positive test results with amphetamine immunoassay

Drug	Comments
Decongestants	Decongestants such as ephedrine, pseudoephedrine, and phenylephrine are most commonly encountered drugs (present in many over the counter cold medications) that cause false positive amphetamine immunoassay screen result
Antihistamine	Brompheniramine and ranitidine may cause false positive test result
Appetite suppressant	Phentermine causes false positive result with amphetamine immunoassay
Antidepressant	Bupropion causes false positive test result. Trazodone also causes false positive test result due to cross-reactivity of its metabolite meta-chlorophenylpiperazine with assay antibody. Desipramine and trimipramine may also cause false positive test result
Antipsychotics	Chlorpromazine and promethazine may cause false positive test result
Beta-blocker	Labetalol may cause false positive test result
Antimalarial	Chloroquine if present in high concentration in urine may cause false positive test result
Antiviral/ antiparkinsonian	Amantadine may cause false positive result with amphetamine immunoassay
Herbal supplement	Dimethylamylamine interferes with amphetamine immunoassay

and heptafluorobutyric anhydride are commonly used. Deuterated amphetamine and methamphetamine can be used as internal standard. MDMA and MDA can be confirmed by GC/MS using similar extraction and derivatization protocol.

Ephedrine/pseudoephedrine if present in urine may cause a false positive test result if injector port temperature at the gas chromatograph is 300°C. This is due to thermal transformation of ephedrine/pseudoephedrine causing an artifact peak which was misidentified as methamphetamine. Lowering injector port temperature can circumvent such a problem [20]. For differentiating d-methamphetamine from l-amphetamine, chiral derivatization using l-N-trifluoroacetyl-1-propyl chloride can be used prior to GC/MS confirmation [21]. Wang et al. reported chiral separation and determination of methamphetamine and its metabolite amphetamine using liquid chromatography electrospray ionization tandem mass spectrometry operating in the positive ion multiple-reaction monitoring mode. The chiral column (Chirobiotic V2) was used to separate optical isomers [22].

Analysis of cocaine as benzoylecgonine

Cocaine abuse is usually confirmed by detecting the presence of benzoylecgonine, an inactive metabolite of cocaine in the urine. In general the antibodies used in cocaine immunoassays are specific for benzoylecgonine and these assays, unlike amphetamine immunoassays, demonstrate good specificity as well as sensitivity. However, life-threatening acute cocaine overdose may not be identified by urine toxicological screenings because sufficient concentration of benzoylecgonine may not be present in urine after severe acute overdose of cocaine. In one case report, where the person died from cocaine overdose, the urine drug test was negative for cocaine using EMIT assay. Later GC/MS analysis confirmed that the concentration of benzoylecgonine was only 75 ng/mL while the concentration of cocaine in the urine was only 55 ng/mL in the urine specimen. The immunoassay cut-off concentration of 300 ng/mL cannot detect such low levels of benzoylecgonine. Moreover, cocaine has poor cross-reactivity with the antibody specific for benzoylecgonine. However, the heart blood concentration of cocaine in the deceased was 18,330 ng/mL, explaining the cause of death as cocaine overdose [23].

Although cocaine and cocaethylene can be analyzed by GC/MS without derivatization, benzoylecgonine must be derivatized prior to analysis by GC/MS. Common derivatives are trimethylsilyl and pentafluoropropionyl derivatives although benzoylecgonine can also be analyzed after methylation. Fluconazole, an antifungal agent, does not produce false negative test results with cocaine immunoassays, but it may cause false negative results in the GC/MS confirmation step using trimethylsilyl derivative because derivatized fluconazole elutes with derivatized benzoylecgonine. However, such interference can be eliminated using a pentafluoropropionyl derivative of benzoylecgonine because derivatized benzoylecgonine elutes before derivatized fluconazole [24].

Importantly, positive cocaine test results, both by immunoassay screening and GC/MS confirmation method, may occur after drinking coca tea. Mazor et al. reported that when five healthy subjects drank a cup of coca tea, all urine specimens tested positive for cocaine (as benzoylecgonine) 2 h after ingestion and three out of five participant's urine specimens remained positive for up to 36 h post ingestion. Mean urinary benzoylecgonine concentration in all specimens was 1777 ng/mL. This was due to the presence of cocaine in coca tea [25].

Analysis of opioids

In order to circumvent false positive test results due to ingestion of poppy seed contained in food in opiate assays, the current SAMHSA guideline recommends a cut-off of 2000 ng/mL for opiate screening tests. However, private employers may still use the old cut-off concentration of 300 ng/mL for opiate and consumption of poppy seed contained in food can easily result in a positive screening as well as confirmation of codeine and morphine by GC/MS. The antibody in the opiate immunoassay targets morphine but can detect codeine. However, many opioids such as oxycodone, oxymorphone, methadone, fentanyl, meperidine, and propoxyphene show poor cross-reactivity with various opiate assays. Smith et al. commented that in general immunoassays for opiates displayed substantially lower sensitivity for detecting 6-keto opioids, and urine specimens containing low to moderate amounts of hydromorphone, hydrocodone, oxymorphone, and oxycodone will likely be negative if analyzed using opiate immunoassays [26]. However, specific immunoassays such as DRI oxycodone assay, DRI hydrocodone/hydromorphone assay, as well as specific immunoassays for detecting methadone, propoxyphene, and fentanyl are commercially for detecting such opioids.

Heroin is first metabolized to 6-acetylmorphine and then further transformed into morphine by a liver enzyme. Presence of 6-monoacetylmorphine (6-acetylmorphine) in urine is considered as confirmation of heroin abuse. Although 6-acetylmorphine is further metabolized into morphine, which can be detected easily by a standard opiate immunoassay, there are also commercially available immunoassays for detection of 6-acetylmorphine in urine at a cut-off concentration of 10 ng/mL.

Buprenorphine is a morphine-based semisynthetic opioid which is a partial antagonist of mu-opioid receptors in the brain. This drug is used in addiction treatment and also has analgesic properties. However, the morphine antibody used in opiate immunoassay does not detect the presence of buprenorphine. In order to monitor compliance of buprenorphine therapy, a specific immunoassay that is designed for detecting buprenorphine in urine must be used. Hull et al. reported that using a 5 ng/mL cut-off concentration, results obtained by using the CEDIA buprenorphine immunoassay agreed 97.9% time with results obtained by using liquid chromatography combined with tandem mass spectrometry (LC/MS/MS) [27].

Opiate immunoassays like other immunoassays also suffer from providing false positive test results due to presence of various cross-reacting substances other than opioids in urine specimens. Certain quinolone antibiotics may cause false positive test results with opiate immunoassay screening. Baden evaluated potential interference of 13 commonly used quinolones (levofloxacin, ofloxacin, pefloxacin, enoxacin, moxifloxacin, gatifloxacin, trovafloxacin, sparfloxacin, lomefloxacin, ciprofloxacin, clinafloxacin, norfloxacin, and nalidixic acid) with various opiate immunoassays (at 300 ng/mL cut-off concentration) and observed that levofloxacin and ofloxacin may cause false positive opiate test results with assays manufactured by Abbot Laboratories for application on the AxSYM analyzer (Abbott Laboratories, Abbott Park, IL). In addition, such interferences were also observed with CEDIA, EMIT II, and Abuscreen ONLINE assay (Roche Diagnostics, Indianapolis, IN). Moreover, pefloxacin administration may cause false positives with CEDIA, EMIT II, and Abuscreen ONLINE assay, gatifloxacin with CEDIA and EMIT II assays, lomefloxacin, moxifloxacin, ciprofloxacin, and norfloxacin with the Abuscreen ONLINE assay [28]. Rifampicin is used in treating tuberculosis and may cause false positive test results with opiate immunoassays such as the (KIMS methods assay on the Cobas Integra analyzer (Roche Diagnostics, Indianapolis, IN). A false positive result may be observed even after 18 h of administration of a single oral dose of 600 mg of rifampicin [29]. Interferences in opiate immunoassays are summarized in Table 10.4.

False positive test results with methadone immunoassays due to the presence of interfering substance in urine have also been reported. In one report, the authors

Table 10.4 Interferences in immunoassays (false positive results) for opiate, methadone, marijuana, phencyclidine, benzodiazepines, and barbiturates

Immunoassay	Interfering drugs
Opiate	Levofloxacin, ofloxacin, pefloxacin, gatifloxacin, lomefloxacin, moxifloxacin, ciprofloxacin, and norfloxacin
Methadone	Quetiapine, diphenhydramine, doxylamine, and verapamil metabolites
Marijuana	Niflumic acid, efavirenz, ibuprofen, and naproxen
Phencyclidine	Dextromethorphan, ibuprofen, metamizole, thioridazine, and venlafaxine
Benzodiazepine	Oxaprozin and sertraline
Barbiturates	Ibuprofen and naproxen

observed false positive methadone test results using the Cobas Integra Methadone II test kit (Roche Diagnostics) in three schizophrenia patients treated with quetiapine monotherapy. The authors used a 300 ng/mL cut-off concentration of methadone in urine specimens for their screening of urine specimens. However, no methadone was detected in the plasma specimen of any patient using LC−MS [30]. Rogers et al. reported positive methadone urine drug test results in a patient using the One Step Multi-Drug, Multi-Line Screen Test Devices (ACON Laboratories, San Diego, CA), a point of care device for urine drug screen. The patient had no history of methadone exposure but ingested diphenhydramine. The GC/MS confirmatory test failed to detect presence of methadone in the urine specimen, confirming that the presumptive methadone test result was a false positive result. When drug free urine specimens were supplemented with diphenhydramine, false positive methadone tests were also observed using the point of care device [31]. Doxylamine intoxication may cause false positive results with both EMIT d.a.u opiate and methadone assays. The urine doxylamine concentration needed to cause positive test result was 50 μg/mL for methadone and 800 μg/mL for opiate [32]. Verapamil metabolites also interfere with methadone assay for the application on Olympus AU5000 analyzer [33]. Interferences in methadone immunoassays are summarized in Table 10.4.

Confirmation of opioids

Codeine is metabolized to morphine and then morphine is conjugated with glucuronic acid to form morphine-3-glucuronide and morphine-6-glucuronide. Other opioids are also metabolized and then conjugated. Therefore, these glucuronide metabolites must be hydrolyzed into free drugs prior to extraction for GC/MS analysis. Both acid hydrolysis and enzymatic hydrolysis can be used to generate free drug but enzyme hydrolysis using beta-glucuronidase may require much longer incubation time unless elevated temperature is used to accelerate enzymatic hydrolysis. Although morphine and codeine can be analyzed after derivatization to respective pentafluoropropionyl or trimethylsilyl derivative, keto opioids such as oxycodone and oxymorphone may cause problems during quantification. One approach to circumvent this problem is to use hydroxylamine to convert keto-opioids into oxime derivative and followed by a second derivatization step. In this approach multiple opioids can be analyzed in one run.

Broussard et al. described a method for simultaneous identification and quantitation of codeine, morphine, hydrocodone, and hydromorphone in urine as trimethylsilyl and oxime derivatives using GC/MS. After adding deuterated codeine, morphine, hydrocodone, and hydromorphone in urine the authors hydrolyzed conjugated metabolites already present in urine using beta-glucuronidase. For achieving complete hydrolysis the specimen was incubated at 56°C for 2 h with beta-glucuronidase. After hydrolysis, aqueous hydroxylamine was added for derivatization of keto opiates. Then derivatized hydrocodone, hydromorphone along with free morphine, codeine, and internal standards were extracted from urine using solid phase bonded silica extraction columns (Varian, Palo Alto, CA). Further derivatization (trimethylsilyl derivatives) was performed using N-O-bis (trimethylsilyl) trifluoroacetamide and trimethylchlorosilane followed by analysis using GC/MS. The mass spectrometer was operated under selected ion monitoring mode and ions selected for codeine were m/z 243, 343, and 371 while ions selected for d_3-codeine were 346 and 374. For quantitation, m/z 371 (for codeine) and 374 (for d_3-codeine) were selected. Similarly for morphine ions selected were m/z 234, 401, and 429 while for d_3-morphine ions selected were 417, and 432. Again m/z 429 and 432 were used for quantitation. For hydrocodone m/z 297, 371, and 386 were selected and for d_3-hydrocodone m/z 300 and 389 were selected. For quantitation, m/z 386 and m/z 389 were selected. For analysis of hydromorphone m/z 355, 429, and 444 were chosen while for analysis of d_3-hydromorphone m/z 358 and 447 were selected. For quantification, m/z 355 and m/z 358 were used [34].

Various opioids can also be analyzed using LC−MS/MS. Cone et al. used LC-MS/MS for analysis of codeine, nor-codeine, morphine, hydrocodone, nor-hydrocodone, hydromorphone, dihydrocodeine, oxycodone, nor-oxycodone, and oxymorphone in urine after hydrolysis of conjugates using beta-glucuronidase [35]. Yang et al. also used LC−MS/MS for analysis of morphine, codeine, hydromorphone, hydrocodone, oxymorphone, oxycodone, 6-acetylmorphine, methadone, buprenorphine, nor-buprenorphine, fentanyl, and nor-fentanyl after hydrolysis of glucuronides conjugates with beta-glucuronidase. The authors used deuterated morphine and fentanyl as internal standards [36].

Analysis of marijuana

The active component of marijuana, Δ^9-tetrahydrocannabinol (THC) is metabolized into 11-nor-Δ^9-tetrahydrocannabinol-9-carboxylic acid (THC-COOH). Then THC-COOH is conjugated with glucuronic acid. The immunoassays for marijuana target THC-COOH. Passive inhalation of marijuana should not cause false positive test results with immunoassays because in one study, the maximum concentration of the THC-COOH was only 7.8 ng/mL after volunteers were exposed to passive inhalation of marijuana smoke [37]. Similarly use of hemp oil should not produce positive marijuana test results because hemp seeds are washed with water prior to extraction of oil, a procedure that removes traces of marijuana from the seed hull. However, prescription use of synthetic marijuana (Marinol) should cause positive marijuana test results. However, marijuana immunoassays do not cross-react with synthetic cannabinoids if present in the urine specimen.

Although uncommon, false positive marijuana test results may occur during the screening step due to cross-reactivity from other compounds which are not illicit drugs. Boucher et al. described a case of a 3-year old girl who was hospitalized because of behavioral disturbance of unknown cause. The only remarkable finding in her medication history was the suppositories of niflumic acid which was initiated 5 days before hospitalization. After admission her urinary toxicology screen was positive for the presence of marijuana metabolite but parents strongly denied such exposure. Further analysis of the specimen using chromatography failed to confirm the presence of marijuana metabolite but niflumic acid was detected in the specimen. The authors concluded that the false positive marijuana test result was due to the presence of niflumic acid in the urine specimen [38]. The antiviral agent efavirenz is known to cross react with marijuana immunoassays. In one study the authors analyzed 30 urine specimens collected from patients receiving efavirenz using the Rapid Response Drugs of abuse test strips, the Beckman Coulter SYNCHRON marijuana immunoassay (Beckman Coulter, Brea, CA), and the Roche Diagnostic's Cannabinoid II assay. Only the Rapid Response test strips demonstrated positive marijuana test results in 28 out of 30 specimens while the 2 other immunoassays did not show any interference from efavirenz. As expected, GC/MS confirmation failed to demonstrate the presence of marijuana metabolite in any of these 30 specimens analyzed [39]. Nonsteroidal drugs naproxen and ibuprofen may cause false positive test results with marijuana immunoassay [40]. Interferences in marijuana immunoassays are summarized in Table 10.4.

Confirmation of THC-COOH

In urine, THC-COOH is mostly present as glucuronic acid conjugate. Therefore hydrolysis of glucuronide derivative is necessary. In one report the authors used d_9-THC-COOH as the internal standard. After adding the internal standard in the urine specimen, hydrolysis of conjugated metabolite of THC was achieved by heating the specimen with 6 M sodium hydroxide solution for 20 min at 56°C. Then free THC-COOH along with the internal standard was extracted using hexane/ethyl acetate (9:1 by vol) followed by derivatization using N-methyl-(N-trimethylsilyl) trifluoroacetamide (MSTFA)/ammonium iodide/ethanethiol (380:1:2 by vol). Then trimethylsilyl-iodide derivative of THC was analyzed by GC/MS [41]. The GC/MS analysis of THC-COOH can be also be achieved by derivatization of THC-COOH with MSTFA alone to produce trimethylsilyl derivative of THC [42]. Another method for derivatization of THC-COOH is using a reagent mixture of tetramethylammonium hydroxide and iodomethane. In addition, absorptive loss of THC-COOH usually takes place upon storage if the urine pH is acidic. Plastic containers also tend to absorb THC-COOH on prolonged storage [43]. LC-MS/MS can also be used for analysis of THC-COOH. Lee et al. described a protocol for analysis of THC-COOH and formoterol in urine using LC-MS/MS after hydrolysis of THC-COOH glucuronide using beta- glucuronidase. The authors used d_9-THC-COOH and d_6-formoterol as internal standards [44].

Analysis of phencyclidine

False positive test results may occur in phencyclidine (PCP) immunoassays due to cross-reactivity of several drugs with various commercially available immunoassays. Dextromethorphan is an antitussive agent which is found in many over the counter cough and cold medications. Ingesting high amounts of dextromethorphan (over 30 mg) may result in positive false positive test results with opiate and phencyclidine (PCP) immunoassays. In one report, the authors observed three false positive phencyclidine tests in pediatric urine specimens using an on-site testing device (Instant-View Multi-Test drugs of abuse panel; Alka Scientific, Designs, Poway, CA). The authors concluded that false positive PCP tests were due to the cross-reactivities of ibuprofen, metamizole, dextromethorphan, and their metabolites with the PCP assay [45]. Thioridazine is known to cause false positive PCP tests with both EMIT d.a.u. and EMIT II phencyclidine immunoassays [46]. Venlafaxine and its metabolites also may cause false positive PCP test with immunoassay [47]. For GC/MS confirmation of phencyclidine, no derivatization is necessary. Deuterated phencyclidine can be used as the internal standard.

Analysis of benzodiazepines

Benzodiazepine immunoassays may use antibodies that recognize oxazepam but cross-react with a variety of other benzodiazepines. However, certain benzodiazepines may have poor cross-reactivity. In addition, many benzodiazepine metabolites are conjugated before being excreted in urine and such glucuronide metabolites may have poor cross-reactivity with the antibody used in the assay design. After therapeutic use, the drug concentration may be below the 200 ng/mL cut-off and result may be false negative using an immunoassay. Therefore, benzodiazepine immunoassay may not be appropriate for monitoring compliance of a patient with a drug in the benzodiazepine class. Dixon et al. reported that even after hydrolysis of glucuronide conjugates using beta-glucuronidase, the EMIT benzodiazepine assay showed a false negative rate of 35% (all specimens showed benzodiazepine level of 200 ng/mL or more using LC-MS/MS) indicating that benzodiazepine immunoassays have limitations for monitoring compliance of patients receiving prescription benzodiazepines [48].

Clonazepam is metabolized to 7-aminoclonazepam. West et al. reported that when urine specimens collected from subjects taking clonazepam were tested using the DRI benzodiazepine immunoassay at 200 ng/mL cut-off, only 38 specimens out of 180 tested positive by the immunoassay (21% positive). However, using LC/MS/

MS, 126 specimens out of 180 specimens tested positive (70% positive) using the same cut-off concentration 200. The authors proposed a lower cut-off level of 40 ng/mL for monitoring patients receiving clonazepam [49].

Flunitrazepam (Rohypnol) although not approved by FDA is encountered in date rape situations. Forsman et al., using a CEDIA benzodiazepine assay at a cut-off of 300 ng/mL, failed to obtain positive results in the urine of volunteers after they received a single dose of 0.5 mg flunitrazepam. In addition, only 22 out of 102 urine specimens collected from volunteers after receiving the highest dose of flunitrazepam (2 mg) showed positive screening test results using the CEDIA benzodiazepine assay [50]. Kurisaki et al. reported that the Triage benzodiazepine assay has low sensitivity in detecting estazolam, brotizolam, and clotiazepam. Therefore, a negative result in a Triage test may not mean the absence of these drugs in the urine specimen [51]. In another report, the authors demonstrated that the Abuscreen ONLINE benzodiazepine assay (Roche Diagnostics) has 96% specificity but only 36% sensitivity because all urine specimens containing lorazepam and lormetazepam (as confirmed by GC/MS) tested negative by the immunoassays due to poor cross-reactivities of these drugs with the antibody used in the assay [52]. However, oxaprozin, a nonsteroidal antiin-flammatory drug may cause false positive test results with CEDIA, EMIT, and FPIA benzodiazepine immunoassays using a cut-off of 200 ng/mL [53]. Sertraline may also cause false positive test results with benzodiazepine immunoassays [54]. Interferences in benzodiazepine immunoassays are summarized in Table 10.4.

Confirmation of benzodiazepines

Benzodiazepines are metabolized followed by conjugation before being excreted in urine. Therefore hydrolysis of conjugate using beta-glucuronidase prior to extraction is recommended. Benzodiazepines and their metabolites can be analyzed by GC/MS as trimethylsilyl derivatives, which can be prepared by using N-O-bis (trimethylsilyl) trifluoroacetamide [55]. Instead of trimethylsilyl derivative, tert-butyl-dimethylsilyl derivatives can also be used for GC/MS analysis and such derivatization can be achieved by using N-methyl-N-(tert-butyldimethylsilyl)-trifluoroacetamide. West and Ritz analyzed oxazepam, nor-diazepam, desalkyl-flurazepam, temazepam, and alpha-hydroxy-alprazolam by GC/MS using tert-butyldimethylsilyl derivatives. The authors used d_5-oxazepam, d_5-nor-diazepam, and d_5-alpha-hydroxyalprazolam as internal standards [56]. LC-MS/MS can also be analyzed for analysis of various benzodiaze-pines. Jeong et al. analyzed various benzodiazepines, zolpidem, and their metabolites using LC−MS/MS where urine specimens were mixed with deuterated internal stan-dards and after centrifugation, an aliquot was directly injected into LC−MS/MS [57].

Analysis of barbiturates

Barbiturate immunoassays can recognize a wide variety of barbiturates including amobarbital, butalbital, pentobarbital, secobarbital, and phenobarbital. Secobarbital is used as a calibrator in several commercially available immunoassays for barbiturates. Acute ingestion of ibuprofen and chronic ingestion of naproxen may cause false positive test results with barbiturate immunoassay [40]. Interferences in barbiturates immunoassays are summarized in Table 10.4.

For GC/MS confirmation of barbiturates, hydrolysis of conjugated metabolites using beta-glucuronidase is carried out prior to extraction using an organic solvent such as ethyl acetate. Solid phase extraction of barbiturates (after adjusting urine pH to 7) using Bond-Elute extraction column has also been described. After extraction, methylation of barbiturates/metabolites can be achieved using iodomethane and tetra-methylammonium hydroxide by using dimethyl sulfoxide as a solvent followed by analysis using GC/MS. The authors used d_5-pentobarbital as an internal standard [58]. Barbiturates can also be analyzed by GC/MS as tert-butyldimethylsilyl deriva-tive using methyl-N-(tert-butyldimethylsilyl) trifluoroacetamide [59]. Johnson and Garg described a GC/MS protocol for analysis of amobarbital, butalbital, pentobarbi-tal, phenobarbital, and secobarbital in urine and serum after extraction of these drugs from urine or serum using acidic phosphate buffer and methylene chloride. The authors used flash methylation technique where the dried organic extract was mixed with trimethylanilinium hydroxide and ethyl acetate and then injected into the GC/MS. The derivatization was achieved at the hot injector port. Barbital was used as the internal standard [60].

Issues with urine adulteration

For medical drug testing, specimen adulteration may not be an issue because a patient overdosed with drugs and being admitted to the hospital is unable to adulter-ate a urine specimen. However, for workplace drug testing, people may try to beat a drug testing in three different ways:

- Substitute the urine with synthetic urine or drug free urine purchased from a clandestine source
- Drink a commercially available product to flush out drugs
- Add adulterants to the urine specimen in vitro to beat drug test

However, drug testing laboratories routinely perform "Specimen Validity Testing" to identify adulterated urine specimens before analysis because many adul-terants are capable of invalidating immunoassay screening steps while some adul-terants may invalidate both immunoassay screening and GC/MS confirmation. At the collection site, the temperature of the urine specimen must be determined and the temperature should be between 90°F and 100°F. SAMHSA guidelines also require further testing of all specimens for specimen integrity starting November 1, 2004. Then in 2008, updated guidelines were published in Federal Register. According to these guidelines, every laboratory involved in Federal workplace drug testing must perform following tests:

- Analysis of creatinine in urine
- Analysis of specific gravity if creatinine is less than 20 mg/dL
- Analysis of pH of every urine specimen

- Performing one or more validity tests for the presence of oxidizing adulterants
- Performing additional tests if the specimen appears abnormal or responses obtained during analytical steps indicate presence of an adulterant

Although initial testing of creatinine, specific gravity, and pH can be measured using specially designed colorimetric urine dipsticks, for establishing a specimen as adulterated or substituted, pH must be measured by a pH meter, specific gravity by a refractometer and urine creatinine by a suitable chemistry analyzer. Refractometers either manual or digital can provide accurate specific gravity readings of up to several decimal points.

Criteria for diluted, substituted, and adulterated urine

The normal creatinine concentration of urine varies from 20 to 400 mg/dL and specific gravity from 1.005 to 1.030. The normal pH of human urine is 4.5−8.0. A specimen is considered diluted when creatinine concentration is greater than 2 mg/dL but less than 20 mg/dL and the specific gravity is greater than 1.0010 but less than 1.0030 on a single aliquot. A specimen is considered substituted if creatinine concentration is less than 2 mg/dL in both initial and confirmatory tests and specific gravity is less than or equal to 1.0010 or greater than or equal to 1.0200 on initial and confirmatory specific gravity test using a refractometer on two separate aliquots. If the pH is less than 3 or greater than 11 (colorimetric tests on the first aliquot and confirmatory test by a pH meter in the second aliquot) the specimen is considered as adulterated. The presence of nitrite at a concentration of 500 μg/mL or higher is considered as adulterated urine. Moreover, chromium (VI) at a concentration of 50 μg/mL or higher is also indicative of adulterated urine. The presence of halogen, glutaraldehyde, pyridine (due to adulteration with pyridinium chlorochromate (PCC)), or surfactant confirmed at a level greater than or equal to the laboratory's limit of detection also indicates adulterated urine.

Urine specimens that do not meet the criteria above but clearly are not normal should be reported as invalid specimens. When creatinine concentration and specific gravity show discrepancy and are not consistent with normal physiological range, specimen is considered as invalid. Moreover, when pH is between 3 and 4.5 or between 9 and 11 where acceptable immunoassay screening of specimen may produce inaccurate results, the specimen is considered invalid. In addition, if nitrite concentration is 200 μg/mL or more but less than 500 μg/mL, the specimen may be considered as invalid. A specimen is also considered invalid if oxidant activity is detected in the specimen but no particular oxidant can be identified [1]. Moreover, if specimen contains a substance that is not a normal constituent of urine, e.g., a high amount of diuretic, the specimen may also be considered invalid.

Analytical methods for detecting adulterant: an overview

The SAMHSA guidelines indicate that initial screening of nitrite can be performed by a nitrite colorimetric test or general adulterant colorimetric test but the confirmation must be conducted using multiwavelength spectrophotometry, capillary electrophoresis, or ion chromatography. The initial presence of chromate may be detected by a general colorimetric chromium test or colorimetric test for oxidants but confirmatory test must be performed using atomic absorption spectrophotometry, multiwavelength spectrophotometry, ion chromatography, capillary electrophoresis, or inductively couple plasma MS. The presence of halogen should be screened by using a general oxidant colorimetric test (500 μg/mL or more equivalent of nitrite/50 μg/mL or more equivalent of chromate) but initial positive tests must be confirmed using multiwavelength spectrophotometry, ion chromatography, or inductively coupled plasma MS. The presence of glutaraldehyde can be determined by an aldehyde test but confirmation is needed and can be achieved by using GC/MS. The presence of pyridine (e.g., PCC) at a concentration of 50 μg/mL must also be confirmed. The presence of surfactant is verified by using a surfactant colorimetric test with an equal or greater than 100 μg/mL dodecylbenzene sulfonate equivalent and confirmation at the same level by using a different analytical method, e.g., multiwavelength spectrophotometry.

For initial screening of a specimen for the presence of oxidants, DRI General Oxidant-Detect test (Microgenics, Fremont, CA) may be used which also can be easily adopted on automated chemistry analyzer. The assay is based on the reaction between the substrate tetramethylbenzidine and oxidant present in the specimen producing color that can be measured spectrophotometrically at 660 nm (DRI General Oxidant-Detect test package insert) and is capable of detecting the presence of nitrite, PCC, and Stealth if present in urine. In addition, initial adulteration checks can also be performed by using specialized urine dipsticks such as AdultaCheck 4, AdultaCheck 6, AdultaCheck 10, or Intect 7. AdultaCheck 10 is available from Sciteck (Asheville, NC) which tests for specific gravity, pH, oxidants, creatinine, nitrite, aldehyde, chromate, peroxidase, and halogen/bleach. Intect 7 test strip for checking adulteration in urine is composed of seven different pads to test for creatinine, nitrite, glutaraldehyde, pH, specific gravity, bleach, and PCC. However, initial results must be confirmed by different analytical methods. Criteria for diluted, substituted, adulterated, and invalid specimens and their effectiveness in identifying adulterated urine specimens are summarized in Table 10.5.

Effectiveness of specimen validity testings in detecting adulterated specimens

People also try to beat drug tests by adulterating urine with a variety of products including household chemicals and urinary adulterants available through Internet sites. Specimen integrity testing is very helpful to identify many such adulterants. For example, adulteration with sodium chloride at a concentration necessary to produce false negative results using immunoassays requires a specific gravity of over 1.035. Vinegar, laundry bleach, hand soap, Drano, sodium bicarbonate, sodium hypochlorite, concentrated lemon juice, if used as adulterants result in pH outside

Table 10.5 Criteria for diluted, substituted, adulterated, and invalid specimen urine specimen

Specimen	Criteria (any one)	Application for detecting adulterated specimen
Diluted specimen	• Creatinine is greater than 2 mg/dL but less than 20 mg/dL and the specific gravity is greater than 1.0010 but less than 1.0030 on a single aliquot	• Ingesting detoxifying agent and drinking lots of water will produce dilute urine with creatinine below 20 mg/dL and low specific gravity • Diluting urine specimen after collection with tap water will have similar effect • Adulterated specimen containing sodium chloride usually shows specific gravity of 1.035 or more
Substituted specimen	• Creatinine is less than 2 mg/dL in both initial and confirmatory test and specific gravity is less than or equal to 1.0010 or greater than or equal to 1.0200 on initial and confirmatory specific gravity test using a refractometer on two separate aliquots	• If urine specimen is substituted these criteria can identify such specimen
Adulterated specimen	• The pH is less than 3 or greater than 11 • Nitrite confirmation test indicates nitrite at a level of 500 µg/mL or more • Chromium (VI) confirmed at 50 µg/mL or higher • Glutaraldehyde is present • Pyridine (pyridinium chlorochromate) is present • Surfactant is present at 100 µg/mL dodecylbenzene sulfonate equivalent or higher	• The pH test is effective in detecting adulterated specimens using household chemicals such as vinegar, lemon juice, laundry bleach, soap, etc. • Nitrite, glutaraldehyde, chromium, and pyridine tests detect commonly available Internet based urinary adulterants except zinc sulfate
Invalid	• Creatinine concentration and specific gravity values are discrepant and outside physiological range • Urine pH is either 3.0–4.5 or 9–11, which may invalidate immunoassay screening step • Nitrite between 200 and less than 500 µg/mL • The presence of oxidant is confirmed but no particular oxidant identified	• These tests are helpful in detecting many Internet based urinary adulterants except zinc sulfate

the acceptable range. However, Visine eye drop is capable of producing false negative tests with marijuana. The presence of Visine eye drops in adulterated urine cannot be determined by urine specimen integrity testing.

Many urinary adulterants are available through the Internet but many such urine adulterants may contain the same active ingredient. Wu et al. reported that the active ingredient of "Urine Luck" was PCC, a strong oxidizer which caused significantly decreased response rate for all EMIT II drug screens indicating the possibility of false negative results. However, Wu et al. also described a simple spot test using 1,5-diphenylcarbazide in methanol (10 gm/L) to detect the presence of PCC in urine (reddish purple color developed in the presence of PCC) [61]. The DRI General Oxidant-Detect test can detect the presence of PCC in urine. In addition, urine dipsticks such as AdultaCheck 10, Intect 7, etc., have specific reaction pads for detecting PCC. However, the presence of PCC should be confirmed by a different analytical method. Other adulterants available through the Internet such as "Clear Choice," "Lucky Lab LL 418," "Randy's Klear II," and "Sweet Pea's Spoiler" also contain PCC and have similar effects on drugs of abuse testing as Urine Luck.

The product "Klear" is supplied in the form of two small tubes containing 500 mg of white crystalline material which Elsohly et al. identified as potassium nitrite and also provided evidence that nitrite adulteration caused interference in both immunoassay screening and GC/MS confirmation of THC-COOH. However, a bisulfite step at the beginning of sample preparation could eliminate such a problem [62]. Spot tests are available for detecting the presence of nitrite in urine. Addition of a few drops of a nitrite adulterated urine specimen to 0.5 mL of 1% potassium permanganate solution followed by addition of a few drops of 2N hydrochloric acid turned the pink permanganate solution colorless with effervescence. Another spot test to detect nitrite used 1% potassium iodide solution. Addition of a few drops of nitrite adulterated urine to 0.5 mL of potassium iodide solution followed by addition of a few drops of 2N hydrochloric acid resulted in immediate release of iodine from the colorless potassium iodide solution. If any organic solvent such as hexane was added the iodine was readily transferred in the organic layer giving the layer a distinct color of iodine [63]. Specialized urine dipsticks have a specific pad for detecting nitrite. The DRI General Oxidant-Detect test is also capable of detecting nitrite if present in the adulterated urine. However, a different analytical method must be used for confirmation.

Stealth is an adulterant which consists of two vials, one containing a powder (peroxidase), and another vial containing a liquid (hydrogen peroxide). Both products should be added to the urine specimen in order to cheat the drug test. Stealth is capable of invalidating immunoassay screening of marijuana, lysergic acid diethylamide, and opiates using both Roche ONLINE assays and CEDIA assays if these drug or metabolites are present in modest concentrations (125–150% of cutoff values). In addition, GC/MS confirmation could also be affected [64]. Valtier and Cody described a rapid spot test to detect the presence of Stealth in urine. Addition of 10 μL of urine to 50 μL of TMB (Tetramethylbenzidine) working solution followed by addition of 500 μL of 0.1 M phosphate buffer solution caused the specimen to turn dark brown. Peroxidase activity could also be monitored by using a spectrophotometer [65]. If Stealth is present, the DRI General Oxidant-Detect test should be able to detect its presence. Moreover, urine dipsticks can also be used for detecting the presence of Stealth in urine.

Glutaraldehyde-containing products such as "UrinAid" are one of the first to appear on the market to invalidate drugs of abuse testing. Glutaraldehyde at a concentration of 0.75% volume could lead to false negative screening results for a cannabinoid test using the EMIT II drugs of abuse screen. At 2% glutaraldehyde concentration almost all EMIT II assays were affected. Wu et al. also described a simple fluorometric method for the detection of glutaraldehyde in urine. When 0.5 mL of urine was heated with 1.0 mL of 7.7 mmol/L potassium dihydrogen phosphate (pH 3.0) saturated with diethyl-thiobarbituric acid for 1 h at 96−98°C in a heating block, a yellow−green fluorophore developed if glutaraldehyde was present. Shaking the specimen with n-butanol resulted in the transfer of this adduct to the organic layer, which could be viewed under long wavelength UV light. Glutaraldehyde in urine could also be estimated using a fluorometer [66]. Specialized urine dipsticks have a pad for detecting glutaraldehyde.

Zinc sulfate has recently been promoted as an effective urinary adulterant to invalidate drug tests by several websites that provide tips to beat drug testing. Zinc sulfate at a concentration 15 ng/mL has been reported to cause false negative test results with EMIT assays for opiates, marijuana, benzoylecgonine, phencyclidine. At a higher concentration of 50 ng/mL all tests except amphetamines were affected. Spot tests are available for detecting the presence of zinc sulfate in urine. Addition of 3−4 drops of 1N sodium hydroxide solution to approximately 1 mL of urine containing zinc sulfate resulted in formation of a white precipitate (zinc hydroxide), which was soluble in excess sodium hydroxide. In the second spot test, addition of 3−4 drops of 1% sodium chromate solution to 1 mL of urine containing zinc sulfate followed by addition of 4−5 drops of 1N sodium hydroxide resulted in formation of a yellow precipitate (zinc chromate) [67]. Although not specifically applied for analysis of adulterate urine, atomic absorption, or inductively coupled plasma MS may be used for confirmation. However, concentration of zinc in adulterated specimens is very high and it must be diluted significantly prior to analysis.

Conclusions

Although immunoassays are widely used for screening purpose, presumptive positive specimens must be confirmed by a different analytical technique preferably GC/MS or LC−MS/MS in legal drug testing. However, confirmation may or may not be performed during medical drug testing. Urine is the most commonly used specimen for drugs of abuse testing and also for monitoring compliance of patients with opioid pain medications or treatment with a drug belonging to benzodiazepine class. Moreover, benzodiazepine immunoassays at a cut-off of 200 ng/mL may not be sensitive enough to monitor compliance of patients with various benzodiazepines, especially clonazepam and lorazepam. For this purpose more sensitive GC/MS or LC−MS/MS methods with a lower cut-off such as 40 ng/mL is more appropriate. Although traditionally GC/MS have been used for confirmation of various drugs in urine more recently LC−MS/MS based methods are gaining popularity. One advantage of LC−MS/MS based methods is that derivatization prior to analysis may not be needed whereas for GC/MS analysis many drugs require derivatization prior to analysis. In addition, LC−MS/MS based methods also offer higher sensitivity and specificity. Urine adulteration is an important issue in workplace drugs testing. Because many adulterants can invalidate drug testing specimen validity testing following SAMHSA guidelines, is essential to avoid false negative test results in workplace drug testing.

References

[1] Bush D. The US mandatory guidelines for Federal workplace drug testing programs: current status and future considerations. Forensic Sci Int 2008;174:111−19.
[2] Montoya ID, Elwood WN. Fostering a drug free workplace. Health Care Superv 1995;14:1−3.
[3] Carpenter CS. Workplace drug testing and worker drug use. Health Serv Res 2007;42L:795−810.
[4] Department of Health and Human Services. Proposed revision to mandatory guidelines for federal workplace drug testing programs. Fed Regist 2015;80:28101−51.
[5] Jaffee WB, Truccp E, Teter C, Levy S, et al. Focus on alcohol and drug abuse: ensuring validity in urine drug testing. Psychiatr Serv 2008;59:140−2.
[6] Eichhorst JC, Etter ML, Rousseaux N, Lehotay DC. Drugs of abuse testing by tandem mass spectrometry: a rapid simple method to replace immunoassay. Clin Biochem 2009;42:1531−42.
[7] Poklis A, Fitzgerald RL, Hall KV, Saddy JJ. EMIT d.a.u monoclonal amphetamine/methamphetamine assay II. Detection of methylenedioxyamphetamine (MDA) and methylenedioxymethamphetamine (MDMA). Forensic Sci Int 1993;59:63−70.
[8] Lekskulchai V, Mokkhavesa C. Evaluation of Roche Abuscreen ONLINE amphetamine immunoassay for screening of new amphetamine analogs. J Anal Toxicol 2001;25:471−5.
[9] Kerrigan S, Mellon MB, Banuelos S, Arndt C. Evaluation of commercial enzyme-linked immunosorbent assays to identify psychedelic phenethylamine. J Anal Toxicol 2011;25:444−51.
[10] Apollonio LG, Whittall IR, Pianca DJ, Kyd JM, et al. Matrix effect and cross-reactivity of select amphetamine-type substances, designer analogues, and putrefactive amines using the Bio-Quant direct ELISA presumptive assays for amphetamines and methamphetamines. J Anal Toxicol 2007;31:208−13.
[11] Petrie M, Lynch KL, Ekins S, Chang JS, et al. Cross-reactivity studies and predictive modeling of "Bath salts" and other amphetamine type stimulants with amphetamine screening immunoassays. Clin Toxicol (Phila) 2013;51:83−91.
[12] Kerrigan S, Banuelos S, Perrella L, Hardy B. Simultaneous detection of ten psychedelic phenethylamine in urine by gas chromatography-mass spectrometry. J Anal Toxicol 2011;35:459−69.
[13] Poklis A, Jortani WSA, Brown CS, Crooks CR. Response of the EMIT II amphetamine/methamphetamine assay to specimens collected following use of Vicks inhalers. J Anal Toxicol 1993;17:284−6.

[14] Dietzen DJ, Ecos K, Friedman D, Beason S. Positive predictive values of abused drug immunoassays on the Beckman SYNCHRON in a Veteran population. J Anal Toxicol 2001;25:174−8.

[15] Casey ER, Scott MG, Tang S, Mullins ME. Frequency of false positive amphetamine screens due to bupropion using the Syva EMIT II immunoassay. J Med Toxicol 2011;7:105−8.

[16] Baron JM, Griggs DA, Nixon AL, Long WH, et al. The trazodone metabolite meta-chlorophenylpiperazine can cause false positive urine amphetamine immunoassay result. J Anal Toxicol 2011;35:364−8.

[17] Yee LM, Wu D. False positive amphetamine toxicology screen results in three pregnant women using labetalol. Obstet Gynecol 2011;117(2 Pt 2):503−6.

[18] Merigian KS, Beowning RG. Desipramine and amantadine causing false positive urine test for amphetamine. Ann Emerg Med 1993;22:1927−8.

[19] Vorce SP, Holler JM, Cawrse BM, Magluilo J. Dimethylamine: a drug causing positive immunoassay results for amphetamines. J Anal Toxicol 2011;35:183−7.

[20] Hornbeck CL, Carrig JE, Czarny RJ. Detection of GC/MS artifact peak as methamphet-amine. J Anal Toxicol 1993;17:257−63.

[21] Wang SM, Wang TC, Giang YS. Simultaneous determination of amphetamine and methamphetamine enantiomers in urine by simultaneous liquid-liquid extraction and diastereomeric derivatization followed by gas chromatography-isotope dilution mass spectrometry. J Chromatogr B Analyt Technol Biomed Life Sci 2005;816:131−45.

[22] Wang T, Shen B, Shi Y, Xiang P, et al. Chiral separation and determination of R/S-methamphetamine and its metabolite R/S-amphetamine in urine using LC-MS/MS. Forensic Sci Int 2015;246:72−8.

[23] Baker JE, Jenkins AJ. Screening for cocaine metabolite fails to detect an intoxication. Am J Forensic Med Pathol 2008;29:141−4.

[24] Dasgupta A, Mahle C, McLemore J. Elimination of fluconazole interference in gas chromatography/mass spectrometric confirmation of benzoylecgonine, the major metab-olite of cocaine using pentafluoropropionyl derivative. J Forensic Sci 1996;41:511−13.

[25] Mazor SS, Mycyk MB, Wills BK, Brace LD, et al. Coca tea consumption causes posi-tive urine cocaine assay. Eur J Emerg Med 2006;13:340−1.

[26] Smith ML, Hughes RO, Levine B, Dickerson S, et al. Forensic drug testing for opiates. VI. Urine testing for hydromorphone, hydrocodone, oxymorphone, and oxycodone with commercial opiate immunoassays and gas chromatography-mass spectrometry. J Anal Toxicol 1995;19:18−26.

[27] Hull MJ, Bierer MF, Griggs DA, Long WH, et al. Urinary buprenorphine concentration in patients treated with suboxone as determined by liquid chromatography-mass spec-trometry and CEDIA immunoassay. J Anal Toxicol 2008;32:516−21.

[28] Baden LR, Horowitz G, Jacoby H, Eliopoulos GM. Quinolones and false positive urine screening for opiates by immunoassay technology. JAMA 2001;286:3115−19.

[29] De Paula M, Saiz LC, Gonzalez-Revalderia J, Pascual T, et al. Rifampicin causes false positive immunoassay results for opiates. Clin Chem Lab Med 1998;36:241−3.

[30] Widschwendter CG, Zernig G, Hofer A. Quetiapine cross-reactivity with urine metha-done immunoassays. Am J Psychiatry 2007;164:172.

[31] Rogers SC, Pruitt CW, Crouch DJ, Caravati EM. Rapid urine drug screens: diphenhy-dramine and methadone cross-reactivity. Pediatr Emerg Care 2010;26:665−6.

[32] Hausmann E, Kohl B, von Boehmer H, Wellhoner HH. False positive EMIT indication for opiates and methadone in doxylamine intoxication. J Clin Chem Clin Biochem 1983;21:599−600.

[33] Lichtenwalner MR, Mencken T, Tully R, Petosa M. False positive immunochemical screen for methadone attributable to metabolites of verapamil. Clin Chem 1998;44:1039−2041.

[34] Broussard L, Presley LC, Pittaman T, Clouette R, et al. Simultaneous identification and quantitation of codeine, morphine, hydrocodone and hydromorphone in urine as trimethylsilyl and oxime derivatives by gas chromatography-mass spectrometry. Clin Chem 1997;43:1029−32.

[35] Cone EJ, Zichterman A, Heltsley R, Black DL, et al. Urine testing for nor-codeine, nor-hydrocodone and noroxycodone facilitates interpretation and reduces false negatives. Forensic Sci Int 2010;198:58−61.

[36] Yang HS, Wu AH, Lynch KL. Development and validation of a novel LC-MS/MS opioid confirmation assay: evaluation of beta-glucuronidase enzymes and sample clean up methods. J Anal Toxicol 2016;40:323−9.

[37] Rohrich J, Schimmel I, Zorntlein S, Becker J, et al. Concentrations of delta-9-tetrahydrocannabinol and 11-nor 9-carboxytetrahydrocannabinol in blood and urine after passive exposure to cannabis smoke in a coffee shop. J Anal Toxicol 2010;34:196−203.

[38] Boucher A, Vilette P, Crassard N, Bernard N, et al. Urinary toxicological screening: analytical interference between niflumic acid and cannabis. Arch Pediatr 2009;16:1457−60. [Article in French].

[39] Oosthuizen NM, Laurens JB. Efavirenz interference in urine screening immunoassays for tetrahydrocannabinol. Ann Clin Biochem 2012;49:194−6.

[40] Rollins DE, Jennison TA, Jones G. Investigation of interference by nonsteroidal anti-inflammatory drugs in urine tests for abused drugs. Clin Chem 1998;36:602−6.

[41] De Cook KJ, Delbeke FT, DeBoer D, Van Eenioo P, et al. Quantitation of 11-nor-delta-9-tetrahydrocannabinol-9-carboxylic acid with GC-MS in urine collected for doping analysis. J Anal Toxicol 2003;27:106−9.

[42] Crockett DK, Nelson G, Dimson P, Urry FM. Solid-phase extraction of 11-nor-delta-9-tetrahydrocannabinol-9-carboxylic acid from urine drug testing specimens with cerex polycrom-THC column. J Anal Toxicol 2000;24:245−9.

[43] Jamerson MH, McCue JJ, Klette KL. Urine pH, container composition and exposure time influence absorptive loss of 11-nor-delta-9-tetrahydrocannabinol-9-carboxylic acid. J Anal Toxicol 2005;29:627−31.

[44] Lee KM, Kim HJ, Son J, Park JH, et al. Simple quantitation of formoterol and 11-nor-Δ^9-tetrahydrocannabinol-9-carboxylic acid in human urine by liquid chromatography-tandem mass spectrometry. J Chromatogr B Analyt Technol Biomed Life Sci 2014;967:8−12.

[45] Marchei E, Pellegrini M, Pichini S, Martin I, et al. Are false positive phencyclidine immunoassay instant-view multi test results caused by overdose concentrations of ibuprofen, metamizol and dextromethorphan?. Ther Drug Monit 2007;29:671−3.

[46] Long C, Crifasi J, Maginn D. Interference of thioridazine (Mellaril) in identification of phencyclidine. Clin Chem 1996;42:1885−6.

[47] Bond GR, Steele PE, Uges DR. Massive venlafaxine overdose resulted in a false positive Abbott AxSYM urine immunoassay for phencyclidine. J Toxicol Clin Toxicol 2003;41:999−1002.

[48] Dixon RB, Floyd D, Dasgupta A. Limitations of EMIT benzodiazepine immunoassay for monitoring compliance of patients with benzodiazepine therapy even after hydrolyzing glucuronide metabolites in urine to increase cross-reactivity: comparison of immunoassay results with LC-MS/MS values. Ther Drug Monit 2015;37:137−9.

[49] West R, Pesce A, West C, Crews B, et al. Comparison of clonazepam compliance by measurement of urinary concentration by immunoassay and LC-MS/MS in patient management. Pain Physician 2010;13:71−8.

[50] Forsman M, Nystrom I, Roman M, Berglund L, et al. Urinary detection times and excretion patterns of flunitrazepam and its metabolites after a single oral dose. J Anal Toxicol 2009;33:491−501.

[51] Kurisaki E, Hayashida M, Nihira M, Ohno Y, et al. Diagnosis performance of Triage for benzodiazepines: urine analysis of the dose of therapeutic cases. J Anal Toxicol 2005;29:539−43.

[52] Augsburger M, Rivier L, Mangin P. Comparison of different immunoassays and GC-MS screening of benzodiazepines in urine. J Pharm Biomed Anal 1998;18:681−7.

[53] Fraser AD, Howell P. Oxaprozin cross-reactivity in three commercial immunoassays for benzodiazepines in urine. J Anal Toxicol 1998;22:50−4.

[54] Nasky KM, Cowan GL, Knittel DR. False positive urine screening for benzodiazepines: an association with streamline? A two year retrospective chart analysis. Psychiatry 2009;6:36−9.

[55] Valentine JL, Middleton R, Sparks C. Identification of urinary benzodiazepines and their metabolites: comparison of automated HPLC, GC-MS after immunoassay screening of clinical specimens. J Anal Toxicol 1996;20:416−24.

[56] West RE, Ritz DP. GC/MS analysis of for five common benzodiazepine metabolites in urine as tert-butyldimethylsilyl derivatives. J Anal Toxicol 1993;17:114−16.

[57] Jeong YD, Kim MK, Suh SI, In MK, et al. Rapid determination of benzodiazepines, zolpidem and their metabolites in urine using direct injection liquid chromatography-tandem mass spectrometry. Forensic Sci Int 2015;257:84−92.

[58] Liu RH, McKeehan AM, Edwards C, Foster G, et al. Improved gas chromatography/mass spectrometry analysis of barbiturates in urine using centrifuged based solid-phase extraction, methylation with d_5-pentobarbital as internal standard. J Forensic Sci 1994;39:1504−14.

[59] Treston AM, Hooper WD. Metabolic studies with phenobarbitone, primidone and their N-alkyl derivatives: quantification of substrate and metabolites using chemical ionization gas chromatography-mass spectrometry. J Chromatogr 1990;526:59−68.

[60] Johnson LL, Garg U. Quantitation of amobarbital, butalbital, pentobarbital, phenobarbital and secobarbital in urine, serum and plasma using gas chromatography-mass spectrometry (GC-MS). Methods Mol Biol 2010;603:65−74.

[61] Wu A, Bristol B, Sexton K, Cassella-McLane G, Holtman V, Hill DW. Adulteration of urine by Urine Luck. Clin Chem 1999;45:1051−7.

[62] ElSohly MA, Feng S, Kopycki WJ, Murphy TP, et al. A procedure to overcome interferences caused by adulterant "Klear" in the GC-MS analysis of 11-nor-Δ9-THC-9-COOH. J Anal Toxicol 1997;20:240−2.

[63] Dasgupta A, Wahed A, Wells A. Rapid spot tests for detecting the presence of adulterants in urine specimens submitted for drug testing. Am J Clin Pathol 2002;117:325−9.

[64] Cody JT, Valtier S, Kuhlman J. Analysis of morphine and codeine in samples adulterated with Stealth. J Anal Toxicol 2001;25:572−5.

[65] Valtier S, Cody JT. A procedure for the detection of Stealth adulterant in urine samples. Clin Lab Sci 2002;15:111−15.

[66] Wu A, Schmalz J, Bennett W. Identification of Urin-Aid adulterated urine specimens by fluorometric analysis [Letter]. Clin Chem 1994;40:845−6.

[67] Welsh KJ, Dierksen JE, Actor JK, Dasgupta A. Novel spot tests for detecting the presence of zinc sulfate in urine, a newly introduced urinary adulterant to invalidate drugs of abuse testing. Am J Clin Pathol 2013;140:572−8.

Analysis of drugs of abuse in serum, hair, oral fluid, sweat, and meconium

Introduction

Currently, the most commonly used specimen for drug abuse testing is urine and approximately 90% of all drug abuse testings are conducted using urine specimens. However, alternative specimens such as serum, hair, oral fluid, sweat, and meconium are also used for drug testings because such alternative matrixes offer different advantages over the testing of urine specimens. For example, during an acute overdose, serum is the preferred specimen. In general, drugs can be detected from a few hours up to 1 day using a serum specimen, up to a day for oral fluid, 2–3 days to up to 30 days in urine (chronic use of marijuana), from weeks to months using meconium, but from months to years for hair specimens. Guidelines are available for screening and confirmation cut-off concentrations of various drugs in alternative matrices from Substance Abuse Mental and Health Services Administration (SAMHSA). Advantages and disadvantages of different specimen types for drugs of abuse testing are summarized in Table 11.1.

Serum/whole blood as specimen for drug testing

Serum specimens are useful for diagnosis of acute overdose in a patient admitted with a suspected drug overdose. Postmortem whole blood is often used in forensic death investigations. However, in contrast to urine specimen, where immunoassays can be used directly without any sample preparation, immunoassays are not readily available for screening of drugs in serum. In general, liquid chromatography combined with tandem mass spectrometry (LC–MS/MS) can be applied for detection of several drugs in serum with minimum sample preparation. Bouzas et al. analyzed opiates (morphine, codeine, and 6-actylmorphine), amphetamine, methamphetamine, 3,4-methylenedioxymethamphetamine (MDMA), 3,4-methylenedioxyamphetamine (MDA), cocaine, benzoylecgonine, methadone, and methadone metabolite in serum using LC–MS/MS. The authors used deuterated analogs of these drugs as internal standards [1]. Bjork et al. used ultra-performance LC–MS/MS for analysis of alprazolam, amphetamine, benzoylecgonine, bromazepam, cathine, cathinone, chlordiazepoxide, clonazepam, 7-aminoclonazepam, cocaine, codeine, diazepam, flunitrazepam, 7-amino flunitrazepam, ketamine, ketobemidone, 6-acetylmorphine, MDA, MDMA, methamphetamine, morphine, nitrazepam, 7-aminonitrazepam, oxazepam, temazepam, tramadol,

Alcohol, Drugs, Genes and the Clinical Laboratory. DOI: http://dx.doi.org/10.1016/B978-0-12-805455-0.00011-7

Table 11.1 **Advantages and disadvantages of different specimens for drugs of abuse testing**

Specimen	Advantages	Disadvantages
Urine (most common specimen)	• Noninvasive collection Quantity of specimen always sufficient • Well documented guidelines for screening and confirmation cut-off for all illicit drugs (and/or their metabolites) • Sufficient concentrations of drugs and/or metabolites in urine for detection • Immunoassay and point of care devices are readily available for screening and no pretreatment of specimen is necessary • Well-researched methods for drug confirmation using GC/MS or LC−MS/MS	• Shorter window of detection (2−3 days to up to 1 month for chronic use of marijuana) • For workplace drug testing, if specimen collection is not observed, adulteration of urine is possible. As a result, an extra step is necessary to document that no adulterant is present prior to analytical step
Blood	• Suitable for detecting recent use of a drug in a suspected overdose patient • Sufficient concentrations of drugs and or metabolites present for detection • Specimen adulteration is not possible	• Specimen collection is invasive • Window of detection is even shorter than urine specimen
Hair	• Longest detection window compared to all other specimen types • Collection process is noninvasive and specimen cannot be adulterated • Drugs are very stable once incorporated into hair	• Cannot detect a recent use of a drug (less than 3−4 days) • Analytical methods need to be very sensitive to detect very low level of drug (ng to pg/mg of hair) • Extensive specimen preparation involving washing and digestion of specimen prior to GC/MS or LC−MS/MS analysis • Hair testing is not readily available and testing is expensive

(Continued)

Table 11.1 (Continued)

Specimen	Advantages	Disadvantages
Oral fluid	• Noninvasive collection and virtually no chance of specimen adulteration • Ability to detect recent abuse • Parent drugs rather than drug metabolites are targeted for detection • Testing methods including point of care devices readily available for detecting various drugs in oral fluid	• Short window of detection • Low sample volume • Requires supervision of the subject 10–30 min prior to collection to ensure nothing is taken through the mouth
Sweat	• Noninvasive specimen collection • Detect recent use of drug • Difficult to adulterate the specimen	• May require two visits, once for putting the sweat patch and one for removing • Limited widow of detection with a sweat swipe but longer detection window with a sweat patch (worn 7–14 days) • Limited sample volume for multiple drug testing • Sweat testings are not readily available
Meconium	• Long detection window (3–6 months) • Easy sample collection with no chance of adulteration	• Not useful for detecting recent use • Extensive sample pretreatment is required before the analytical step • Testing not readily available

O-desmethyltramadol, zolpidem, and zopiclone in whole blood. The authors used deuterated analogs of drugs as internal standards and a robotic system based on automatic sample handling for fast analysis of specimens [2].

Drugs in serum can also be analyzed using gas chromatography combined with mass spectrometry (GC/MS) but derivatization may be required for analysis of most drugs. Lerch et al. used GC/MS for analysis of cocaine, benzoyl-ecgonine, methadone, morphine, codeine, 6-acetylmorphine, dihydrocodeine, and 7-aminoflunitrazepam in serum, urine, heart blood, and tissue samples. The authors used protein precipitation, and solid phase extraction followed by derivatization with N-methyl-N-trimethylsilyl-trifluoroacetamide prior to GC/MS analysis [3].

Hair as specimen for drug testing

Hair consists of the hair follicle and the hair shaft. Drugs if present in the blood are trapped into hair shaft (matrix cells present at the base of hair follicle move upward and become hair shaft as hair grows) and once trapped, drugs are very stable in hair. Drugs can also be entrapped into hair from sweat, sebum, and the external environment. One major advantage of hair testing is that it provides the longest window of drug abuse detection (3 days to many years) [4]. Hair grows approximately 1 cm per month and as a result segmental testing of hair provides a history of drug abuse in the past. However, a major challenge in hair testing is the very low concentration of drug (ng/mg of hair to pg/mg of hair), which is analytically challenging. Nevertheless, hair drug testing has many applications including workplace drug testing, military drug testing (especially return to duty after vacation), forensic drug testing, occupational medicine, and determination of possible drug exposure to fetus due to maternal drug abuse (fetal hair grows in the last trimester and positive neonatal hair indicates maternal drug use during late pregnancy).

Specimen collection for hair analysis is not well standardized, and varies significantly among collection facilities and laboratories. Hair collection from the area of the back of the head called the vertex posterior is most common. Generally a 100–300 mg sample is sufficient for screening and confirmation of drugs of abuse. The distance from the hair root reflects the time elapsed since drug use. SAMHSA-proposed guidelines recommend the use of ~1.5″ long hairs which represent a time period of ~90 days. Due to sample collection under direct supervision, hair collection is considered less prone to adulteration than urine. Bush discussed US mandatory guidelines for drug testing including testing using alternative specimens [5]. Proposed screening and confirmatory cut-off concentrations of drugs in hair by SAMHSA are summarized in Table 11.2. Although it was initially speculated that hair color may impact the concentration of drug incorporated into hair (black hair

Table 11.2 **Screening and confirmation cut-off of various drugs in hair according to SAMHSA guidelines**

Drug	Screening cut-off (pg/mg of hair)	Confirmation cut-off (pg/mg of hair)
Amphetamine/methamphetamine[a]	500	300
MDMA/MDEA/MDA	500	300
Cocaine	500	500
Benzoylecgonine (cocaine metabolite)	500	50
Morphine/codeine	200	200
6-Acetylmorohine	200	200
Phencyclidine	300	300
Marijuana metabolite	1	0.05

[a]For confirmation of methamphetamine in hair, amphetamine must also be confirmed at a concentration of 50 pg/mg or higher.

may be most absorptive but light color hair may be less absorptive for drugs), newer experiments as well as large population-based studies indicate that such differences may be insignificant for interpretation of results [4].

One advantage of hair analysis is that specimen cannot be adulterated. Since the hair samples are collected under direct supervision, the chances of sample adulteration are minimal. However, questions have been raised about sample adulteration since the donor can treat hair before the sample collection. A number of products are listed on the Internet which guarantee to beat hair drug tests. Examples of these products include "Ultra Clean," "Hair Follicle Shampoo & Purifier Treatment Pack," "Hair Purifying Shampoo," "Hair Detox," and "Clean Zone." However, published papers in the literature indicate that these products are ineffective in removing drugs from hair.

Hair drug analysis

After collection, hair specimens must be washed to remove external contaminants, dirt, and grease from the specimen. For this purpose, hair is generally washed with organic solvents such as acetone, methanol, methylene chloride, or isopropanol. Aqueous solutions such as water and phosphate buffer are not very effective. Before drug extraction, the sample is dried and cut into 1−3 mm long pieces or grounded by mechanical beating using metal or glass beads. Then drugs and/or metabolites are removed from the hair specimen by a digestion/extraction procedure. Digestion of hair specimen may be carried out using alkali (e.g., digesting hair with sodium hydroxide overnight at 37°C), acid (e.g., digestion with hydrochloric acid at room temperature or at 37°C overnight), or a suitable enzyme (beta-glucuronidase/arylsulfatase, protease, etc.). Then drugs are extracted from hair using appropriate solvents. Although immunoassays can be used for initial screening of drugs present in hair, chromatographic methods such as GC/MS and LC−MS/MS are more suitable analytical techniques for drug analysis using hair specimens. In general, derivatization is required for analysis of most drugs and/or metabolites using GC/MS but for the LC−MS/MS method drugs can be analyzed either without derivatization or after derivatization. In general chromatographic methods used for urine drug confirmation can be used for analysis of drugs in other specimens including hair, provided such methods are sensitive enough to detect very low amounts of drugs present in hair or other matrices.

Analysis of amphetamine

Amphetamines and other sympathomimetic amines incorporate into hair. GC/MS method for simultaneous determination of amphetamine, methamphetamine, MDA, MDMA, 3,4-methylenedioxyethylamphetamine (MDEA), and N-methyl-1-(1,3-benzodioxy-5-yl)-2-butylamine (MBDB) has been described. The authors used deuterated amphetamine, methamphetamine, MDA, and MDMA as internal standards. The hair specimen (3 cm) was digested with sodium hydroxide, followed by solid phase extraction and derivatization with pentafluoropropionic anhydride.

The concentrations of amphetamine in 20 volunteers studied varied from 0.1 to 4.8 ng/mg of hair (17 specimens) while methamphetamine concentrations varied from 0.05 to 0.89 ng/mg of hair (16 specimens) [6]. There are many other published methods for analysis of amphetamine and related drugs in hair specimens.

Analysis of cocaine and benzoylecgonine

Cocaine and its metabolites accumulate in hair. Immunoassays and GC/MS are commonly used techniques for the detection of cocaine and its metabolites in hair. Due to the question of external contamination, cocaine metabolite (most commonly benzoylecgonine) is measured in hair specimens to ensure cocaine abuse by the subject. Cocaine accumulates in hair in a concentration-dependent manner. Graham et al. correlated benzoylecgonine concentration in subjects with heavy and occasional use of cocaine. The concentration of benzoylecgonine was 0.64−29.1 ng/mg in heavy users and 0.032−1.21 ng/mg in occasional users [7]. A study on maternal urine and neonatal hair testing for cocaine showed hair analysis for gestational cocaine exposure had a sensitivity of 88%, specificity of 100%, and positive and negative predictive values of 100% and 85%, respectively [8]. LC−MS/MS methods are also used for analysis of cocaine and its metabolites in hair. Morris-Kukoski et al. used LC−MS/MS method for simultaneous analysis of cocaine, benzoylecgonine, nor-cocaine, cocaethylene, and hydroxycocaine after extensively washing hair specimens for removing external contamination. The authors detected cocaine along with its metabolites (cocaethylene, nor-cocaine, and hydroxycocaine metabolites) in the hair of cocaine abusers but cocaine metabolites were not present in research chemists who worked with cocaine but never abused it [9].

Analysis of opiates

GC/MS is commonly used for analysis of morphine, codeine, and 6-acetylmorphine (also known as 6-monoacetylmorphine, a metabolite of heroin) in hair after extraction and derivatization. Moller et al. analyzed codeine, morphine, and 6-acetylmorphine in hair after extracting drugs with methanol (18 h incubation at 56°C) and derivatization using N-O-bis-(trimethylsilyl)-trifluoroacetamide (BSTFA) containing 1% trimethylchlorosilane. The authors used deuterated analogs of these compounds as internal standards and mass spectrometer was operated in selected ion mode monitoring m/z 429 and 414 for morphine, m/z 432 and 417 for morphine-d_3, m/z 371 and 343 for codeine, m/z 374 and 436 for codeine-d_3, m/z 399 and 340 for 6-acetylmorphine, and m/z 402, 343 for 6-acetylmorphine-d_3. The limit of quantification was 0.01 ng/mg of hair for both morphine and 6-acetylmorphine and 0.005 ng/mg of hair for codeine [10].

Fucci et al. described a case of a 3-year old boy who on admission to the hospital tested positive for opiates during immunoassay screening but parents claimed that the boy accidentally ingested a white powder contained in a plastic wrapper that was found in a park. His hair specimen (20 mg) was pulverized and was digested with 0.1N hydrochloric acid overnight at 40°C. Then deuterated morphine and deuterated 6-acetylmorphine were added (internal standards) followed by extraction with chloroform/isopropanol (9:1). Finally after derivatization with pentafluoropropionic anhydride, the specimen was analyzed by GC/MS. The authors confirmed the presence of 6-acetylmorphine and morphine in 1.5 cm of hair indicating chronic heroin intake for 1−2 months. The court ordered supervision of the boy and the boy's family was involved with social services for a period of observation and 6 months letter his hair specimen was negative for both morphine and 6-acetylmorphine [11].

Analysis of cannabinoids

The major psychoactive cannabinoid found in marijuana is Δ^9-tetrahydrocannabinol (THC), which is metabolized into 11-hydroxy-Δ^9-tetrahydrocannabinol (11-OH-THC; active) and 11-nor-9-carboxy-Δ^9-tetrahydrocannabinol (THC-COOH) (inactive). Although THC-COOH is found at a much higher concentration in urine compared to THC, in hair THC is present a much higher concentration than THC-COOH. However, detection of THC-COOH in hair is considered as better proof of drug use because THC-COOH is absent in marijuana smoke thus ruling out environmental contamination of hair. Uhl and Sachs reported a case in which hair samples from a couple living together tested positive for THC and cannabinol. However, the hair sample from the male who used marijuana tested positive for THC-COOH, whereas the sample from the female subject who did not use marijuana tested negative [12]. Although Cannabio shampoo and hemp shampoo may contain very small amounts of cannabinol, cannabidiol, or even THC, normal use of such shampoo should not cause false positive hair testing for THC-COOH.

Several methods have been described for the detection THC and THC-COOH in hair. Kintz used GC coupled with MS operated in negative chemical ionization mode (GC/MS−NCI) for detection of THC-COOH in hair. In their method, hair samples were decontaminated with methylene chloride and pulverized in 1 mL of 1N sodium hydroxide for 30 min at 95°C. The digest was acidified and the drug was extracted with *n*-hexane/ethyl acetate and derivatized with pentafluoropropionic anhydride/pentafluoropropanol. The concentration of THC-COOH in the hair ranged from 0.02 to 0.39 ng/mg [13]. Wilkins et al. analyzed THC-COOH along with THC and 11-OH-THC in hair using deuterated analogs as internal standards. The authors digested hair specimen with 1N sodium hydroxide overnight at 37°C followed by extraction and derivatization of drugs along with internal standard prior to analysis by GC/NCI/MS [14].

Analysis of other drugs

Many other drugs including opiates, phencyclidine (PCP), benzodiazepines, barbiturates, gamma-hydroxybutyrate, ketamine, anabolic steroids, and zolpidem have been analyzed in hair specimens using either GC/MS or LC−MS/MS. Baumgartner et al. also analyzed PCP in hair from seven subjects admitting the use of PCP. All subjects showed the presence of PCP in hair (0.3−2.8 ng/mg of washed hair) but only one subject showed positive PCP in urine toxicology analysis [15]. In another study using psychiatric patients, hair analysis detected PCP in 11 out of 47 patients. Blood and urine tests were negative in all these 47 patients [16].

Although GC/MS is widely used for analysis of various drugs in hair, LC−MS/MS are gaining popularity to be the method of choice because many different drug classes can be analyzed in one run even without derivatization. Shah et al. analyzed nandrolone, stanozolol, testosterone, boldenone, cocaine, benzoylecgonine, cocaethylene, amphetamine, methamphetamine, MDMA, MDA, desmethyl-selegiline, ephedrine, THC, 11-hydroxy-THC, THC-COOH, ketamine, nor-ketamine, clenbuterol, propranolol, terbutaline, salbutamol, morphine, codeine, and phencyclidine in hair specimens after washing with dichloromethane, digesting with 1M sodium hydroxide and then extracting drugs along with internal standards for analysis using LC−MS/MS. The authors used stanozolol-d_3, cocaine-d_3, MDMA-d_5, THC-d_3, codeine-d_3, ketamine-d_4, and PCP-d_5. The authors analyzed 233 human hair specimens using this method and 70 volunteers were confirmed positive for some drugs but mostly drugs of abuse and steroids. Although 56 volunteers showed the presence of 1 drugs, other volunteers showed the presence of multiple drugs (1 volunteer was positive for 5 drugs) [17].

Koster et al. also used LC−MS/MS for simultaneous analysis of amphetamine, methamphetamine, MDMA, MDA, MDEA, methylphenidate, cocaine, benzoylecgonine, morphine, codeine, heroin, 6-monoacetylmorphine, methadone, 2-ethylidene-1,5-dimethyl-3,3-diphenylpyrrolidine (EDDP, methadone metabolite), THC, nicotine, and cotinine in human hair. The authors applied their method to analyze hair samples from patients who were monitored for drug abuse. Hair specimens from 47 patients showed the presence of MDMA, methylphenidate, cocaine, benzoylecgonine, codeine, methadone, EDDP, THC, nicotine, and cotinine at concentrations above the analytical cut-off. One patient showed the presence of high amounts of cocaine (38,762 pg/mg of hair), benzoylecgonine (6052 pg/mg of hair), methadone (14,402 pg/mg of hair), and EDDP (1573 pg/mg of hair) [18].

Oral fluid as specimen for drug testing

Oral fluid containing saliva, mucosal transudate, crevicular fluid, and other substances present in the oral cavity is gaining popularity as an alternative matrix to urine for drug testing because the presence of a drug in oral fluid is indicative of recent drug use. Oral fluid testing is widely used in European countries to identify impaired drivers. Moreover, drug concentrations in oral fluid correlate better with blood levels compared to urinary levels. For example, concentration of amphetamine in oral fluid correlates with whole blood amphetamine concentration but for certain drugs, e.g., cocaine, the concentration may be higher in oral fluid than in serum. The parent drug is usually found in the oral fluid at higher concentration than its metabolites. Oral fluid can be collected using commercially available devices. Moreover, point of care testing devices is also available for screening of drugs in the oral fluid at the site of collection. However, for legal drug testing the specimen must be shipped to a certified laboratory for drug confirmation using GC/MS. Many studies

Table 11.3 Screening and confirmation cut-off concentrations of various drugs in oral fluid according to 2015 SAMHSA guidelines

Drug	Screening cut-off (ng/mL)	Confirmation cut-off (ng/mL)
Amphetamine/methamphetamine[a]	25	15
MDMA/MDEA/MDA	25	15
Cocaine	15	8
Benzoylecgonine (cocaine metabolite)	15	8
Morphine/codeine	30	15
6-Acetylmorohine	3	2
Oxycodone/oxymorphone	30	15
Hydrocodone/hydromorphone	30	15
Phencyclidine	3	2
Marijuana	4	2

MDMA, 3,4-methylenedioxymethamphetamine; MDA, 3,4-methylenedioxyamphetamine; MDEA, 3,4-methylenedioxyethylamphetamine.
[a]For confirmation of methamphetamine in oral fluid, amphetamine must also be confirmed at a concentration above the confirmation cut-off.

also validated use of oral fluid as an alternate specimen for drug of abuse testing. Cone et al. analyzed 77,218 oral fluid specimens collected using Intercept Oral Collection device (OraSure Technologies, Bethlehem, PA), screened using immunoassays and if necessary confirmed by gas chromatography combined with tandem mass spectrometry (GC−MS/MS). Of 77,218 samples tested, 3908 (5.06%) confirmed positive. The frequency of positivity was THC (3.22%) > cocaine (1.12%) > amphetamines (0.47%) > opiates (0.23%) > PCP (0.03%). Oral fluid positivity rates, for amphetamine and cocaine, were 60% higher as compared to urine, suggesting that these drugs are more efficiently accumulated in oral fluid compared to urine [19]. SAMHSA-proposed screening and confirmation cut-off values in oral fluid for various drugs of abuse in 2015 and these cut-offs are given in Table 11.3 [20].

The main advantage of using oral fluid for drug testing is that it is difficult to adulterate such specimens. Moreover, a person is watched for 10−20 min to make sure nothing is taken through the mouth. Although many products are available for beating oral fluid drug testing, no product is effective in invalidating oral fluid drug testing. However, some people have dry mouth and some medications may also cause dry mouth where collection of oral fluids may be difficult or time consuming. Another limitation of oral fluid testing is the narrow window of detecting drugs in oral fluid even compared to urine. If more than 24 h has passed after abusing a drug, oral fluid may not be a suitable specimen for drug testing.

Analysis of specific drugs

GC/MS or LC−MS/MS can be used for analysis of drugs in oral fluid. Gunnar et al. described a solid phase extraction, long-column fast gas chromatography/

electron impact mass spectrometry (GC/EI−MS) method for simultaneous determination of 30 drugs of abuse including amphetamines, opiates, methadone, cocaine, THC, alprazolam, midazolam, fentanyl, and zolpidem after proper derivatization. Amphetamine-type stimulant drugs were derivatized with heptafluorobutyric anhydride, benzodiazepines, and THC with N-methyl-N-(tert-butyl-dimethylsilyl)-trifluoroacetamide and benzoylecgonine, codeine, ethylmorphine, 6-monoacetylmorphine, morphine, pholcodine, buprenorphine, and nor-buprenorphine with N-methyl-N-(trimethylsilyl)trifluoroacetamide [21].

Although THC may be present in higher concentration in oral fluid, analysis of THC-COOH is important because it eliminates false positive test result due to passive exposure to THC smoke. Choi et al. analyzed THC and THC-COOH in oral fluid using GC/MS after derivatization with BSTFA with 1% trimethylchlorosilane. The authors used deuterated THC and THC-COOH as internal standards. Applying this method, the authors analyzed oral fluid collected from 12 drug abusers. Two subjects showed the presence of only THC in oral fluid (13.4 and 1.4 ng/mL) while one subject showed the presence of both THC (9.8 ng/mL) and THC-COOH (25.1 ng/mL) [22]. THC-COOH in oral fluid can also be analyzed by LC−MS/MS using solid phase extraction and C-18 reverse phase chromatographic column. THC-COOH was monitored in negative mode electron ionization and multiple reaction monitoring MS. Deuterated THC-COOH was used as the internal standard [23].

Various opioids and their metabolites are also present in oral fluid. For GC/MS analysis of morphine, codeine, and 6-monoacteylmorphine, extraction of these compounds from oral fluid either by solid phase extraction or liquid/liquid extraction followed by a single derivatization step is sufficient for sample preparation. Campora et al. analyzed codeine, morphine, and 6-acetylmorphine by GC/MS in oral fluid after liquid/liquid extraction and derivatization with BSTFA containing 1% trimethylchlorosilane. The mass spectrometer was operated in positive chemical ionization mode using methane as the reagent gas. The authors used morphine-d_3, codeine-d_3, and 6-acetylmorphine-d_3 as internal standards. The authors also analyzed 80 oral fluid specimens collected from volunteers under heroin addiction treatment. Codeine was detected in all 80 specimens (mean: 62.4 ng/mL, morphine in 78 specimens (mean: 202.2 ng/mL), and 6-acetylmorphine in 77 cases (mean: 484.4 ng/mL). Interestingly, oral fluid from 75 cases tested positive for all 3 compounds [24]. However, for simultaneous analysis of codeine, morphine, 6-acetylmorphine, along with hydrocodone, hydromorphone, and oxycodone, the keto-opioids must be derivatized first followed by a second derivatization for other compounds. Jones et al. used aqueous methoxyamine hydrochloride (also known as O-methylhydroxylamine) to form methoxime derivative of keto-opiate in oral fluid followed by extraction of all drugs and second derivatization using BSTFA. The authors used morphine-d_3, codeine-d_3, 6-acetylmorphine-d_3, hydrocodone-d_3, and oxycodone-d_3 as internal standards. The authors also applied the same GC/MS method for analysis of opioids in hair specimen [25].

Although GC/MS is widely used for analysis of various drugs in oral fluid, LC−MS/MS methods are also very useful for analysis of drugs in oral fluid with an added advantage of analyzing different drug class in a single run. Concheiro et al. developed two different LC−MS protocol for analysis of 11 drugs or metabolites in oral fluid. The first LC–MS/MS method was validated for analysis of morphine, 6-acetylmorphine, amphetamine, methamphetamine, MDA, MDMA, MBDB, cocaine, and benzoylecgonine in oral fluid. This method required only 100 μL of oral fluid. Another method requiring 200 μL oral fluid was developed for analysis of THC. The authors also compared LC–MS/MS results with results obtained by point of care devices OraLab and Drager. Out of 160 valid results in oral fluid (during roadside testing) obtained by using OraLab devices, 21 cases were positive for cocaine. Other positive cases were THC (5 cases), opiates (2 cases), amphetamine (1 case), a combination of cocaine and THC (7 cases), and a combination of cocaine and opiates (3 cases). The OraLab results compared well with LC–MS/MS for opiates and cocaine. For Drager devices, out of 230 valid results 104 tested positive but most common drugs present were cocaine and THC. The Drager oral fluid results compared well with LC–MS/MS for cocaine only showing good sensitivity and specificity. The authors commented that for other drugs, there is room for improvement for both point of care oral fluid testing device [26]. Montesano et al. analyzed amphetamine, methamphetamine, MDMA, MDA, MDEA, cocaine, benzoylecgonine, ecgonine-methyl ester, nor-cocaine, buprenorphine, nor-buprenorphine, codeine, morphine, heroin, 6-acetylmorphine, methadone, phencyclidine, and mescaline, in oral fluid by LC–MS/MS after microextraction on packed sorbent. The authors used deuterated analogs of amphetamine, methamphetamine, MDMA, cocaine, benzoylecgonine, ecgonine-methyl ester, buprenorphine, morphine, and phencyclidine as internal standards. The lower limit of quantitation varied from 0.5 to 30 ng/mL [27].

Flood et al. analyzed 3608 oral fluid specimens (collected from 921 patients undergoing treatment at outpatient addiction treatment centers) using LC–MS/MS and compared the impact of new lower cut-off levels for cocaine, benzoylecgonine, 6-caetylmorphine, and morphine on interpretation of test results. The authors used deuterated cocaine, benzoylecgonine, codeine, morphine, and 6-acetylmorphine as internal standards. The authors observed that cocaine was detected more often than its metabolite benzoylecgonine in oral fluids (154 specimens showed only cocaine but no benzoylecgonine). Overall 662 specimens were positive for cocaine (range: 2.0–13,047 ng/mL; median: 15.2 ng/mL) or benzoylecgonine (range: 2.0–2797 ng/mL, median: 52.4 ng/mL), and 603 specimens were positive for opiates. The median morphine concentration was 19.0 ng/mL (range: 2.0–11,894 ng/mL), codeine concentration was 14.7 ng/mL (range: 2.0–620 ng/mL), and 6-acetylmorphine was 14.0 (2.0–43,205 ng/mL). The authors concluded that cocaine not benzoylecgonine is the dominant low concentration oral fluid analyte in an addiction medicine treatment settings [28].

Sweat as specimen for drug testing

Sweat produced by eccrine and apocrine glands is an alternative specimen for drug testing. Sweat testing is gaining popularity in various situations including outpatient drug rehabilitation programs, criminal justice, and workplace drugs testing due to the developments of reliable sweat collection devices and sensitive analytical methods. Passive diffusion is the mechanism by which drugs accumulate in sweat. The advantages of sweat analysis for drugs of abuse include continuous drug monitoring for a longer period of time (from 3 days to 14 days) and noninvasive procedure to collect sweat. Sweat may be collected as liquid perspiration on sweat wipes or with a suitable sweat patch. Commercially available sweat patches are waterproof, tamper resistant, and are comfortable to wear. For putting a sweat patch, the skin should be cleaned with soap and water, followed by alcohol swab. Then a staff member should put the patch and at the end of the period, a staff member should remove the patch for analysis. The swab must be visually inspected by the staff member in order to eliminate any possibility of tampering. Sweat is less susceptible to tampering or adulteration compared to urine specimen. Contaminants applied to the outer surface of the sweat patch usually do not affect drug testing in sweat specimen. In general parent drugs are found in sweat although metabolites may also be present. SAMHSA guidelines are available for screening and cut-off concentrations of various drugs present in sweat.

Analysis of specific drugs in sweat

Various drugs including amphetamine, methamphetamine, MDMA, THC, opiates, cocaine, and phencyclidine are present in sweat. Drugs present in the sweat patch must be extracted prior to analysis using immunoassay or a chromatographic method. Because drugs are present in nanogram quantities in the sweat patch, both GC/MS and LC−MS/MS are suitable for confirmation of drugs in the sweat patch. In general, chromatographic methods developed for analysis of various drugs in oral fluid or hair specimens can also be applied to analysis of drugs using sweat specimen.

The presence of amphetamines in sweat has been reported in several studies. Fay et al. collected sweat, using a Federal Food and Drug Administration approved device PharmChek (PharmChem, Inc., Haltom City, TX) sweat patch, from volunteers dosed with 10, 20, and 25 mg methamphetamine. The drugs were eluted from the collection pad of the patch and tested using EIA and GC−MS. Sweat primarily contained parent methamphetamine [29]. Preston et al. studied cocaine concentrations in sweat collected from 44 patients undergoing methadone maintenance program. Paired sweat patches were removed weekly (on Tuesday) and three to five consecutive urine specimens collected Monday, Wednesday, and Friday. The authors used both immunoassays and GC/MS for analysis of drugs. Cocaine was confirmed by GC/MS in 99% immunoassay positive sweat specimens. The median concentrations of cocaine, benzoylecgonine, and ecgonine-methyl ester were 378, 78.7, and 74 ng/mL respectively, indicating that cocaine is the major drug present in the sweat. The authors concluded that sweat patches can be used for monitoring cocaine in suspected drug users [30].

Opiates are excreted in sweat and the parent drug is found as the predominant analyte in sweat. Opiate concentrations in sweat accounts for only 1−2% of the dose. Fogerson et al. used PharmChek patches for sweat collection, and immunoassay as well as GC−MS for opiates analysis in sweat collected from human volunteers who received known amounts of opiates (codeine or heroin). The authors observed that sweat primarily contained parent opiates such as heroin or codeine, as well as lipophilic metabolite 6-monoacetylmorphine, the metabolite of heroin in case of heroin administration but little amount of morphine [31]. Studies on sweat PCP testing are limited. Using radioactive PCP, Perez-Reyes et al. found that PCP is excreted in sweat. After intravenous administration, PCP was detectable in sweat for 54 h. PCP was found to be highly concentrated in sweat as compared to blood during heavy exercise [32].

THC is also excreted in sweat but THC metabolites may not be detected in sweat due to very low concentration. Huestis et al. analyzed THC in sweat collected from 11 daily marijuana users using PharmChek after cessation of drug use. The authors used deuterated THC as the internal standard which was directly added to the sweat patch and after drying. Then THC and the internal standard present in the sweat patch were extracted with organic solvent followed by derivatization with trifluoroacetic anhydride prior to GC/MS analysis. The mean THC concentration was 3.85 ng/patch during the first week of monitored abstinence in these 11 daily marijuana users. However, 8 out of 11 users showed no detectable THC in the second week of monitoring using sweat patches. One subject was still positive after 4 weeks [33]. Kintz et al. used cosmetic pads for sweat collection from foreheads and tested for THC using GC/MS. Out of 198 impaired drivers tested, 22 subjects were positive for THC-COOH in urine, 14 subjects tested positive for THC in oral fluid (1−103 ng/Salivette) and 16 showed positive THC in sweat (4−152 ng/pad). However, no THC metabolite (11-hydroxy-THC or THC-COOH was detected in oral fluid as well as sweat [34].

LC−MS/MS methods are also widely used for determination of concentrations of drugs and metabolites in sweat. Koster et al. analyzed amphetamine, methamphetamine, MDMA, MDA, MDEA, methylphenidate, cocaine, benzoylecgonine, morphine, codeine, heroin, 6-acetylmorphine, methadone, EDDP, nicotine, and cotinine in PharmChek sweat patches using LC−MS/MS. The drugs present in the patch were extracted with 1.5 mL of 20 mmol/L ammonium formate (pH 7) and methanol (50:50 by vol), followed by a clean up by filtering through Whatman Mini-UniPrep syringeless filter vials before injection into the LC−MS/MS. The run time was 9.6 min and analytical measurement range was 3.0−300 ng/patch except for nicotine (30−3750 ng/patch). All drug/metabolites were stable in the patch for 7 days at room temperature except heroin [35].

Meconium as specimen for drug testing

Drug abuse by a pregnant woman may have devastating effects on the fetus because like alcohol many drugs can pass through the placenta causing injury to the fetus. Cocaine abuse during pregnancy is associated with an increased risk of prematurity, small fetus for gestational age status, microcephaly, congenital anomalies including cardiac and genitourinary abnormalities, necrotizing enterocolitis, and central nervous system stroke or hemorrhage. Similarly, intrauterine exposure to amphetamine and methamphetamine is associated with low birth weight, premature delivery, and congenital brain hemorrhage.

Due to the negative consequences of admitting illicit drug abuse, maternal self-reporting of possible drug abuse is not reliable. Maternal urine drug testing is useful to identify mothers who may be using drugs but such testing may underestimate drug exposure due to short window of detection of drugs in urine. Meconium has been shown to be a reliable source for detection of fetal drug exposure with higher sensitivity than urine drug testing. Meconium starts forming between the 12th and 16th week of gestation and accumulates until after birth. It is a complex mixture of epithelial and squamous cells, amniotic fluid, and many other products. The disposition of drugs in meconium is not well understood. It is proposed that the fetus excretes drugs into bile and amniotic fluid, and drugs accumulate in meconium either by direct deposition or through swallowing of amniotic fluid [36].

Analysis of specific drugs in meconium

Although meconium is easily collectable from a newborn, drugs must be extracted from meconium prior to analysis by immunoassays or GC/MS or LC–MS/MS. Meconium is a nonhomogenous gelatinous material, and meconium first must be homogenized followed by extraction using organic solvents. Common methods include using 100–500 mg of meconium and extraction of drugs with 1–2 mL of acetonitrile and methanol by vigorous agitation of the sample with a vortex mixer. The specimen is then centrifuged at high speed ($\sim 10,000 \times g$), and supernatant is used for analysis using immunoassays. Some laboratories evaporate the organic solvent extract and reconstitute the residue into a buffer prior to analysis [37]. However, the metabolism of abused drugs as well as accumulation of drug metabolites in meconium may be different compared to urine or blood. ElSohly et al. showed that many meconium samples which tested positive by immunoassay, tested negative by GC–MS when benzoylecgonine was used as the target analyte. However, when hydroxy metabolites of cocaine were included in the target analytes during confirmation, more immunoassay positive specimens could be confirmed for the presence of cocaine and its metabolites [38].

Mantovani et al. analyzed anhydroecgonine methyl ester, a marker compound for abuse of crack cocaine (produced during pyrolysis) along with cocaine, benzoylecgonine, ecgonine-methyl ester, cocaethylene, and m-hydroxybenzoylecgonine in meconium using GC/MS after extraction and derivatization using pentafluoropropionic anhydride and pentafluoro-1-propanol. The authors used cocaine-d_3, cocaethylene-d_3, benzoylecgonine-d_3, and ecgonine-methy esters-d_3 as internal standards. The method was applied for analysis of 342 meconium samples and cocaine/cocaine metabolites were detected in 19 specimens (5.6% specimens). The m-hydroxybenzoylecgonine was the most commonly detected metabolite (94.7% specimens) followed by ecgonine-methyl ester (84.2% specimens), benzoylecgonine (78.9% specimens), and cocaine (73.7% specimens) in specimens tested positive for cocaine/metabolites. In one positive specimen only m-hydroxybenzoylecgonine was present. In 5 out of 19 specimens anhydroecgonine methyl ester (highest concentration: 181.6 ng/g) was present indicating abuse of crack cocaine by mothers. Cocaethylene was detected (highest concentration: 113.3 ng/g) in only 3 specimens [39].

Marchei et al. analyzed THC and its two metabolites THC-COOH and 11-OH-THC in meconium using GC/MS and deuterated THC as well as THC-COOH as internal standards. The meconium was subjected to liquid/liquid extraction after enzymatic hydrolysis to de-conjugate glucuronide metabolites followed by derivatization using BSTFA containing 1% trimethylchlorosilane prior to analysis by GC/MS. The authors analyzed 300 meconium specimens out of which 27 specimens showed positive results for the presence of THC and or its metabolites. Within positive specimens THC-COOH and 11-OH-THC were present in most of the specimens while THC was present in only five specimens including two specimens showing the presence of THC alone [40]. Tenon et al. analyzed marijuana metabolites; 11-OH-THC and THC-COOH in meconium after extraction and derivatization with BSTFA containing 1% trimethylchlorosilane. The detection limit for both analytes was 5 ng/g. The authors analyzed 183 meconium specimens and confirmed the presence of THC-COOH (mean: 55.0 ng/g; range: 5−265 ng/gin 123 specimens. In addition, 11-OH-THC was present in four specimens (mean: 8.25 ng/g; range: 5−15 ng/g) [41].

Many investigators used LC−MS/MS method for analysis of various drugs in meconium. Launiainen et al. analyzed amphetamine, methamphetamine, MDMA, MDA, buprenorphine, nor-buprenorphine, morphine, codeine, 6-acetylmorphine, oxycodone, methadone, tramadol, and THC-COOH in meconium using LC−MS/MS. Out of 143 meconium specimens analyzed 57 specimens (40%) showed positive for at least 1 drug/metabolite. The drugs used in opioid substitution treatment (methadone and buprenorphine) together with other medicinal opioids comprised both expected/admitted and unexpected/denied findings in meconium. THC-COOH was detected in only two meconium specimens [42].

Conclusions

Urine is the most common specimen for drug testing but other matrices such as blood, hair, oral fluid, sweat, and meconium offer certain advantages over testing of conventional urine specimen. Testing of whole blood or serum for drugs is very useful in diagnosis of a recent drug overdose. In contrast, hair has the longest window of detection for any drug and is very useful in evaluating history of drug abuse. Oral fluid is very popular for evaluating impaired drivers in some European countries because oral fluid can be collected noninvasively and drug concentration in oral fluid may reflect blood concentration and is correlated with degree of impairment. Meconium is a very useful specimen for evaluating exposure of drugs by the fetus due to maternal drug abuse. Several other matrices including amniotic fluid, vitreous fluid, breast milk, nails, semen, sebum, cerumen, breath, fat, and placental tissue have been studied as potential alternative matrices for drug testing.

Although drug testing in urine is a straightforward procedure where urine specimens can be analyzed by immunoassays without any specimen preparation, preanalytical steps are necessary for using alternative matrices for drug testing except for oral fluid. In addition, relatively low quantitates of drugs in alternative matrices also pose additional analytical challenges for drug testings in alternative matrices.

References

[1] Bouzas NF, Dresen S, Munz B, Weinmann W. Determination of basic drugs in human serum by online extraction and LC-MS/MS. Anal Bioanal Chem 2009;395:2499–507.

[2] Bjork MK, Simonsen KW, Andersen DW, Dalsgaard PW, et al. Quantification of 31 illicit drugs and medicinal drugs and metabolites in whole blood by fully automated solid phase extraction and ultra-performance liquid chromatography-tandem mass spectrometry. Anal Bioanal Chem 2013;405:2607–17.

[3] Lerch O, Temme O, Daldrup T. Comprehensive automation of the solid phase extraction gas chromatographic mass spectrometric analysis (SPE-GC/MS) of opioids, cocaine, and metabolites from serum and other matrices. Anal Bioanal Chem 2014;406: 4443–51.

[4] Boumba VA, Ziavrou KS, Vougiouklakis T. Hair as a biological indicator of drug abuse or chronic exposure to environmental toxins. Int J Toxicol 2006;25:143–63.

[5] Bush DM. The U.S. mandatory guidelines for federal workplace drug testing programs: current status and future considerations. Forensic Sci Int 2008;174:111–19.

[6] Rothe M, Pragst F, Spiegel K, Harrach T, et al. Hair concentrations and self-reported abuse history of 20 amphetamine and ecstasy users. Forensic Sci Int 1997;89:111–28.

[7] Graham K, Koren G, Klein J, Schneiderman J, Greenwald M. Determination of gestational cocaine exposure by hair analysis. JAMA 1989;262:3328–30.

[8] Katikaneni LD, Salle FR, Hulsey TC. Neonatal hair analysis for benzoylecgonine: a sensitive and semiquantitative biological marker for chronic gestational cocaine exposure. Biol Neonate 2002;81:29–37.

[9] Morris-Kukoski CL, Montgomery MA, Hammer RL. Analysis of extensively washed hair from cocaine users and drug chemists to establish new reporting criteria. J Anal Toxicol 2014;38:628–36.

[10] Moller M, Aleksa K, Walasek P, Karaskov T, et al. Solid phase microextraction for the detection of codeine, morphine and 6-monocetylmorphine in human hair by gas chromatography-mass spectrometry. Forensic Sci Int 2010;196:64–9.

[11] Fucci N, Vetrugno G, De Giovanni N. Drugs of abuse in hair: application in pediatric patients. Ther Drug Monit 2013;35:411–13.

[12] Uhl M, Sachs H. Cannabinoids in hair: strategy to prove marijuana/hashish consumption. Forensic Sci Int 2004;145:143–7.

[13] Kintz P, Cirimele V, Mangin P. Testing human hair for cannabis. II. Identification of THC-COOH by GC-MS-NCI as a unique proof. J Forensic Sci 1995;40:619–22.

[14] Wilkins D, Haughey H, Cone E, Huestis M, Foltz R, Rollins D. Quantitative analysis of THC, 11-OH-THC, and THCCOOH in human hair by negative ion chemical ionization mass spectrometry. J Anal Toxicol 1995;19:483–91.

[15] Baumgartner AM, Jones PF, Black CT. Detection of phencyclidine in hair. J Forensic Sci 1981;26:576–81.

[16] Sramek JJ, Baumgartner WA, Tallos JA, Ahrens TN, Heiser JF, Blahd WH. Hair analysis for detection of phencyclidine in newly admitted psychiatric patients. Am J Psychiatry 1985;142:950—2.

[17] Shah I, Petroczi A, Uvacsek M, Ranky M, et al. Hair-based rapid analyses of multiple drugs in forensic and doping: application of dynamic multiple reaction monitoring with LC-MS/MS. Chem Cent J 2014;8:73.

[18] Koster RA, Alffenaar JW, Greijdanus B, VanDernagel JE, et al. Fast and highly selective LC-MS/MS screening for THC and 16 other abused drugs and metabolites in human hair to monitor patients with drug abuse. Ther Drug Monit 2014;36:234—43.

[19] Cone EJ, Presley L, Lehrer M, Seiter W, Smith M, Kardos KW, et al. Oral fluid testing for drugs of abuse: positive prevalence rates by Intercept immunoassay screening and GC-MS-MS confirmation and suggested cutoff concentrations. J Anal Toxicol 2002;26: 541—6.

[20] Department of Health and Human Services. Proposed revision to mandatory guidelines for federal workplace drug testing programs. Fed Regist 2015;80:28054—101.

[21] Gunnar T, Ariniemi K, Lillsunde P. Validated toxicological determination of 30 drugs of abuse as optimized derivatives in oral fluid by long column fast gas chromatography/electron impact mass spectrometry. J Mass Spectrom 2005;40:739—53.

[22] Choi H, Baeck S, Kim E, Lee S, et al. Analysis of cannabis in oral fluid specimens by GC-MS with automatic SPE. Sci Justice 2009;49:242—6.

[23] Scheidweiler KB, Himes SK, Chen X, Liu HF, et al. 11-Nor-9-carboxy-Δ^9-tetrahydrocannabinol in human oral fluid by liquid chromatography-tandem mass spectrometry. Anal Bioanal Chem 2013;405:6019—27.

[24] Campora P, Bermejo AM, Tabernero MJ, Fernandez P. Use of gas chromatography/mass spectrometry with positive chemical ionization for the determination of opiates in human oral fluid. Rapid Commun Mass Spectrom 2006;20:1288—92.

[25] Jones J, Tomlinson K, Moore C. The simultaneous determination of codeine, morphine, hydrocodone, hydromorphone, 6-acetylmorphine and oxycodone in hair and oral fluid. J Anal Toxicol 2002;26:171—5.

[26] Concheiro M, de Castro A, Quintela O, Cruz A, et al. Confirmation by LC-MS of drugs in oral fluid obtained from roadside testing. Forensic Sci Int 2007;170:156—62.

[27] Montesano C, Simeoni MC, Curini R, Sergi M, et al. Determination of illicit drugs and metabolites in oral fluid by microextraction on packed sorbent coupled with LC-MS/MS. Anal Bioanal Chem 2015;407:3647—58.

[28] Flood JG, Khaliq T, Bishop KA, Griggs DA. The new substance abuse and mental health services administration oral fluid cutoffs for cocaine, and heroin related analytes applications to addiction medicine settings: important unanticipated findings with LC-MS/MS. Clin Chem 2016;62:773—80.

[29] Fay J, Fogerson R, Schoendorfer D, Niedbala RS, Spiehler V. Detection of methamphetamine in sweat by EIA and GC-MS. J Anal Toxicol 1996;20:398—403.

[30] Preston KL, Huestis MA, Wong CJ, Umbricht A, et al. Monitoring cocaine use in substance abuse treatment patients by sweat and urine drug testing. J Anal Toxicol 1999;23:313—22.

[31] Fogerson R, Schoendorfer D, Fay J, Spiehler V. Qualitative detection of opiates in sweat by EIA and GC-MS. J Anal Toxicol 1997;21:451—8.

[32] Perez-Reyes M, Di Guiseppi S, Brine DR, Smith H, et al. Urine pH and phencyclidine excretion. Clin Pharmacol Ther 1982;32:635—41.

[33] Huestis MA, Scheidweiler KB, Satio T, Fortner N, et al. Excretion of delata-9-tetrahydrocannabinol in sweat. Forensic Sci Int 2008;174:173—7.

[34] Kintz P, Cirimele V, Ludes B. Detection of cannabis in oral fluid (saliva) and forehead wipes (sweat) from impaired drivers. J Anal Toxicol 2000;24:557−61.

[35] Koster RA, Alffenaar JW, Greijdanus B, VanDerNagel JE, et al. Application of sweat patch screening for 16 drugs and metabolites using a fast and highly selective LC-MS/MS method. Ther Drug Monit 2014;36:35−45.

[36] Ostrea Jr. EM, Brady MJ, Parks PM, Asensio DC, Naluz A. Drug screening of meconium in infants of drug-dependent mothers: an alternative to urine testing. J Pediatr 1989;115:474−7.

[37] Ryan RM, Wagner CL, Schultz JM, Varley J, DiPreta J, Sherer DM, et al. Meconium analysis for improved identification of infants exposed to cocaine in utero. J Pediatr 1994;125:435−40.

[38] ElSohly MA, Kopycki W, Feng S, Murphy TP. Identification and analysis of the major metabolites of cocaine in meconium. J Anal Toxicol 1999;23:446−51.

[39] Mantovani Cde C, Lima MB, Oliveira CD, Menck Rde A, et al. Development and practical applications of accelerated solvent extraction for the isolation of cocaine/crack biomarkers in meconium samples. J Chromatogr B Analyt Technol Biomed Life Sci 2014;957:14−23.

[40] Marchei E, Pellegrini M, Pacifici R, Palmi I, et al. Quantification of delta-9-tetrahydrocannabinol and its metabolites in meconium by gas chromatography-mass spectrometric assay: assay validation and preliminary results of the "meconium project". Ther Drug Monit 2006;28:700−6.

[41] Tynon M, Porto M, Logan BK. Simplified analysis of 11-hydroxy-delta-9-tetrahydrocannabinol and 11-carboxy-delta-9-tetrahydrocannabinol in human meconium: method development and validation. J Anal Toxicol 2015;39:35−40.

[42] Launiainen T, Nupponen I, Halmesmaki E, Ojanpera I. Meconium drug testing revealed maternal misuse of medicinal opioids among addicted mothers. Drug Test Anal 2013;5:529−33.

Index

Note: Page numbers followed by "*f*" and "*t*" refer to figures and tables, respectively.

Printed in the United States
By Bookmasters